SPINAL CORD INJURY

Clinical Outcomes from the Model Systems

Samuel L. Stover, MD
Professor Emeritus
Department of Rehabilitation Medicine
University of Alabama at Birmingham
Birmingham, Alabama

Joel A. DeLisa, MD, MS
Professor and Chairman
Department of Physical Medicine and Rehabilitation
UMDNJ– New Jersey Medical School
Newark, New Jersey

Gale G. Whiteneck, PhD
Director of Research
Rocky Mountain Regional Spinal Injury System
Craig Hospital
Englewood, Colorado

An Aspen Publication®
Aspen Publishers, Inc.
Gaithersburg, Maryland
1995

Library of Congress Cataloging-in-Publication Data

Spinal cord injury: clinical outcomes from the model systems/
[edited by] Samuel L. Stover, Joel A. DeLisa, Gale G. Whiteneck.
p. cm.
Includes bibliographical references and index.
ISBN 0-8342-0697-8
1. Spinal cord—Wounds and injuries—Longitudinal studies.
2. Spinal cord—Wounds and injuries—Complications—
Longitudinal studies. 3. Spinal cord—Wounds and injuries—
Patients—Rehabilitation—Longitudinal studies.
I. Stover, S.L. (Samuel L.)
II. DeLisa, Joel A. III. Whiteneck, Gale G.
[DNLM: 1. Spinal Cord Injuries. WL 400 S75696 1995]
RD594.3.S6653   1995
617.4'82004—dc20
DNLM/DLC
for Library of Congress
94-49602
CIP

Aspen Publishers, Inc., grants permission for photocopying for limited personal or internal use.
This consent does not extend to other kinds of copying, such as copying for general
distribution, for advertising or promotional purposes, for creating new collective
works, or for resale. For information, address Aspen Publishers, Inc., Permissions
Department, 200 Orchard Ridge Drive, Suite 200, Gaithersburg, Maryland 20878.

Editorial Resources: Jane Colilla
Library of Congress Catalog Card Number: 94-49602
ISBN: 0-8342-0697-8

Printed in the United States of America

1 2 3 4 5

This book is fondly dedicated to:

John S. Young, MD
(1919–1994)

A true pioneer of spinal cord injury management in the United States. He was also the first director of the Model Spinal Cord Injury Systems database.

He was a teacher and a scholar, endowed with vision, leadership, a warm generous personality, and an infectious sense of humor. Dr. Young was an inspiration and a role model, and is truly missed.

Table of Contents

Contributors

Michelle Buda Abela, MA
Research Coordinator
Rehabilitation Institute of Michigan
Detroit, Michigan

Rodney H. Adkins, PhD
Co-Director
SCI Project
Rancho Los Amigos Medical Center
Downey, California

David F. Apple, Jr., MD
Medical Director
Shepherd Spinal Center
Atlanta, Georgia

Diana D. Cardenas, MD
Professor
Department of Rehabilitation
   Medicine
University of Washington
Project Director
Northwest Regional SCI System
Seattle, Washington

R. Edward Carter, MD
Professor of Clinical Rehabiliation
Department of Physical Medicine
   and Rehabilitation

Baylor College of Medicine
Houston, Texas

Edgar D. Charles, Jr., MS, PhD
Former Professor of Public Health
   and Medicine
University of Alabama at
   Birmingham
Birmingham, Alabama

Michelle E. Cohen, PhD
Assistant Director of Research
Regional Spinal Cord Injury Center
   of Delaware Valley
Thomas Jefferson University
Philadelphia, Pennsylvania

Theodore M. Cole, MD
Professor
Department of Physical Medicine
   and Rehabilitation
University of Michigan
Ann Arbor, Michigan

Barry Corbet
Writer
Research Department
Craig Hospital
Englewood, Colorado

Jerome M. Cotler, MD
The Everett J. and Marian Gordon
  Professor
Vice Chairman
Department of Orthopaedic Surgery
Jefferson Medical College
Thomas Jefferson University
Philadelphia, Pennsylvania

Joel A. DeLisa, MD, MS
Professor and Chairman
Department of Physical Medicine
  and Rehabilitation
UMD-NJ New Jersey Medical
  School
Newark, New Jersey
Senior Vice President and Chief
  Medical Officer
Kessler Rehabilitation Corporation
  and Other Affiliated Organizations
West Orange, New Jersey
Chairman
Physical Medicine and Rehabilita-
  tion
Saint Barnabas Medical Center
Livingston, New Jersey

Michael J. DeVivo, DrPH, MBA
Associate Professor
Manager of Analytic Services
Department of Rehabilitation
  Medicine
University of Alabama at Birming-
  ham
Birmingham, Alabama

Marcel P. Dijkers, PhD
Director of Research
Rehabilitation Institute of Michigan
Associate Professor

Department of Physical Medicine
  and Rehabilitation
Wayne State University
Detroit, Michigan

John F. Ditunno, Jr., MD
Michie Professor of Rehabilitation
  Medicine
Chairman
Department of Rehabilitation
  Medicine
Thomas Jefferson University
  Hospital
Philadelphia, Pennsylvania

William H. Donovan, MD
Clinical Professor and Chairman
Department of Physical Medicine
  and Rehabilitation
University of Texas—Houston
  Medical School
Houston, Texas

Lisa Farrell-Roberts, RN, MN
Neuroscience Clinical Nurse
  Specialist
Northwest Hospital
Seattle, Washington

Christopher Formal, MD
Assistant Medical Director of
  Educational Programs
Magee Rehabilitation Hospital
Philadelphia, Pennsylvania

Bruce M. Gans, MD, MS
President
Rehabilitation Institute of Michigan
Chairman and Professor
Department of Physical Medicine
  and Rehabilitation

Wayne State University
Detroit, Michigan

Bette K. Go
Manager
National Spinal Cord Injury
  Statistical Center
Birmingham, Alabama

Wayne A. Gordon, PhD
Professor and Associate Director
Department of Rehabilitation
  Medicine
Mount Sinai Medical Center
New York, New York

Karyl M. Hall, MA, MFCC, EdD
Director of Rehabilitation Research
Co-Director of SCI and TBI Model
  Systems of Care
Santa Clara Valley Medical Center
San Jose, California

Karen A. Hart, PhD
Assistant Professor
Baylor College of Medicine
Vice President for Education
The Institute for Rehabilitation and
  Research
Houston, Texas

Allen W. Heinemann, PhD
Associate Professor
Department of Physical Medicine
  and Rehabilitation
Northwestern University Medical
  School
Chicago, Illinois

Lesley M. Hudson, MA
Director of Research
Project Co-Director
Georgia Regional Spinal Cord Injury
  Care System
Department of Clinical Research
Shepherd Spinal Center
Altanta, Georgia

Rosalie S. Karunas, MPH
Health Science Research Associate
Department of Physical Medicine
  and Rehabilitation
University of Michigan
Ann Arbor, Michigan

Patricia B. Lazarus
Data Collection Manager
Spain Rehabilitation Center
Birmingham, Alabama

Frederick M. Maynard, MD
Professor of Medicine
Case Western Reserve University
Chairperson
Department of Physical Medicine
  and Rehabilitation
Medical Director
MetroHealth Center for
  Rehabilitation
Cleveland, Ohio

Robert R. Menter, MD
Project Director
Rocky Mountain Spinal Injury
  System
Principal Investigator

Spinal Cord Injury Aging
Rehabilitation Research and Training
  Center
Craig Hospital
Englewood, Colorado

Paul R. Meyer, Jr., MD, MM
Professor of Orthopaedic Surgery
Northwestern University Hospital
Chicago, Illinois

Kristjan T. Ragnarsson, MD
Dr. Lucy G. Moses Professor
Chairman
Department of Rehabilitation
  Medicine
Mount Sinai School of Medicine
New York, New York

J. Scott Richards, PhD
Professor
Director of Research
Director of Psychology
Department of Rehabilitation
  Medicine
University of Alabama at
  Birmingham
Birmingham, Alabama

Deborah Rubner
Staff Research Associate
Department of Physical Medicine
  and Rehabilitation
University of California, Davis
Sacramento, California

Richard D. Rutt
Systems Analyst
Spain Rehabilitation Center
Birmingham, Alabama

Marca L. Sipski, MD
Medical Director
Kessler Institute for Rehabilitation
Associate Professor
UMD-New Jersey Medical School
Newark, New Jersey

Samuel L. Stover, MD
Professor Emeritus
Department of Rehabilitation
  Medicine
University of Alabama at
  Birmingham
Birmingham, Alabama

J. Paul Thomas
Former Director
Medical Sciences Programs
National Institute on Disability and
  Rehabilitation Research
Washington, DC

William P. Waring III, MD
Director of Physical Medicine and
  Rehabilitation
St. Francis Health Care Centre
Green Springs, Ohio

Robert L. Waters, MD
Clinical Professor of Orthopaedic
  Surgery
University of Southern California
Rancho Los Amigos Medical Center
Downey, California

Gale G. Whiteneck, PhD
Director of Research
Rocky Mountain Regional Spinal
  Injury System
Craig Hospital
Englewood, Colorado

Conal B. Wilmot, MD, MRCPI
Chairman
Department of Rehabilitation
  Medicine
Santa Clara Valley Medical Center
San Jose, California
Clinical Associate Professor
Department of Functional
  Restoration
Stanford University
Palo Alto, California

Gary M. Yarkony, MD
Vice President
Clinical Program Development
Schwab Rehabilitation Hospital and
  Care Network
Former Director
Spinal Cord Injury Rehabilitation
Midwest Regional Spinal Cord
  Injury Care System
Chicago, Illinois

Foreword

The National Institute on Disability and Rehabilitation Research (NIDRR) takes pride in supporting the Model Spinal Cord Injury Systems. The Model Systems embodies NIDRR's vision of a comprehensive, interdisciplinary service delivery system in which the finest talent in medicine, rehabilitation engineering, and the social sciences work with the primary consumer—the spinal cord injured person—to achieve his or her maximum potential through individual empowerment, independence, and community integration. Today, the Model Spinal Cord Injury System projects are experiencing particularly serious challenges. Some of these challenges are medical, but the most serious appear to be socioeconomic.

To exemplify the dramatic change in the results of treatment for spinal cord injury, authors often cite the ancient Egyptian physicians who referred to spinal cord injury as "an ailment not to be treated." By the middle of the twentieth century, treatment had become increasingly successful. Now, nearing the end of the twentieth century, service delivery has been integrated into a comprehensive system. In the words of one physician, "The Model Spinal Cord Injury System has as its ideal a service delivery system with an enduring core value of life-long commitment to the patient."

Today, there are dramatic changes affecting the System which are both medical and nonmedical. The etiology of the condition has changed increasingly from unintentional injury to intentional injury. The patient profile is also changing. Many patients have neither conventional families nor conventional social support structures in their communities. A third major change is in financing approaches. Health care providers and primary consumers are voicing concern that new approaches to health care financing threaten the ideal of lifetime commitment to the patient. NIDRR and the Model System are working to meet these challenges so that future observers will find that they are as addressable as the medical challenges of the Egyptian period.

These challenges can be stated in more specific terms. Changes in the patient profile present a serious challenge to developing effective interventions. Changes in the length of rehabilitation from 6 months to 6 weeks present extraordinary challenges in identifying optimum nontraditional settings, including independent living and community-based home health strategies. Changes in the financing of health care will require data that show the cost-effectiveness of model service and treatment strategies.

There are a number of opportunities that, if harnessed, can help to transform these challenges into new and innovative possibilities for individuals with spinal cord injury, their families, and health care providers. The Model Systems may have the opportunity to mine the present and future resources generated by the Americans with Disabilities Act, the Technology-Related Assistance for Individuals with Disabilities Act, and other legislation adopted over the past 20 years. These laws should result in improved employment opportunities, including accessible workplaces. However, in a very real sense, proof of the cost-effectiveness of the Model System will be a function of its ability to generate compelling data. The Model System database can be a powerful tool with which to illustrate the problem, demonstrate cost-effectiveness, and identify successful strategies and support system advocacy. The apparent success of the Model Spinal Cord Injury System has inspired the development of other model systems in burn and traumatic brain injury treatment. These systems may also provide useful data on cost-effectiveness.

Finance of health care and intentional injury certainly do not exhaust the list of issues that challenge the Model System! Medical success creates challenges such as those related to secondary conditions, aging with a disability, substance abuse, and the availability of accessible housing and work, to name a few. Professionals and consumers must regard the disability unemployment rate as a tremendous challenge. In addition, training of professional personnel and primary consumers requires innovative and thoughtful instructional designs as a response to changes in research, finance, patient profile, the law, and other key issues.

The information exchanged through this publication will be of great interest to our colleagues throughout the world. This book is a major step forward in our understanding of human physical function and in addressing issues in spinal cord injury in the late twentieth century.

Katherine D. Seelman, PhD
Director
National Institute on Disability Rehabilitation and Research
Washington, DC

Preface

The Model Spinal Cord Injury Systems program has been at the heart of the dramatic change in service delivery for persons with spinal cord injury over the past two decades. Model Systems in different parts of the United States work together to demonstrate improved care, maintain a national database, participate in independent and collaborative research, and provide continuing education relating to spinal cord injury.

This book provides some of the data from the Model Systems Uniform Database which is believed to be the largest longitudinal dataset on spinal cord injuries in the world covering almost the past two decades (June 1973 to June 1992). Most chapters have been arranged to include: a short introductory statement, data from the National Spinal Cord Injury Statistical Center, data from collaborative studies conducted by the Model Systems, an interpretation of the findings from the database and collaborative studies, and other appropriate information from the literature including independent and personal studies. The chapters do not provide an extensive literature review, but they include pertinent information to supplement data from the Model Systems.

Chapter 1 provides general background on the development and implementation of the Model Spinal Cord Injury System concept, and Chapter 2 highlights the specific history of the collaborative research which has produced the National Spinal Cord Injury Database. An understanding of the evolution of the National Spinal Cord Injury Collaborative Database and its current operation is necessary to fully appreciate the nuances and limitations which must be considered when interpreting the many findings presented throughout the remainder of the book. Chapter 3 describes the epidemiology of spinal cord injury and addresses the issue of the representativeness of 14,791 new cases of spinal cord injury in the dataset. Chapters 4 through 8 describe data pertaining to the management of spinal cord injury on an organ system basis, while Chapters 9 and 10 describe functional and psychosocial outcomes. Chapter 11 emphasizes the importance of consumer involvement in the research process, while Chapter 12 itemizes the economic impact of spinal cord injury. The long-term medical complications and survival after spinal cord injury are addressed in Chapters 13 and 14. The final two chapters of the book highlight the demonstrated benefits of a comprehensive system of care and discuss implications for the future of spinal cord injury care.

Throughout this book, the term tetraplegia is synonymous with the term quadriplegia. This was done to conform with the revised 1992 International Standards for Neurological and Functional Classification of Spinal Cord Injury, published by the American Spinal Injury Association (ASIA) and the International Medical Society of Paraplegia. Although the International Standards now recommend the ASIA Impairment Scale for incomplete injuries, the formerly used Frankel Scale is reported throughout this book. For precision, a glossary of selected terms is provided at the end of the book. Definitions of variables are given only when they differ from definitions in standard medical dictionaries or may be difficult to find in other source books.

We wish to thank all of the authors for their efforts to evaluate and analyze the data presented in these chapters. Personnel of the National Spinal Cord Injury Statistical Center (NSCISC) have assisted the authors and prepared data for some of the chapters. A special thanks must be given to Mrs. Paula Fulton who helped with many of the editing responsibilities prior to the publishing contract with Aspen Publishers, Inc.

It has been impossible to try to analyze all of the data in the database. Other publications have and will continue to provide additional information from the Model Systems Database. The whole Spinal Cord Injury Model Systems effort has been funded and supported by the National Institute on Disability and Rehabilitation Research (NIDRR). The project officers for NIDRR, J. Paul Thomas and Toby Lawrence, have helped greatly in coordinating and advising the Model Systems over the years, enabling us to achieve this dissemination milestone. Appendix B is a list of the Spinal Cord Injury Model Systems that have contributed data to the database since 1973. Those identified with an asterisk are currently funded Model Systems which participated in the preparation of this book.

Samuel L. Stover, MD
Joel A. DeLisa, MD, MS
Gale G. Whiteneck, PhD

1

The Model Spinal Cord Injury Concept: Development and Implementation

J. Paul Thomas

INTRODUCTION

The practice of medicine traditionally has been organized around specific body systems. This phenomenon has stimulated the development of numerous medical specialties focused largely on single-body-system clinical pathology and therapeutics. The narrowing of concentration by these medical specialties has been further advanced by the acquisition of significant new molecular and cellular biologic knowledge and technical skills resulting from the phenomenal explosion of scientific discovery over the past 50 years.

Some clinical entities, however, are so complex as to not lend themselves to single-specialty medical management. These entities usually affect multiple body systems and require the coordinated skills and knowledge of many different disciplines working as a team to provide effective and coordinated care. Spinal cord injury (SCI) is such an entity.

HISTORY

From a historical perspective, SCI dates from the Edwin Smith surgical papyrus written about 5000 years ago by an unknown Egyptian physician. This earliest reference to spinal cord trauma contains a cogent description of the major symptoms of a complete lesion of the cervical cord following dislocation or fracture of the spinal column. In discussing the prognosis and therapy of such patients (cases 31 and 33 of the papyrus), the comment of the unknown author is as brief as it is significant: "an ailment not to be treated."

Source: Adapted with permission from J. Paul Thomas, Opportunities for Cooperation, *Paraplegia News,* Vol. 48, No. 9, pp. 34–39, copyright © 1994, Paralyzed Veterans of America.

The most significant modern-day development in categorical care for SCI was the radical approach advanced by the British Medical Research Council during the Second World War. It was decided to gather spinal cord casualties in special care units within the Ministry of Pension hospitals throughout Great Britain. This policy was precipitated by the many civilian air raid casualties, in addition to large numbers of military personnel receiving spinal cord trauma for war injuries and accidents.

In 1943, British authorities established a new spinal care unit at the ministry hospital, Mandeville in Aylesbury. With the opening of this unit on February 1, 1944, and with the medical leadership of Sir Ludwig Guttmann, a concept of comprehensive treatment and rehabilitation was introduced. By 1951, when Stoke Mandeville Hospital was acquired by the National Health Service, the unit had grown with a complement of 160 beds. With the designation as the National Spinal Injuries Centre, admitting patients from all parts of the United Kingdom, the bed capacity increased to 195.

Concurrently in the United States, several significant developments were taking place in categorical SCI care. At the Boston University Hospital, Dr. Donald Munro, with the sponsorship of Liberty Mutual Insurance Company, established a 10-bed spinal injury unit. Dr. Munro was also a consultant to the Veterans Administration. This federal agency established six specialized spinal injury units throughout the United States. It was under Veterans Administration sponsorship that Dr. Ernst Bors made his significant categorical care advances at the Long Beach Veterans Hospital. Also to be recognized in this momentous venture were Drs. Estin Comarr and Herbert Talbot.

All of these specialized programs, while rudimentary, had several common features. These included the following:

- supervision of the unit by an experienced and dedicated physician or surgeon who had sacrificed full-time practice
- nursing and other allied health personnel sufficient in number to cope with the many details involved in care
- adequate technical facilities such as laboratories and workshops for the rehabilitation of long-term patients
- arrangements for community placement and vocational rehabilitation
- after-care, including regular medical follow-up of patients after discharge from the hospital

Thus it was through the combined efforts of dedicated and tenacious physicians that the first hope was generated that the extensive medical, psychologic, social, and vocational needs of persons with SCI could be addressed effectively.

In 1968, the U.S. Congress received eloquent testimony on the unmet rehabilitation needs of persons with SCI from Drs. Howard Rusk, Frank Krusen, and Murray Freed. This set in motion a new federal initiative by the Rehabilitation Services Administration (RSA) spearheaded by James F. Garrett, Associate Commissioner for Research and Demonstrations. Effective advocacy and leadership were jointly provided from the rehabilitation community by Dr. John S. Young. It was Dr. Young who provided both government and the developing spinal injury rehabilitation field with the visionary concept of comprehensive, coordinated centers of care for victims of SCI.

After several working conferences and targeted research projects, the RSA proposed to Congress an innovative and experimental service delivery model. It was decided that a national demonstration project would be initiated at one site to serve as a replication model. The model provided for rapid case finding and referral, early rehabilitation coordinated by a sophisticated team, a mechanism for using all essential community resources to facilitate rehabilitation success, and a long-term health maintenance and follow-up program to ensure that gains achieved during intensive rehabilitation were maintained. In essence, this model embodied a comprehensive system of services covering all aspects of care from point of injury through lifelong follow-up.

In June 1970, the RSA awarded a grant to the Good Samaritan Hospital in Phoenix, Arizona, to serve as the first national Model SCI System. The project was known as the Southwest Regional System for Treatment of Spinal Cord Injury. The grant brought together the combined resources of the SCI service of Good Samaritan Hospital; the intensive neurosurgical and acute care capabilities of Barrow Neurological Institute of St. Joseph's Hospital, the Arizona State University, and the Arizona Division of Vocational Rehabilitation; and the air evacuation and emergency medical services of the Arizona State Highway Patrol.

Given the importance of the problem, it was soon determined by RSA that more projects were needed to provide regional coverage for study of local service delivery variations and for replication modeling. In 1972, six additional Model SCI Systems were funded. The seven federally designated Model Systems very early recognized their important role in providing scientific leadership to the field.

The collective power of the seven Model Systems projects was maximized by the collection and analysis of standardized data following a jointly agreed-upon protocol. In 1975, after development of a preliminary database, the National Spinal Cord Injury Data Research Center (NSCIDRC) was established in Phoenix, Arizona, at the site of the original Model System project. The purpose of the NSCIDRC was to serve as the coordinating center for the collection and analysis of standardized data contributed by all seven projects. The center was imaginatively and dynamically led by Dr. John S. Young, who also continued to serve as project director of the Southwest Regional Model System.

In 1984, under support from the National Institute on Handicapped Research (NIHR), the predecessor agency of the NIDRR, the data coordination center was geographically moved and became known as the National Spinal Cord Injury Statistical Center at the University of Alabama at Birmingham. This data coordination center continues to provide national and international scientific leadership under the capable direction of Dr. Samuel L. Stover.

The NIDRR has supported a number of Model SCI Systems on a research and demonstration basis. Currently, there are 13 such projects geographically distributed throughout the United States. Besides measuring and analyzing the effectiveness and outcomes of the Model Systems approach, these projects also evaluate regional and local variations in service delivery modeling.

These federal designations are routinely re-competed, usually on a 5-year basis. This competition process provides an objective scientific-technical peer review of the service delivery capabilities and progress of each applicant. This provides the opportunity for all possible qualified institutions to fairly compete for, and participate in, the program. In the most recent 1990 competition, for example, there were four incumbent projects replaced by new-applicant institutions.

In 1992, with the reauthorization of the Rehabilitation Act, Congress reaffirmed its support of, and confidence in, the Model SCI Systems program by including the following language regarding program purpose and objectives:

> Any agency or organization carrying out a project or demonstration project assisted by a grant under this paragraph that provides services to individuals with spinal cord injuries shall
>
> 1. establish on an appropriate regional basis, a multidisciplinary system of providing vocational and other rehabilitation services, specifically designed to meet the needs of individuals with spinal cord injuries, including acute care as well as periodic inpatient or outpatient follow-up and services
> 2. demonstrate and evaluate the benefits to individuals with spinal cord injuries served in, and the degree of cost-effectiveness of, such a regional system
> 3. demonstrate and evaluate existing, new, and improved methods and equipment essential to the care, management, and rehabilitation of persons with spinal cord injury
> 4. demonstrate and evaluate methods of community outreach for persons with spinal cord injury and community education in connection with the problems of such individuals in areas such as

housing, transportation, recreation, employment, and community activities.

CLINICAL SERVICE COMPONENTS OF A MODEL SYSTEM

There are five clinical service components of a Model System. These include emergency medical services, the traumatology-intensive/acute care phase, comprehensive medical rehabilitation, psychosocial and vocational preparation and services, and long-term health maintenance and medical follow-up. This range of services is essential to the Model System and must be included in any application for federal support. In addition, other nonclinical features, discussed later in this chapter, are required that offer important capabilities and resources enabling the Model System to achieve a dynamic and influential service delivery continuum.

Emergency Medical Services

Accessibility to care in the Model System begins at the point of injury and is ensured through a communication network that links emergency treatment and transportation units in the field with a predesignated Level I trauma center or other appropriate medical care facility. Field unit personnel must be qualified in advanced life support and proper handling and extrication techniques, and must be under medical supervision during emergency transport. Life support, resuscitation, and other treatment protocols should be preplanned and well established. Emergency medical services personnel trained in specific methods of emergency stabilization and handling are routinely provided by the medical and nursing staff of the Model System.

Intensive/Acute Medical Care

The intensive/acute medical care component requires the immediate availability of all appropriate medical specialists to control urgent life-threatening emergencies and provide lifesaving resuscitation and medical-surgical critical care. This highly technologic environment must be adequately equipped and staffed to provide appropriate diagnostic, evaluative, and therapeutic services. The experienced trauma team requires the physical facilities, equipment, and sophistication to move quickly between urgent medical emergencies. Standardized protocols for emergency, intensive care, and acute spinal injury units ensure high quality and consistent care in a preplanned and organized manner.

Acute Medical Rehabilitation

Acute medical rehabilitation is fully coordinated with the acute/intensive care team and ensures optimal recovery of function and achievement of potential in all areas of productive living. This comprehensive program of services usually includes rehabilitation nursing with an emphasis on prevention of complications and patient-family education, physical and occupational therapy leading to improved mobility and performance of activities of daily living, bowel and bladder care and training, the fitting and use of orthotic and adaptive equipment, psychologic assessment and counseling, family and social adjustment services, early vocational rehabilitation counseling with timely vocational-educational exploration, recreational therapy, and other services as appropriate. Multispecialty medical consultation should be available to lead intervention efforts in the prevention and treatment of secondary medical complications that prove problematic.

Psychosocial and Vocational Rehabilitation

Awareness and availability of psychosocial and vocational rehabilitation services begin early in the acute rehabilitation phase and become predominant as inpatient medical rehabilitation needs are satisfied. The purpose of these services is to provide the patient and family with the full armamentarium of coping skills and resources to (1) maintain personal adjustment and family cohesion and (2) achieve successful community reintegration and the productive pursuit of educational and/or vocational goals. Typically, these services begin in the rehabilitation hospital, are conducted mainly in community-based agencies and organizations, and continue as long as needed to achieve maximal social and economic independence. All necessary facilities and resources are utilized in the community, including training and educational facilities, social service agencies, sheltered workshops, vocational evaluation and work adjustment programs, private business and commercial establishments, and community colleges and technical and trade schools.

Long-Term Follow-Up

The long-term follow-up should emphasize health maintenance, community placement, vocational and social adjustment, and regular monitoring by trained interdisciplinary follow-up personnel. Special attention is to be given to (1) the aggressive prevention and treatment of secondary medical complications and (2) the maintenance of functional gains achieved during the acute rehabilitation phase. Periodic inpatient medical evaluation and diagnostic procedures are to be encouraged. Other kinds of follow-up services may be conducted at the home or work site of the persons with SCI. These numerous follow-up contacts and services will generate the opportunity for the collection of useful up-to-date information, including periodic status evaluations of all persons with SCI discharged from the various subsystems. Aside from the major consulting role played by Model System physicians, local physicians in the community frequently may be utilized for routine medical care and supervision. Formal opportunities should be developed by Model System medical personnel for the orientation and training of these community physicians.

ATTITUDINAL AND BEHAVIORAL COMPONENTS OF A MODEL SYSTEM

Other essential features that contribute to the optimal functioning of a Model SCI System include a number of broadly based attitudinal and behavioral components. While these do not comprise specific clinical or service delivery subsystems, they influence the total viability and effectiveness of the service delivery system and have a significant bearing on ultimate patient outcome. These include accessibility to care, coordination of services, volume of patients, research and evaluation, education and training, and community outreach and advocacy.

Accessibility to Care

All patients within a specific catchment area or region of natural patient flow must be provided direct and automatic access to the Model System through a well-developed emergency evacuation and transportation subsystem. This access should be available regardless of source of economic sponsorship. The catchment area must be predetermined and drawn to provide an optimal level of services across all System components.

Coordination of Services

Coordination of services includes appropriate program leadership and advocacy administered and guided by a lead physician who has recognized, specialized training and experience in SCI rehabilitation. It is expected that this lead physician will coordinate the services of all Model System components through effective supervision and liaison. Particularly vulnerable linkages include the acute care rehabilitation interface and the immediate posthospital discharge period, when many patients are at risk for being lost to the System in returning to the community.

Volume of Patients

The volume of patients is essential because an adequate and substantial critical mass of patients is necessary to support the expertise and quality of care expected of a Model System. For a 20- to 40-dedicated-bed SCI program, a minimum of 50 to 70 new cases per year must be available. Prior rates of admission, readmission, and discharge are utilized to evaluate this criterion.

Research and Evaluation

Research and evaluation dramatically affect program effectiveness through the continued scrutiny of disciplined on-site data collection and appropriate data analysis. It is expected that a Model System will develop the interest in, and environment for, clinical research and program evaluation. This requires sophisticated data collection and analysis capability for each subsystem and the total collective service delivery system. Aside from clinical research on a variety of topics, cost-effectiveness and systems analysis studies will evaluate the benefits and outcomes of the various subsystems and the total system in terms of regional variations and differences in individual project structure and design.

Education and Training

Neurologic trauma lends itself to an effective and relevant medical teaching model because of the extensive body system involvement and multidisciplinary nature of medical management. A Model System builds a critical mass of specialty and allied health expertise. Most important, the Model becomes a demonstration showcase for the innovation of its new programs and services by other localities. Frequently, satellite centers develop in outlying geographic areas that build their own expertise based on the leadership and guidance of the Model System. Also, the Model System resources and facilities are a focal point for public education and primary prevention programs.

Community Outreach and Advocacy

A Model System with its concentrated personnel and resources has the unique potential to influence effectively the development and implementation of public advocacy for disability-oriented programs and services. This will serve to demonstrate purposefully methods of community outreach and advocacy for persons with SCI in such areas as housing, transportation, recreation, employment, and other community needs.

CONCLUSION

The medical management and ultimate successful rehabilitation of SCI is a complex, multidisciplinary challenge. Acutely injured patients routinely have multiple trauma resulting from high-velocity injuries. Subsequent to the injury, they are prone to develop medical complications that involve all major body systems and mitigate the timely achievement of rehabilitation goals. The medical and surgical management of these complex cases requires a highly coordinated program involving a variety of medical, surgical, and allied health professionals.

All of these requirements are best achieved in a coordinated, dedicated SCI service delivery system that includes properly trained and equipped emergency medical services personnel; a designated, highly sophisticated neurotrauma center; a fully comprehensive medical rehabilitation program; appropriate psychosocial, educational, and vocational services to provide for return to the community and a productive lifestyle; and an aggressive and effective follow-up program to maintain rehabilitation gains, prevent further complications, and provide essential support services in the community.

2

The National Spinal Cord Injury Collaborative Database

J. Scott Richards, Bette K. Go,
Richard D. Rutt, and Patricia B. Lazarus

HISTORY

In 1970, the Rehabilitation Services Administration funded a demonstration project called the Southwest Regional System for Treatment of Spinal Cord Injury at the Good Samaritan Hospital in Phoenix, Arizona. One of the objectives of this program was to develop a database to document the results of a system of care including rehabilitation outcomes and cost-effectiveness.

The initial set of variables developed for this purpose was proposed by a multidisciplinary team of rehabilitation consultants and staff, all of whom apparently felt compelled to have the interests of their profession well represented in the database. Input was obtained from professionals in the fields of physiatry, orthopedics, neurosurgery, psychiatry, plastic surgery, urology, pulmonary medicine, social work, and vocational counseling and from insurance case managers, consumers, and others, in an attempt to answer a wide variety of questions pertaining to the process and outcomes of care provided to persons with SCI. During the first year it became clear that the amount of information to be collected (472 variables) was unmanageable and, in many cases, uncollectible.[1]

Six additional Model SCI Systems were funded in 1972 with a mandate to contribute to data collection efforts. This process was begun in 1973. As a consequence, the seven federally designated Model Systems held a series of meetings from 1972 to 1975 to reduce and refine the set of variables. As much as possible, variables selected were objective, collectible, and designed to answer specific clinical or research questions. The resulting 1975 common database contained 108 variables.

The National Spinal Cord Injury Data Research Center (NSCIDRC) was established in Phoenix, Arizona, in 1975 with Dr. John Young as director. The function of the NSCIDRC was to serve as the repository and coordinating center for the common database adopted by the Model Systems. To ensure uniformity of data collection across centers, a detailed syllabus was written precisely defining each variable. Reporting forms were designed and field tested, and data collection was started in 1976. A few variables, including some of the demographic variables, have not required any change in definition over time and have been continued in the database since 1973.

Data collection included two separate instruments referred to as Form I and Form II. Form I was completed at the time of initial discharge and included epidemiologic and demographic data along with descriptive information describing events relating to the initial hospitalization(s) occurring prior to the first definitive discharge. Form II was completed annually on the anniversary date of injury and was confined to events occurring in that reporting period. Technically, the first Form II covered the time between the definitive discharge and the first anniversary date of injury. Subsequent Form IIs covered events occurring during each follow-up year.

On December 31, 1981, funding for the NSCIDRC and national data collection efforts was eliminated as part of a federal austerity initiative. At that time there were 6014 cases in the database. Some of the results of this database were reported by Dr. Young and colleagues in the publication *Spinal Cord Injury Statistics: Experience of the Regional Model Spinal Cord Injury Systems.*[1]

Despite the federal cutback, the project directors and project officer continued to feel very strongly that ongoing collection, maintenance, and analyses of a common nationally oriented database should be continued. The University of Alabama at Birmingham (UAB) developed a proposal to establish an entity to be known as the UAB Spinal Cord Injury Data Management Service to continue as many of the activities of the NSCIDRC as possible. Revisions in the database were made to streamline the data collection and analysis process based on experience with data to that time. By March 1, 1983, 16 of the 17 federally sponsored Model Systems had agreed to utilize the data management services offered by UAB, and data collection was implemented. A computer tape of the final version of the NSCIDRC was transferred to Birmingham, Alabama.

During the hiatus between January 1, 1982, and March 1, 1983, some of the Model Systems had continued to collect the database variables. All of the participating Model Systems were encouraged to collect as much information as possible during this interim. In October 1984, after the Model Systems demonstrated a successful operation for 19 months, the National Institute of Handicapped Research again endorsed the value of the collaborative SCI database by funding the UAB National Spinal Cord Injury Statistical Center (NSCISC). Since 1970, 21 different Model Systems have contributed data to the common database. There are 13 Model Systems reporting data at the present time.

Although this extensive database represents a very significant undertaking, it cannot be expected to answer all questions concerning the outcomes of persons with SCI or the effectiveness of the Model Systems. A realistic goal is to provide quality information, general in nature but with emphasis on medical data, so that the benefits of this specialized care approach can be demonstrated. More specific research questions requiring specialized data collection methods are assigned to intra-System and inter-System collaborative research efforts for which participation is voluntary. An analysis of the information contained in the database reveals variables reflective of the demographics, medical characteristics and complications, etiology, and outcomes for persons treated in these Model Systems.

CHANGES IN THE COLLABORATIVE DATABASE

Since the National SCI Database continues to be a dynamic entity, one of the responsibilities of the NSCISC is to investigate and recommend additions, deletions, and refinements of the current variables. At various times, subcommittees composed of System professionals have also been involved in the modification of variable definitions. Currently, a database subcommittee of the project directors assists the NSCISC staff with the refinement process.

There are 76 variables in the current version of the National SCI Database. Seventy-two percent of today's variables have been a part of the database since 1975. Over the years there have been deletions and major changes in those variables that attempted to document the economics of SCI, medical complications, and operative procedures. In 1986, for example, major revisions were made in the database. In general, the demographic variables remained unchanged, but many of the more specific medical variables were modified to provide much more specific definitions and data collection methods to ensure more accuracy in reporting. The major reasons for deletion of variables have been difficulty in collection, changes in research and clinical outcome interests of the project directors and the funding agency, the accumulation of sufficient data for a particular research question, and/or poor inter-rater reliability.

Poor inter-rater reliability is a particularly vexing problem in collaborative data projects. There are numerous opportunities for error in the data collection process that could compromise the integrity of the data. Figure 2–1 details a number of potential opportunities for error and some of the NSCISC and individual System strategies that have been and are being used to minimize those sources of error. The extensive quality control checks currently in use by the NSCISC are described later in this chapter. The NIDRR and the Model System project directors have viewed the collection of *valid* data to be of the utmost importance and have therefore made surveillance of data a key function for the NSCISC staff.

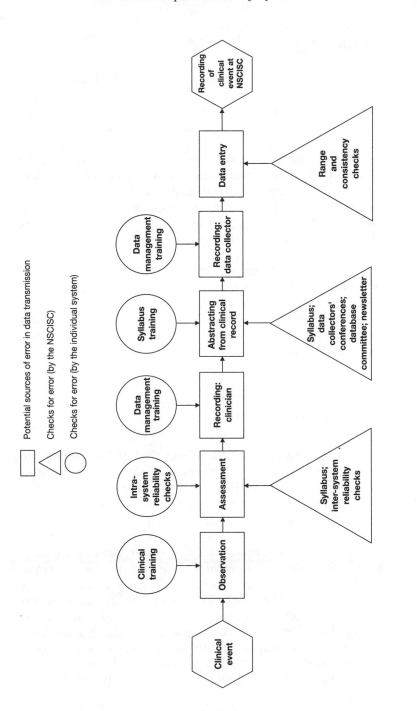

Figure 2–1 Sources of and Checks against Error in the National SCI Database

PATIENT ELIGIBILITY

Most of the criteria used to enter cases into the National SCI Database have remained unchanged over the years. Only traumatic SCIs are reported. Persons must, for the most part, be hospitalized continuously between the time of injury and System admission, and they must be discharged from the System having completed rehabilitation (or expired). Those who have minimal neurologic deficit or are normal neurologically at discharge are also eligible for complete initial hospitalization (Form I) data submission. Eligibility criteria for entry into the database initially included any person with traumatic SCI who was admitted to a Model System within 365 days after injury, remained in the hospital until definitive discharge, and resided in a geographical area as approved by the federal project officer. In 1987, a major change in the eligibility criteria limited entry into the database to those who were admitted to a Model System within 60 days of injury. A Registry data form with a few demographic variables was added to provide minimal data on those individuals admitted between 61 and 365 days of injury. Additionally, individual Systems have at various times adjusted their catchment areas in an effort to improve the quality and quantity of follow-up (Form II) data. Efforts have been made to include only those persons who, for various reasons, will most likely return to the Model System for follow-up care.

THE QUALITY CONTROL PROCESS

To ensure accuracy in the National SCI Database, the NSCISC continues to utilize a quality review process similar to but more detailed than that established by the NSCIDRC in the 1970s. Prior to the implementation of the NSCISC's current personal computer (PC) data entry system, quality checks were performed by the NSCISC and discrepancy lists sent to each system. Currently, comprehensive quality control (QC) programs have been incorporated into the NSCISC's PC data management software, and each system may check its data at any time. The QC checks are divided into three categories: range checks, cross-variable checks, and cross-form checks. Range checks performed during data entry allow only legal values to be entered for each variable. For example, the data entry program will not allow a code of "6" to be entered for Variable 106 (sex) because only codes "1" (male), "2" (female), and "9" (unknown) are valid.

Cross-variable checks ensure that data in different variables on a single record agree with each other. For example, if the date of death is coded "alive," then the cause of death and autopsy variables should also be coded "alive."

The third type of checking is performed across forms to compare data in the same variable for the same person on one record with those of a previous record. For example, if an individual's latest Form II record indicates that he or she is "single, never married," all earlier records should be coded "single, never married."

There are more than 350 such checks performed on each Form I record and more than 120 checks on each Form II record. It is the current NSCISC policy that a record must pass all QC checks before it is allowed into the National SCI Database.

The NSCISC applies other mechanisms to ensure the integrity of the National SCI Database. Computer-generated variables (such as the number of days between two dates) eliminate the possibility for mathematical errors. The NSCISC statistical reports frequently present and evaluate the variability among Systems in reporting selected variables. Periodic data collectors' conferences attended by representatives of each contributing System and the NSCISC staff consist of syllabus review, special sessions for new personnel, open discussions of data problems, and the sharing of different data collection methods. "Test cases" have often been used in these conferences to highlight and/or clarify ambiguities in definitions of variables with high levels of inter-System variability. The NSCISC staff members are regularly consulted regarding data collection and software problems and interpretation of the syllabus.

LOGISTICS OF DATA COLLECTION

Obtaining accurate and complete information for a comprehensive database requires the cooperation and coordination of a team. A clearly defined set of procedures and lines of responsibility must be established by each System to ensure that the required data are collected by qualified staff, familiar with the variable definitions, who will collect the data within the guidelines of the study. Internal data collection forms are frequently developed for use by staff members to document those data items they are most qualified to assess. Comprehensive internal forms, complete medical records, and required test results are among the many items needed by the primary data collector to ensure complete data submission on all study patients.

LOGISTICS OF DATA ENTRY AND DATA SUBMISSION

Until 1990, data for the National SCI Database were submitted on hard copy data forms and entered by the NSCIDRC or NSCISC staff. In December 1990, the NSCISC's PC data management software streamlined the data submission process by enabling each System to enter its own data and submit records to the NSCISC on floppy disks or cassette tape, or via modem transmission. More than 120 software functions (e.g., quality control and the generation of lists of missing follow-up records) provide each System an efficient mechanism for the data management and data submission process.

DISSEMINATION

Two major NSCISC responsibilities are to provide accurate data for System investigators to pursue clinical and research questions and to disseminate information about the outcomes and benefits of the Model Systems to non-System individuals. It is not surprising, therefore, that many of the dissemination activities of the NSCISC and its predecessor NSCIDRC have been directed to professionals, either those within the Model Systems network or those interested in learning about its outcomes. A list of the primary dissemination activities of the NSCIDRC and the NSCISC and their intended audiences may be found in Table 2–1.

This is the third book derived from the database. Its predecessors were *Spinal Cord Injury Statistics* (1982)[1], and *Spinal Cord Injury: The Facts and Figures* (1986).[2] Another publication, the proceedings from the 1990 National Consen-

---

Table 2–1   National SCI Data Research Center and National SCI Statistical Center Dissemination Activities

| | Distribution | | |
Activities	Within Systems	Consumers	Professionals
Spinal Cord Injury Statistics	X		X
Spinal Cord Injury: The Facts and Figures	X	X	X
Model Systems' SCI Digest*	X		X
Model Systems' SCI News Brief*	X		
NSCISC Newsletter*	X		
NSCISC Fact Sheet	X	X	X
NSCISC Quarterly and Annual Statistical Reports	X		
Presentations and Publications	X	X	X
Data Collection Syllabus	X		X
Technical Assistance	X	X	X

*No longer published.

sus Conference, S*pinal Cord Injury: The Model*,[3] utilized some of the national data as well. All these publications have been widely disseminated to consumers, professionals, and government officials. Throughout the years the NSCISC staff and staff from other Systems have used the national data for numerous scientific presentations and peer-reviewed publications. NSCISC staff members also provide daily technical assistance to consumers and professionals who have questions about the epidemiology of SCI and its treatment and outcomes. A copy of the National SCI Database on computer tape may be purchased from the NSCISC by any currently participating System. This mechanism provides each System, in addition to the staff of NSCISC, the opportunity to analyze the current database and disseminate findings.

Attempts will continue to refine and revise the database so as to maximize its validity and utility. Collaborative data collection is a time-intensive and therefore costly endeavor. However, without it, no individual System would likely be able to generate sufficient data to allow a rigorous analysis of the utility of the Model Systems' approach. Therefore, NIDRR and the project directors remain committed to a viable collaborative data effort and the use of those data for public dissemination of the benefits of the Model Systems.

FOLLOW-UP

A major goal of the Model Systems is to provide hands-on follow-up care to all persons treated in a System on at least an annual basis. This goal is part of the system-of-care concept: to provide a continuum of care from time of injury, through the rehabilitation process, and for the remainder of the person's life. The success of System follow-up, therefore, reflects the effectiveness of the continuum-of-care concept, and it also provides the data source to evaluate long-term clinical outcomes of persons treated in a System. Accurate follow-up data can help identify potential areas for follow-up intervention.

It is important to know what sources of bias might be present in a follow-up dataset. For example, those who return to the System for follow-up care may not be representative of the entire SCI population who were rehabilitated, which would affect interpretation of the follow-up data (see Figure 2–2 for trends in follow-up data collection over the past 19 years). For this reason, an analysis of the characteristics of the National SCI Form II Database is presented.

The following analysis compared two groups of persons: (1) those who returned for a follow-up visit in follow-up years 1, 5, and 10 or who were followed in those years by telephone or correspondence, and (2) those who were not followed by one of the Model Systems in those years. Data from deceased individuals were deleted from the analysis at the time of their death. Of those eligible, 78.8% were seen in person or evaluated by telephone or via correspon-

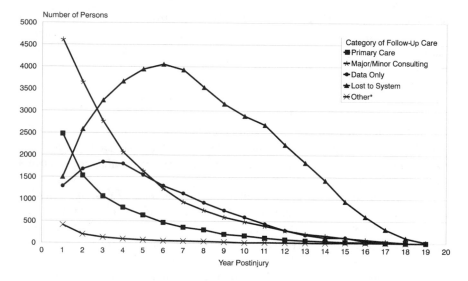

Number of Persons

Category of Follow-Up Care
- ■ Primary Care
- ✦ Major/Minor Consulting
- ● Data Only
- ▲ Lost to System
- ✕ Other*

Year Postinjury

*Other includes the following categories: Transferred, Minimal Deficit, Normal Neuro, Unknown, and Missing Form.

Figure 2–2 Trends in Follow-Up Data Collection over the Past 19 Years

dence for the first annual follow-up visit, 48.4% for the fifth year, and 29.0% for the tenth year. Technical reasons for the drop-off in return rates include the fact that persons followed by telephone or correspondence for 3 consecutive years now fall into the "lost to follow-up" category for purposes of this analysis. Changes in Model System designation (new Systems coming on line; older Systems not being re-funded) and the fact that no follow-up data were collected on any persons from 1973 to 1975 also have affected the follow-up success rate. Possible nontechnical reasons for the drop-off in follow-up rates include cost to the person with SCI, distance, transportation limitations, geographical reloca-tion, lack of complications that require attention, and the availability of alternative local primary health care. It is also possible that persons with minimal neurologic impairment who are doing well medically choose not to return for follow-up or may not be scheduled for yearly follow-up visits.

To determine whether there are any consistent patterns over time for those who have follow-up data versus those who do not, three logistic regression analyses were conducted, again contrasting those persons with and without follow-up data at each of the three follow-up periods. The results are presented in Table 2–2.

For the most part, demographic characteristics are not consistently predictive of those who do or do not have follow-up data. Level of education is an

Table 2–2 A Comparison of Likelihood of Obtaining Annual Follow-Up Data on Persons with Predictive Characteristics Compared to Persons Having Reference Characteristics

Predictive Characteristic*	Odds Ratios		
	Annual 1 (n = 12,100)	Annual 5 (n = 9,480)	Annual 10 (n = 5,325)
Age	1.00	1.00	1.00
Male	1.11	0.88†	1.14
White	1.07	1.09	1.04
Married	0.96	1.12†	1.22†
High School Graduate	1.14†	1.07	0.80†
College Graduate	1.13	1.05	0.87
Employed	1.08	1.15†	1.18
Insurance/Workers' Compensation/DVR	1.37†	1.80†	1.87†
Tetraplegia	1.08	1.23†	1.12
Frankel A, B, C	1.35†	1.31†	1.70†
Neurogenic Bladder	1.88†	2.53†	2.53†

*Reference characteristics in order: female; nonwhite; not married at injury; less than high school graduate at injury; neither employed nor student at injury; no private insurance, workers' compensation, or Department of Vocational Rehabilitation (DVR) sponsorship; paraplegia; Frankel D; normal bladder function.
†$P < 0.05$.

inconsistent predictor. Persons with neurologic impairment assessed as Frankel grade A (complete absence of motor and sensory function), grade B (sensory sparing only), or grade C (motor, nonfunctional) are more likely to have follow-up data in all years than those with Frankel grade D (motor functional). Those with a neurogenic bladder, which correlates both with level and extent of injury and with the type and number of medical complications (see Chapter 7), are also more likely to have follow-up data. Specifically, persons using any artificial method for bladder voiding are more likely to have follow-up data in all 3 years postinjury than those who had achieved normal bladder function. Those with private insurance, workers' compensation, or Department of Vocational Rehabilitation sponsorships are somewhat more likely to have follow-up data.

However, the impact of many of these statistically signficant findings is relatively small when an overall predictive model is considered (Table 2–3). The overall predictive validity of the models developed for each of the 3 years is neither statistically significant (goodness of fit, χ^2) nor a great deal better than chance (50:50, those with data versus those lost to follow-up). The fact that persons with less neurologic involvement are somewhat less likely to have follow-up data may not necessarily represent a self-selection process but clinical

Table 2-3   Sensitivity and Specificity of a Model To Predict Returnees and
Nonreturnees at Annual Follow-Up Years 1, 5, and 10

	Annual 1	Annual 5	Annual 10
Sensitivity	55.9	61.5	56.7
Specificity	59.5	57.8	63.2
Total	56.7	59.6	61.3

practice: managing physicians may not be requesting that such persons return every year for follow-up. From that perspective, then, the follow-up data used for analysis in this book can be taken as consistent with the characteristics of the National SCI Database as a whole.

REFERENCES

1. Young JS, Burns PE, Bowen AM, McCutchen R. *Spinal Cord Injury Statistics: Experience of the Regional Model Spinal Cord Injury Systems.* Phoenix, Ariz: Good Samaritan Medical Center; 1982.

2. Stover SL, Fine PR, eds. *Spinal Cord Injury: The Facts and Figures.* Birmingham, Ala: University of Alabama at Birmingham; 1986.

3. Apple DR, Hudson LM, eds. *Spinal Cord Injury: The Model.* Proceedings of the National Consensus Conference on Catastrophic Illness and Injury, December 1989. Atlanta: Shepherd Center for Treatment of Spinal Injuries; 1990.

3

The Epidemiology of Spinal Cord Injury

Bette K. Go, Michael J. DeVivo, and J. Scott Richards

INTRODUCTION

Since there are substantial physical, emotional, and economic consequences of SCI, and since there is no known cure for SCI at this time, increased emphasis must be placed on the primary prevention of this catastrophic injury. The development of cost-effective primary prevention programs requires detailed information on who is at greatest risk, as well as when, where, and how these injuries occur. In this chapter, detailed information is presented on the characteristics of persons enrolled in the National SCI Database as well as how these characteristics compare with those of "population-based" and other "hospital-based" samples reported in the literature. Basic information on neurologic levels, degree of injury completeness, the occurrence of associated injuries, and the existence of concomitant major medical conditions is presented in this chapter because of the impact these factors have on both the rehabilitation potential of the injured person and the rehabilitation outcome that is ultimately achieved. Biases in the Database are discussed, along with their potential impact on results contained in other chapters. The information provided in this chapter should also be useful in conducting cost-benefit analyses of alternative primary prevention programs.

INCIDENCE AND PREVALENCE

Because the National SCI Database includes only persons treated at Model Systems, it is not designed to determine either the incidence (number of new cases of SCI occurring in the United States each year) or prevalence (number of existing cases of SCI in the United States at any given time) of SCI. However, many studies of both incidence and prevalence have been published.[1-21]

21

Perhaps the most frequently cited study of SCI incidence was conducted in northern California during 1970 and 1971 by Kraus et al.[1] These investigators determined that the annual incidence rate for SCI with survival long enough to reach the hospital was 32.2 cases per million population. They also found that an additional 21.2 cases per million population per year died before reaching the hospital. Similar overall results were obtained by Griffin et al.[5] for Olmsted County, Minnesota, during the period from 1935 to 1981 (34.2 and 20.6, respectively). However, a strongly increasing trend over time was noted in the Olmsted County study during the 1975-1981 time period, when the annual hospitalized incidence rate of SCI had risen to 49.6 cases per million population. This trend did not appear to result from declining numbers of deaths prior to hospitalization, because the annual incidence rate for those who died before reaching the hospital remained relatively constant at 21.2 cases per million population.

In 1981, Clifton[13] conducted a hospital discharge survey in the 13-county area surrounding both Houston and Galveston, Texas. The incidence of SCI in this area was reported to be approximately 60 cases per million population, considerably higher than that reported for other locations. Unfortunately, the survey methodology was not reported in sufficient detail to evaluate this rather exceptional finding.

The annual hospitalized incidence rate of SCI in Alabama was estimated by Fine et al.[4] for the period from 1973 to 1977 to be 29.4 per million population. This study included only persons treated at the Model System in Birmingham who were both residents of and injured in Alabama. Other eligibility criteria included essentially continuous hospitalization from injury until rehabilitation discharge, either death during acute care or an injury severe enough to require rehabilitation, and hospitalization at the Model System within 1 year of injury. As a result, the derived incidence rates are likely to be substantial underestimates of the true incidence of SCI in Alabama. However, this study does provide useful information on the demographic and epidemiologic profile of persons in this "hospital-based" sample.

Two national studies of the incidence of SCI have been conducted.[2,6] Anderson et al. conducted a multistage random sampling based on geographical units, hospitals within the geographical units, and finally, patient records from the selected hospitals.[22] The records were sampled based on discharge ICDA-8 codes that were deemed either probable or possible cases of SCI. However, despite the inclusion of 247 hospitals, only 31 new cases of SCI were ultimately identified.[6] Given the sampling scheme that was used, this corresponded to an incidence rate for the 1974 calendar year of approximately 50 hospitalized cases per million population. Although this figure is somewhat higher than other published estimates, it must be interpreted as consistent with those estimates because of its high standard error.[1,2,5] Nonetheless, the validity of the study by Kalsbeek et al. has been questioned because the demographic profile of identified cases is largely inconsistent with every other study of SCI (e.g., 90% white and 60% women).

Another often-cited study of national incidence of hospitalized SCI was conducted by Bracken et al.[2] These authors identified cases from the National Hospital Discharge Survey for calendar years 1970 through 1977 by searching for specific ICDA-8 codes and subsetting by length of stay to eliminate both prevalent cases being hospitalized for acute medical conditions and double counting resulting from transfers between hospitals. However, it has been demonstrated that the subsetting approach utilized did not adequately address either of these two problems, and as a result the annual incidence rate of 40.1 cases per million population is thought to be somewhat overestimated.[23]

Because of the lack of high-quality national data on the incidence of SCI, several statewide registries have been developed with the idea of eventually pooling these data at a single site such as the Centers for Disease Control and Prevention.[24,25] Using such registry data, the annual hospitalized SCI incidence rate in Florida was reported to decrease from 40.3 to 33.1 cases per million population between 1980 and 1984, while a similar decrease from 33.1 to 29.5 cases per million population occurred in Virginia between 1979 and 1984.[3] More recent data from Virginia suggest that the SCI incidence rate has remained constant since that time. During the 1990–1992 period, the hospitalized SCI incidence rate in Virginia was 29.6 cases per million population.[16] A slight decrease in the annual hospitalized SCI incidence rate was reported in Arkansas from 32.4 cases per million population in 1980 to 26.6 cases per million population in 1989.[12]

Somewhat higher annual hospitalized SCI incidence rates have been reported by other states. In New York, the overall annual hospitalized SCI incidence rate for the years 1982 through 1988 was 43 cases per million population, with a significant decrease over this time period being reported for women but not men.[7] In Louisiana, annual hospitalized SCI incidence rates of 37.7 and 46.0 cases per million population were reported for the years 1990 and 1991, respectively.[17,18] In Georgia, the annual hospitalized SCI incidence rate from June 1991 to June 1992 was 46.1 cases per million population.[15] Finally, annual hospitalized SCI incidence rates of 36.5, 42.8, 33.7, and 37.7 cases per million population were reported in Colorado for the years 1989 through 1992, respectively.[8]

The Utah and Oklahoma registries include both hospitalized cases and those persons who die prior to hospitalization.[10,14] Between 1989 and 1991, the annual hospitalized SCI incidence rate in Utah was reported to be approximately 35 cases per million population. An additional eight cases per million population died prior to hospitalization.[14] Between 1988 and 1992, the annual hospitalized

SCI incidence rate in Oklahoma was reported to be approximately 41 cases per million population, with an additional six cases per million population dying prior to hospitalization.[10] Although a separate hospitalized SCI incidence rate was not reported, the 1990 incidence rate of SCI fatalities in Delaware was reported to be approximately 30 cases per million population, but this figure apparently included both pre- and posthospitalization deaths.[26] Interestingly, the Utah and Oklahoma rates were remarkably constant over time, and when compared with the results reported by both Kraus et al.[1] and Griffin et al.,[5] provide some evidence that the prehospital mortality rate may have declined during the past 20 years.

Variation in reported incidence rates among states is undoubtedly due to a combination of differences in reporting procedures; differences in underlying population characteristics such as age, gender, race, and education levels; and differences in geographic and inter-related social factors such as climate, degree of urbanization, driving patterns, road conditions, gun ownership, and alcohol consumption. Nonetheless, in view of these statewide statistics, it appears that the annual hospitalized SCI incidence rate in the United States as a whole remains in the range of 30 to 40 cases per million population. At this point, it is still too early to tell whether there is a trend over time in the incidence rate of SCI. Some states are reporting increases, others are reporting decreases, and still others are reporting relatively constant SCI incidence rates.

Since the statewide registries are generally designed to collect information only on new injuries, they are not suited to determination of SCI prevalence, unless long-term follow-up information on these individuals is also collected. Kalsbeek et al.[6] estimated the 1974 prevalence of SCI to be about 28,000 persons, or about 130 persons per million population. However, this estimate included only persons injured during the previous 4 years, and is therefore relatively meaningless. In 1975, Kurtzke[27] estimated the prevalence of SCI in the United States to be approximately 525 persons per million population based on an annual incidence rate of 30 new cases per million population and average life expectancy of 17.5 years. In 1980, this estimate was revised upward by DeVivo et al.[21] to 906 persons per million population based on an improved average life expectancy estimate of 30.2 years. Applying the prevalence rate determined by DeVivo et al. to 1992 population data, Gibson[28] estimated the prevalence of SCI in the United States to be approximately 230,000 persons.

The approach used in these studies assumes that both incidence and life expectancy are relatively constant over a long period of time. However, life expectancy has increased over the past few decades. Therefore, since current life expectancy estimates were used to make prevalence projections, these studies have most likely overestimated SCI prevalence slightly.

Since SCI is relatively rare, attempts to determine prevalence by actually counting individuals are generally not practical because of the considerable time and resources that would be required. Nonetheless, Griffin et al.[29] followed all persons enrolled in their study of SCI incidence in Olmsted County, Minnesota, until 1980 and found a prevalence rate of 473 persons per million population. When net population migration was taken into consideration, the 1980 SCI prevalence rate for their county increased to 583 persons per million population because a substantial number of persons with SCI moved into the county after their injuries.

More recently, an area sampling of the United States was funded during 1988 by the Paralyzed Veterans of America, and the results were published by Harvey et al.[19] Applying their prevalence rate of 721 persons per million population to 1992 population data would result in a prevalence estimate for SCI in the United States of almost 183,000 persons. Since Harvey et al. noted several reasons that their estimate is likely to be conservative, the true prevalence probably lies somewhere between 183,000 and 230,000 persons.

NATIONAL CAPTURE

One of the ways that Model System effectiveness is measured is by assessing the percentage of persons with new SCIs who are treated in Model Systems. Gibson[30] conservatively estimated that Model Systems "capture" approximately 15% of all new cases of SCI in the United States. Moreover, within individual Model System catchment areas, estimates of capture ranged from 67% to 74%.[30] While these estimates are only as precise as the underlying estimates of incidence on which they are based, their magnitude is likely a measure of recognition of the high quality of care provided by Model Systems.

THE NATIONAL SPINAL CORD INJURY DATABASE

As of June 1992 the Model Systems' National Spinal Cord Injury Database contained comprehensive (i.e., Form I) initial hospitalization records on 14,791 individuals. Additionally, 2249 Registry records with minimal data were also present in the database. The number of initial hospitalization records by year of injury is presented in Table 3–1. The decline in patients entered into the database in both 1981 and 1982 is the result of an interruption in data management services during these years (see Chapter 2). The decline in patients enrolled in the database since 1984 is the result of fewer systems being funded than in previous years. New eligibility criteria in 1987 account for the further decline in the number of Form I records.

Table 3–1   Number of Records in the National Spinal Cord Injury Database As of June 1992

Year of Injury	Initial Hospitalization Records (Registry and Form I)		Follow-up Records (Form II)	
	No. of Registry Records	No. of Form I Records	Follow-up Year	No. of Form II Records
1973	—	224	1	12,793
1974	—	402	2	10,678
1975	—	579	3	8,813
1976	—	685	4	7,344
1977	—	823	5	6,036
1978	—	852	6	4,859
1979	—	1,009	7	3,883
1980	—	1,132	8	3,107
1981	—	820	9	2,456
1982	—	762	10	1,944
1983	—	1,189	11	1,472
1984	1	1,147	12	1,030
1985	7	1,006	13	692
1986	105	964	14	480
1987	474	698	15	358
1988	417	678	16	188
1989	450	673	17	85
1990	485	606	18	19
1991	299	530	19	1
1992	11	12		
Total	2,249	14,791		66,238

Follow-up (Form II) records total 66,238. Table 3–1 presents the number of these records by follow-up year.

DEMOGRAPHICS

Before proceeding to a detailed discussion of the demographics of SCI, it is important to review the distinction between incidence and prevalence alluded to in the previous discussion. Because Model System data collection is based on new injuries, these data reflect the demographic profile of an incidence series of cases. The demographic profile of all persons with SCI alive today (prevalence) will be different because of differential survival rates among SCI population subgroups. For example, the percentage of all persons with SCI who are alive today and who have paraplegia is considerably higher than the percentage of new SCIs that result in paraplegia. Similarly, the mean age at injury should be slightly younger, and the percentage of whites, females, and persons with neurologically incomplete injuries will be somewhat higher among all existing cases than among new cases. The current average age of all existing cases will be substantially higher than the average age at injury among new cases. A more detailed discussion of the demographic profile of the SCI prevalence population is beyond the scope of this chapter; however, interested readers can refer to the results of the national sample conducted by Berkowitz et al.[20]

Age at Injury

Population-based studies have revealed that SCI occurs most frequently in teenaged persons and young adults between 16 and 30 years of age.[1,5,8–16,18] A similar age pattern is observed for persons enrolled in the National SCI Database. In fact, Figure 3–1 shows that among persons enrolled in the National SCI Database, more SCIs occur in the 16 to 30 age group than all other age groups combined. The average (mean) age at injury is 30.7 years, the median age at injury is 26 years, and the most frequently occurring age at injury (mode) is 19 years. Therefore, the National SCI Database sample appears to be relatively unbiased with respect to age, although it does appear to contain a slightly lower percentage of persons injured at age 60 or greater than population-based studies.[8,11] This issue is discussed in greater detail in Chapter 13.

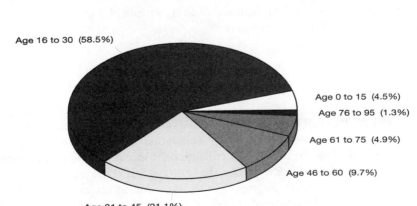

Age 16 to 30 (58.5%)

Age 0 to 15 (4.5%)

Age 76 to 95 (1.3%)

Age 61 to 75 (4.9%)

Age 46 to 60 (9.7%)

Age 31 to 45 (21.1%)

Figure 3–1 Age at Injury

The mean age at injury is slightly higher for females (32.2 years) than for males (30.3 years). Among racial/ethnic groups, Asians have the highest mean age at injury (35.0 years), while Hispanics have the lowest mean age at injury (27.3 years). The mean age at injury for African-Americans is 33.2 years, while for whites it is 30.3 years.

Since 1973 there has been an increase of 4.9 years in mean age at time of injury. Those who were injured between 1973 and 1977 had a mean age of 28.5 years, while those injured between 1990 and 1992 had a mean age of 33.4 years. By comparison, persons with new traumatic SCIs enrolled during 1991 in the Uniform Data System (UDS) for Medical Rehabilitation dataset had a somewhat higher mean age of 40.0 years.[31] In 1991, the UDS dataset contained information from 139 medical rehabilitation hospitals and units from 35 states. Overall, 1160 new cases of traumatic SCI were reported to the UDS in that year. However, the UDS dataset does not represent a national random sample of all SCIs.

In conjunction with the increase in mean age, the proportion of persons enrolled in the National SCI Database who were at least 61 years of age at time of injury increased from 4.5% for the 1973 to 1977 period to 8.5% since 1990. These trends are not surprising, since the median age of the general population has increased from 27.9 years in 1970 to 33.1 years in 1991.[32,33] However, changes in underlying age-specific incidence rates, referral patterns to Model Systems, or survival rates at the injury scene might also explain part of this trend.[34] Nonetheless, this trend has important implications, since older persons who incur SCI have more pre-existing major medical conditions and are more likely to have tetraplegia, develop secondary medical complications during acute care and rehabilitation, require placement in a nursing home, and have more frequent rehospitalizations than their younger counterparts.[35-37] A more complete discussion of the implications of aging with an SCI appears in Chapter 13 and has been published elsewhere.[38]

Gender

Overall, 82.2% of all persons enrolled in the National SCI Database are males. This greater than four-to-one male-to-female ratio has varied little throughout the 19 years of Model Systems' data collection.[39] Since population-based samples range from 69.1% to 80.6% male, the National SCI Database appears to be slightly biased toward the disproportionate inclusion of males.[1,5,8,10-12,14-16,18,40] Only the 1981 population-based sample of the Houston-Galveston area had a higher percentage of males (88.5%) than the National SCI Database.[13]

There was a slight increase in the proportion of males from 81.9% in the years between 1973 and 1977 to 84.2% in the 1984 to 1986 period. When this analysis was confined to six Model Systems in existence throughout this time frame, a virtually identical trend was observed.[34] However, the proportion of males decreased to 80.8% during the 1987–1989 period and has subsequently remained at that level. During 1991, 75% of persons with new traumatic SCI enrolled in the UDS dataset were male.[31]

Since these figures are proportions, they must be interpreted cautiously. Even if one makes the reasonable assumption that no changes in referral patterns occurred with respect to gender, one still cannot infer from these data that the incidence of SCI among males has decreased in recent years. A similar decrease in the male-to-female ratio after 1986 could be obtained if the incidence among females increased while the incidence among males remained constant, or if the incidence among males increased after 1986 but at a slower rate than it did among females. In fact, the increase in the percentage of males during the earlier time periods is consistent with findings from the New York registry of no trend in the incidence rate among males, coupled with a decrease in the incidence rate among females between 1982 and 1988.[7] Therefore, each of these alternative explanations should be kept in mind when interpreting other trends in proportional data throughout the remainder of this chapter.

The preponderance of injuries occurring among males is related, in large part, to both age at injury and cause of injury (i.e., young males are more often involved in high-risk activities), and should come as no surprise since the mortality rate due to all unintentional injuries in the general population is about three times higher for males than females in the 15 to 24 age group and almost four times higher for males than females in the 25 to 44 age group.[41] More specific information about the relationship between gender and etiology of injury is addressed later in this chapter.

Racial/Ethnic Groups

Figure 3–2 compares the racial/ethnic distribution of persons with SCI who are enrolled in the National SCI Database to the overall 1990 United States population. The proportion of persons with SCI who are white is lower than the proportion of whites in the 1990 U.S. general population (70.1% versus 80.3%). Conversely, the proportion of African-Americans is higher among persons with SCI (19.6% versus 12.1%). The proportion of Asians (including Pacific Islanders) is slightly lower, while the proportion of American Indians is slightly higher in the National SCI Database than in the general population.

Part of the racial difference between the SCI and general populations observed in Figure 3–2 results from an inconsistency in definition between the National SCI Database and the Bureau of the Census. In the National SCI Database, persons of Hispanic origin are coded as a separate racial/ethnic group exclusive

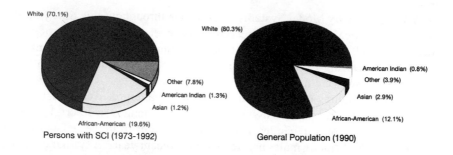

Figure 3–2 Racial Distribution of Persons with SCI and the General Population

of all other groups. However, the Bureau of the Census uses a separate question to assess whether a person is of Hispanic origin. As a result, persons of Hispanic origin are included in the white, African-American, Asian, and American Indian categories in the general population, but are included in the "other" race category for the SCI population. Since most persons of Hispanic origin are also white, the difference between the percentages of whites in the two populations is somewhat overestimated. In fact, persons of Hispanic origin comprise virtually all of the "other" race category in the SCI population (7.5% of all persons with SCI). By contrast, 9.0% of all persons in the 1990 U.S. general population were of Hispanic origin.[33]

Part of the differences seen in Figure 3–2 also result from the geographic locations of the Model Systems and the characteristics of the populations they serve. Most Model Systems are located in large urban areas with heavy concentrations of minorities. Therefore, although it would be difficult to confirm, it seems reasonable to assume that a slight bias exists in the National SCI Database toward the disproportionate inclusion of minorities.

Nonetheless, several studies have shown that although the majority of new SCIs occur among persons who are white, the incidence rate of SCI is actually somewhat higher among African-Americans.[1,4,10–12,15,18] This is consistent with unintentional injury mortality rates for the general U.S. population that are considerably higher for African-Americans than for whites.[42]

Recently, a very significant trend over time was reported in the racial distribution of persons enrolled in the National SCI Database between 1973 and 1986.[34] Since then, the trend has continued. During 1973 through 1977, 76.9% of persons enrolled in the National SCI Database were white, 14.0% were African-American, 6.2% were Hispanic, 2.1% were American Indians, and 0.8% were Asians. However, between 1990 and 1992, only 56.3% of persons enrolled in the National SCI Database were white, while 29.9% were African-American,

11.2% were Hispanic, 1.6% were Asian, 0.4% were American Indians, and 0.6% were classified as "other" races. Moreover, these trends have been very consistent during each successive time period since 1973.

A small portion of this trend is undoubtedly due to similar trends in the U.S. general population. Between 1980 and 1990, the proportion of white persons in the U.S. general population decreased from 83.1% to 80.3%, while the proportion of African-Americans increased slightly from 11.7% to 12.1%, and the proportion of Asians almost doubled from 1.5% to 2.9%.[33] Moreover, the proportion of persons from the U.S. general population who are of Hispanic origin increased from 6.4% to 9.0% during that same period.[33]

Since racial trends in the U.S. general population are insufficient to account for the observed trend in the SCI population, alternative explanations are necessary. Given the magnitude and consistency of the change in the racial composition of the SCI population, it is probably not entirely due to the periodic changes in either the identities of participating Model Systems or the eligibility criteria for inclusion in the National SCI Database.[34] While a change in overall referral patterns to Model Systems might account for at least a portion of these trends, these data suggest that underlying incidence rates for each racial group have changed. However, the exact nature of these changes cannot be determined from the Model Systems' data.

Level of Education

Table 3–2 presents the level of education completed at the time of injury. Since the median age of this population is 26 years, it is not surprising that most (59.3%) have at least completed high school. Nonetheless, education levels for the SCI

Table 3–2 Percentage Distribution of Education Levels Completed at Time of Injury

Level of Education	%
Eighth Grade or Less	12.4
Grades 9 to 11	28.3
High School Diploma	49.8
Associate's Degree	1.3
Bachelor's Degree	5.8
Master's Degree	1.3
Doctorate	0.7
Other	0.4

population are somewhat below those of persons in the U.S. general population of comparable age. For example, 66% of persons with SCI admitted between the ages of 18 and 21 years are at least high school graduates.[43] However, the comparable figure for the U.S. general population is 86%.[33] Although only 2.7% of persons in the National SCI Database are less than 15 years of age when injured, 12.4% have education levels of eighth grade or below. Moreover, only 9.8% of persons enrolled in the National SCI Database are between 15 and 17 years of age at injury, while 28.3% have education levels between the ninth and eleventh grades. These figures represent only the number of grades of school completed; they do not necessarily reflect the level of academic achievement.

Fortunately, the percentage of persons with SCI who are at least high school graduates at the time of injury has increased substantially over time, perhaps due to the increased average age noted earlier.[34] This trend is important because relatively low education levels are one of the many reasons re-employment rates after SCI are so low.[44,45] Additional information on persons who return to school after rehabilitation is contained in Chapter 10 and has been published elsewhere.[43]

Interestingly, there is a strong correlation between education level and age at time of injury among older individuals who presumably have completed their educations. In a Birmingham, Alabama, hospital-based series of persons with SCI, 50.8% of 16- to 30-year-olds were at least high school graduates, compared with 42.4% for the 31- to 45-year-old age group, 30.1% for the 46- to 60-year-old age group, and 18.9% for persons at least 61 years of age.[35] This suggests that there was somewhat less emphasis placed on completing formal education 50 years ago than there is today. It also makes re-employment among older individuals with SCI more difficult to achieve and may in part explain the fact that younger persons are much more likely to become employed after injury than are older persons.[44,45]

To date, only three statewide registries have reported detailed information on education levels. Findings from the Colorado registry are consistent with the National SCI Database in that, among persons over 25 years of age, those with SCI have somewhat lower education levels than the Colorado general population.[8] In general, the Colorado SCI population has higher education levels than persons enrolled in the National SCI Database; however, the Colorado general population is better educated than the U.S. population as a whole. In both Georgia[15] and Virginia,[16] the reported distribution of education levels for persons who incur SCIs is similar to that reported by the Model Systems. Although additional registry data are needed from other locations before a definitive statement can be made, it appears from the Colorado, Georgia, and Virginia data that any potential bias in the National SCI Database with respect to education levels should be relatively small or nonexistent.

Primary Occupational, Educational, or Training Status at the Time of Injury

Most persons with SCI are employed at the time of injury (Table 3–3). However, 14.3% of persons with SCI are unemployed at the time of their injury. This figure is about twice the average unemployment rate for the U.S. general population over the past 20 years. Although this figure is not surprising given the locations of many of the Model Systems (i.e., in large urban areas where unemployment is typically above the national average), it is, once again, important because of the strong relationship between previous employment history and return to work after SCI.[44,45]

According to the Colorado registry, 46% of all SCIs occur among persons who are students, retired, or unemployed.[8] Occupational data have not been reported for other statewide registries. Therefore, based on this somewhat limited information, it appears that the National SCI Database is relatively unbiased with respect to occupational status at the time of injury.

Since 1973, trends in occupational status include a decrease in the percentage of students and homemakers at the time of injury, with a concomitant increase in the percentage of retired and unemployed persons.[34] These trends are consistent with the previously noted changes in age and gender.

Marital Status

It is not surprising, given the young age at which most injuries occur, that most persons with SCI are single (never married) at the time of injury (Figure 3–3). However, when persons who die prior to hospitalization are included, the incidence rate of SCI is actually slightly higher among divorced persons than

Table 3–3 Percentage Distribution of Occupational Status at Time of Injury

Occupational Status	%
Working	59.6
Homemaker	2.4
On-the-Job Training	0.2
Sheltered Workshop	0.1
Retired	4.3
Student	18.5
Unemployed	14.3
Other	0.6

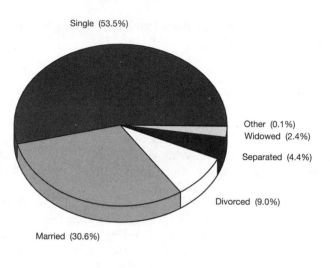

Single (53.5%)

Other (0.1%)
Widowed (2.4%)

Separated (4.4%)

Divorced (9.0%)

Married (30.6%)

Figure 3–3 Marital Status at Time of Injury

either never-married or separated persons, while married and widowed persons have the lowest SCI incidence rates.[1]

Despite the increased average age at time of injury, no trend was observed in marital status.[34] This combination of findings is consistent with trends in the U.S. general population between 1970 and 1988. During this period, the median age at time of first marriage increased 3 years.[33] Therefore, a comparable change in average age of the SCI population would result in no change in marital status at the time of injury.

Marital status at the time of injury was reported by Kraus et al.[1] for their population-based study of 18 northern California counties that was conducted in 1970 and 1971. If all ages are included and persons with unknown marital status are excluded, then just over 40% of persons with SCI included in the northern California study were single at the time of injury. However, this figure includes persons who die prior to hospitalization, most of whom are older and more likely to be married. More recently, 43.3% of persons enrolled in the Georgia registry, 48% of persons enrolled in the Colorado registry, and 50.1% of persons enrolled in the Virginia registry were reported to be single (never married) at the time of injury.[8,15,16] Also, 51% of persons with SCI enrolled in a large hospital-based series in Louisiana between 1965 and 1984 were single at the time of injury.[46] Therefore, the National SCI Database appears to be relatively unbiased with respect to marital status at the time of injury. Additional information on changes in marital status after SCI is contained in Chapter 10 and has been published elsewhere.[43,47,48]

Etiology

The National SCI Database documents 38 causes of injury. For convenience, these 38 specific causes are often grouped into five major categories: motor vehicle crashes, falls, acts of violence, recreational sporting activities, and other causes not fitting into any of these categories.

Almost half (44.5%) of all persons enrolled in the National SCI Database were injured in motor vehicle crashes, the majority of which were automobile crashes (Figure 3–4). The second most common etiology of SCI is falls, followed by acts of violence (primarily gunshot wounds or stabbings) and recreational sporting activities.

More specific information on causes of SCI appears in Table 3–4. Automobile crashes are the leading individual cause of SCI, followed by falls, gunshot wounds, diving incidents, motorcycle crashes, and being hit by a falling object. Closer inspection of the sports category reveals that almost two thirds of all sports-related SCIs are due to diving incidents. Injuries due to all-terrain vehicles/all-terrain cycles are under-reported, since this category was not added to the Database until 1986. Prior to that time, these injuries were documented as either motorcycle or other vehicular crashes.

The information contained in Table 3–4 should not be interpreted to reflect either the absolute or relative risk of SCI associated with participating in these

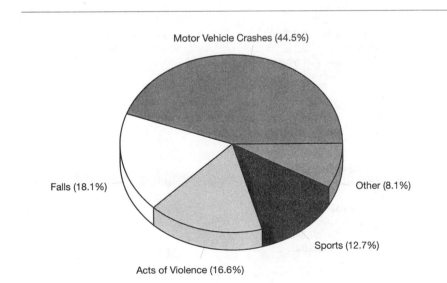

Figure 3–4 Grouped Etiology

Table 3–4 Percentage Distribution of Specific Causes of SCI

Etiology	%
Motor Vehicle Crashes	
Automobile	35.8
Motorcycle	6.1
Bicycle	0.9
Other Vehicular	0.7
Fixed-Wing Aircraft	0.4
All-Terrain Vehicles and Cycles	0.2
Rotating Wing Aircraft	0.2
Boat	0.1
Snowmobile	0.1
Sports	
Diving	8.5
Football	0.7
Snowskiing	0.5
Horseback Riding	0.4
Surfing, Body Surfing	0.4
Gymnastics	0.3
Trampoline	0.3
Wrestling	0.3
Other Winter Sports	0.3
Other Sports, Unclassified	0.3
Field Sports	0.2
Hang Gliding	0.2
Waterskiing	0.2
Baseball, Softball	0.1
Rodeo	<0.1
Basketball, Volleyball	<0.1
Air Sports	<0.1
Track and Field	<0.1
Skateboarding	<0.1
Falls	18.1
Acts of Violence	
Gunshot Wound	14.6
Other Penetrating Wound	1.0
Personal Contact	0.9
Explosion	0.1
Other	
Hit by Falling Objects	3.7
Pedestrian	1.7
Medical/Surgical Complication	1.7
Other, Unclassified	1.0

activities. Before any such conclusions can be made, actual incidence rates for each cause must be known. Incidence rates can only be calculated based on a more complete enumeration of cases, coupled with knowledge of levels of general-population participation in each activity. For example, although more SCIs were reported to the National SCI Database as being secondary to playing football (n = 102) than to participating in wrestling events (n = 48), it has also been reported that during the 1985–1986 sports season, there were about 1,300,000 high school and 75,000 college football players, compared with only 250,000 high school and 8,000 college wrestlers.[49] Therefore, although SCIs are more common among football players than among wrestlers, it would appear that the risk of SCI might be higher for wrestling than for football. However, more detailed information on numbers of participants outside of organized high school and college athletics programs, as well as frequency and duration of participation, would be necessary before final conclusions could be made.

Although further details concerning the exact nature of the injury-producing events listed in Table 3–4 are not contained in the National SCI Database, this information is occasionally available from other published studies. For example, Fine et al.[50] reported a detailed accounting of a series of 48 SCIs resulting from gunshot wounds, including the exact nature of each event as well as an epidemiologic profile of the entire series. Similar data on SCI secondary to gunshot wounds were included in the latest report from the Louisiana state registry.[18] Kraus et al., Wigglesworth, and both the Utah and Louisiana state registries have reported extensive analyses of neurologic outcomes as well as vehicle and crash factors in motor vehicle–related SCIs.[14,18,51,52] Separate analyses of SCIs secondary to motorcycle crashes and falls have been reported.[53–55] Information on alcohol and drug involvement as well as safety belt usage at the time of injury has also been reported.[8,10–12,14,18]

Some interesting trends in the causes of SCI have developed since the inception of the Model System program in 1973. The proportion of SCIs due to motor vehicle crashes has declined from a peak of 47.2% between 1978 and 1980 to only 38.1% since 1990. The proportion of SCIs due to sports activities has also declined from 14.8% prior to 1978 to only 8.8% since 1990. Conversely, the proportion of SCIs due to falls has increased slightly from 15.3% between 1978 and 1980 to 20.2% since 1990, while the proportion of SCIs due to acts of violence has increased from only 13.9% prior to 1978 to 25.1% since 1990. Interestingly, the latter trend has been limited to African-Americans and Hispanics. Among African-Americans, the percentage of SCI due to acts of violence has increased from 39.5% prior to 1978 to 45.7% since 1990, while among Hispanics, the comparable increase has been from 24.9% to 52.4%. In fact, acts of violence are now the leading cause of SCI among both these racial/ ethnic groups. These trends could be due at least in part to any combination of changes in referral patterns, locations of Model Systems, or survival rates at the injury scene.

The trend toward a greater percentage of new cases of SCI due to acts of violence and a lower percentage of new cases of SCI due to motor vehicle crashes is consistent with recently reported general population mortality trends in both Louisiana and Texas.[56] In Louisiana, the motor vehicle–related death rate decreased by 30% between 1970 and 1990, while in Texas, it decreased by 42% over the same time period. Conversely, the firearm-related death rate remained relatively constant during this period. Therefore, changes in the underlying cause-specific incidence rates are likely to be causing at least part of this proportional trend in SCI etiologies.

Most population-based studies of SCI have included information on the causes of these injuries. However, the results vary considerably across locations. Nonetheless, motor vehicle crashes are always the leading cause of SCI, accounting for about half of all cases.[1,5,8,10–16,18,40] Falls usually rank second, accounting for between 13% and 23% of cases. Violence ranges from 3% to 17%, except in Louisiana, where violence ranks as the second leading cause of SCI and accounts for 32% of cases. Sports ranges from 6% to 17%, and being hit by falling objects ranges from 1% to 5%. Therefore, although no valid national studies of the etiology of SCI have been conducted, it appears that the National SCI Database has a slight bias toward the inclusion of more cases of SCI due to acts of violence and fewer cases caused by motor vehicle crashes than would be expected based on the results of population-based studies. Once again, this is not surprising given the locations of the Model Systems in predominantly large urban areas.

Interestingly, the causes of SCI differ substantially by age, gender, and race. Figure 3–5 illustrates grouped etiologies by age at time of injury. Vehicular crashes are the leading cause of SCI up to 45 years of age. After age 45, falls are the leading cause of SCI. Both the proportions of SCIs due to sports activities and acts of violence decline steadily with advancing age at injury, while the reverse is true for falls. Motor vehicle crashes cause 48.5% of all SCIs among 16- to 30-year-olds but only 29.8% among persons over 75 years of age. Both population- and hospital-based studies have revealed similar relationships between age at time of injury and cause of SCI.[1,10–12,35]

Population-based studies have shown that cause-specific incidence rates of SCI are always higher for men than for women.[1,11,12,18] Differences in the proportionate distribution of SCI etiologies by gender are illustrated in Figure 3–6. Not surprisingly, the most striking difference between genders is in the proportion of sports-related SCIs: 14.1% among males versus 6.6% among

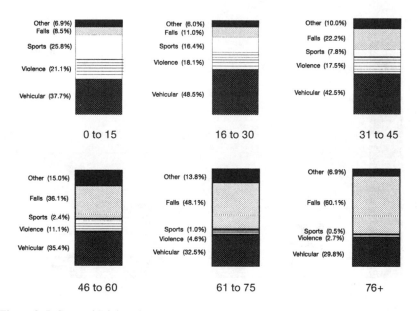

Figure 3–5 Grouped Etiology by Age at Injury

females. Additionally, motor vehicle crashes account for 56.3% of SCIs among females but only 41.9% among males. These differences between genders are similar to those observed in population-based studies.[11,12,18]

The distribution of SCI etiologies by racial/ethnic group appears in Table 3–5. Motor vehicle crashes are the leading cause of SCI among whites, American Indians, Asians, and "others." However, among African-Americans and Hispanics, acts of violence account for a plurality of injuries, with motor vehicle crashes ranking second. In fact, since 1973, acts of violence have accounted for 42.5% of all SCIs among African-Americans and 37.4% of all SCIs among Hispanics, but only 7.1% of all SCIs among whites. As indicated previously, since 1990, the percentages of SCI due to acts of violence among African-Americans and Hispanics are even higher. Falls are the second leading cause of SCI for whites and American Indians, and tied for second with acts of violence for Asians. The third leading cause of SCI among whites is sports, while falls ranks third for African-Americans and Hispanics, and acts of violence ranks third for American Indians.

Population-based studies have shown that the incidence rate of SCI due to acts of violence is between six and nine times higher among African-Americans than among whites.[11,12,18] Kraus et al.[1] also found an excess of SCIs due to firearms among African-Americans. This finding is not surprising, given that the homi-

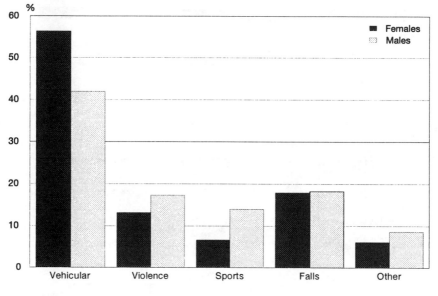

Figure 3–6 Grouped Etiology by Gender

cide rate in the general population is 6.5 times higher among African-Americans than among whites.[42] There are no significant racial differences in any other cause-specific SCI incidence rates.[11,12,18] Therefore, the trend toward an increasing percentage of African-Americans in the National SCI Database that was noted previously explains, at least partially, the concomitant trend toward an increasing share of SCIs enrolled in the National SCI Database being caused by acts of violence.

Table 3–5 Distribution of SCI Etiologies by Racial/Ethnic Group

Racial/Ethnic Group	Grouped Etiology (%)					
	Motor Vehicle Crashes	Falls	Acts of Violence	Sports	Other	Total
White	49.9	18.4	7.1	16.0	8.6	100.0
African-American	26.6	19.6	42.5	4.1	7.2	100.0
American Indian	67.4	12.8	9.1	4.8	5.9	100.0
Hispanic	34.4	13.3	37.4	7.5	7.4	100.0
Asian	50.3	17.7	17.7	7.4	6.9	100.0
Other	59.5	11.9	19.0	4.8	4.8	100.0

Day and Month of Injury

SCIs occur in cycles, with the fewest injuries occurring in February, followed by a steady increase until July and a steady decline until the next February (Figure 3–7). Given the injury etiologies identified previously, it is not surprising that SCI incidence increases as daylight hours increase and temperatures rise. The same monthly pattern has been observed for U.S. general population overall injury mortality rates.[41] In fact, except for the time period between 1984 and 1986, when most SCIs occurred during the month of August, and between 1973 and 1977, when the fewest SCIs occurred during January, there has been no deviation from this cycle since 1973.

Seasonal variation in SCI incidence is reduced slightly in areas of the United States where there is less temperature fluctuation from month to month.[4,8,10,12,18,28,46] Among Model Systems located in the northern United States, the distribution of new SCIs ranges from 5.8% in February to 12.0% in July, while the comparable range for Model Systems located in the South is from 6.7% to 10.2%. Moreover, virtually the entire trend appears to be due to sports-related injuries. Among

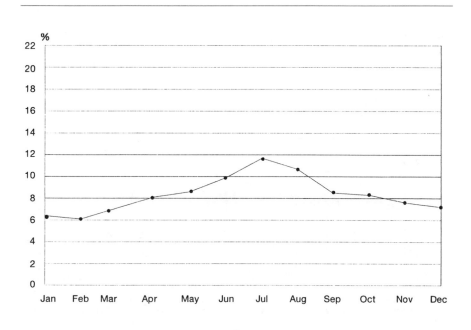

Figure 3–7 Percentages of Reported SCI Cases by Month of Injury

Model Systems located in the North, 2.4% of sports-related injuries occur in November, while 29.2% occur in July. However, among southern Model Systems, the range for new cases of sports-related SCI is from 1.5% in December to 19.5% in July.

Figure 3–8 shows the percentages of reported SCIs by day of occurrence. More SCIs occur on Saturday (20%) than on any other day. The next most common day of occurrence for SCI is Sunday (18.6%), followed by Friday (14.5%). Population-based studies have revealed a similar pattern.[8,10,12,18] The pattern shown in Figure 3–8 is virtually identical to that of U.S. general population motor vehicle crash fatalities.[41] Interestingly, one small hospital-based series revealed that 52% of all SCIs due to gunshot wounds occurred on either Saturday or Sunday.[50]

Pre-Existing Major Medical Conditions

Since October 1986, the National SCI Database has contained information on nine major medical conditions in existence at the time of injury that have the

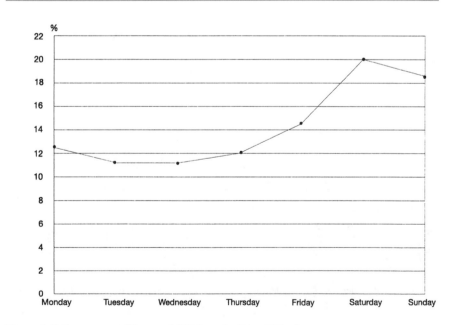

Figure 3–8 Percentages of Reported SCI Cases by Day of Injury

capacity to inhibit or impair the rehabilitation potential of a person with SCI. The definitions of each condition are contained in Appendix A.

Table 3–6 shows the overall prevalence of each condition. The overall prevalence of each condition is slightly higher for females than for males with the exception of chronic obstructive pulmonary disease (COPD) and renal/ureteral calculi. Excluding American Indians because of their small sample size, the prevalence of ankylosing spondylitis/rheumatoid arthritis, COPD, heart disease, and renal/ureteral calculi is highest among whites; the prevalence of degenerative joint diseases, hypertension, diabetes mellitus, and spinal canal stenosis is highest among African-Americans. The prevalence of cervical spondylosis is highest among persons of Asian descent. However, these differences are relatively small and generally not statistically significant.

Given the nature of these medical conditions, it is not surprising that their prevalence increases substantially with advancing age at time of injury. Overall, 84.9% of those who had at least one condition were older than 30 years of age at the time of injury. Additional information on the relationship between age at time of injury and the prevalence of pre-existing major medical conditions, as well as the clinical implications of this relationship, is contained in Chapter 13 and has been published elsewhere.[35]

Associated Injuries

Since SCIs are the result of traumatic physical impact (car crashes, gunshot wounds, falls, etc.), it is not surprising they are often accompanied by other

Table 3–6   Prevalence of Pre-Existing Major Medical Conditions for All Persons Enrolled in the National SCI Database since 1986

Medical Condition	*Prevalence (%)*
Hypertension	8.6
Cervical Spondylosis	4.4
Heart Disease	4.0
Degenerative Joint Disease	4.0
Spinal Canal Stenosis	3.9
Chronic Obstructive Pulmonary Disease	3.0
Diabetes Mellitus	2.9
Ankylosing Spondylitis, Rheumatoid Arthritis	1.9
Calculus in Kidney or Ureter	0.8
None of the Documented Conditions	79.1
One or More Conditions	20.9

associated injuries. The number and severity of these associated injuries affect not only the length of initial hospitalization (and therefore hospitalization expenses), but also the initial rehabilitation outcome.[57] Moreover, some associated injuries can have long-term consequences affecting functional capabilities.

Since 1986, the occurrence of eight associated injuries that could severely affect the treatment course for a person with SCI has been documented in the National SCI Database (see Appendix A for definitions). Of the 4107 persons enrolled in the Database since that time, 44.8% had none of the documented injuries. Table 3–7 presents the percentages of all persons with each associated injury by grouped etiology of SCI. The percentages do not sum to 100 because some persons have more than one associated injury.

The most common injuries (occurring in more than one fourth of the population) are fractures (29.3%) and loss of consciousness (28.2%). Traumatic pneumothorax or hemothorax occurs in 17.8% of all persons with SCI, while head injuries of sufficient severity to affect either cognitive or emotional functioning are reported in 11.5% of all cases. Only rare occurrences of the remaining four types of associated injuries were reported.

Persons injured in motor vehicle crashes were at greatest risk for fractures (39.7%), head injuries (18.4%), and loss of consciousness (42.5%), and were the most likely persons to have at least one reportable associated injury. Not surprisingly, since most persons whose injuries result from gunshot wounds are

Table 3–7 Occurrence of Associated Injuries by Grouped Etiology for All Persons Enrolled in the National SCI Database since 1986

Associated Injury	Grouped Etiology (%)					
	Motor Vehicle Crashes	Falls	Acts of Violence	Sports	Other	Total
Brachial Plexus Injury	1.2	0.8	1.8	0.2	2.8	1.3
Fracture(s)	39.7	30.5	16.0	5.7	35.4	29.3
Head Injury	18.4	10.3	2.5	4.2	11.4	11.5
Loss of Consciousness	42.5	24.0	8.1	22.4	26.2	28.2
Amputation	0.6	0.2	0.2	0.0	2.8	0.6
Major Burn	0.5	1.2	0.0	0.0	0.6	0.5
Peripheral Nerve Injury	1.1	0.8	2.2	0.2	1.6	1.2
Traumatic Pneumothorax/ Hemothorax	16.6	10.1	35.9	2.7	16.6	17.8
None of the Above	33.3	48.1	50.2	69.4	51.1	44.8

shot in the chest rather than the neck, persons injured in acts of violence are most likely to have a pneumothorax and/or hemothorax (35.9%). With the exception of head injuries and loss of consciousness, persons injured in sports-related incidents were least likely to have any of the associated injuries, with 69.4% of these individuals having none of the reportable associated injuries.

Neurologic Level of Injury at Discharge

Severity of the SCI is evaluated by several variables in the National SCI Database. Neurologic level of injury documents the most caudal (lowest) segment of the spinal cord with normal sensory and motor function on both sides of the body. Persons with tetraplegia have injuries affecting any of the eight cervical segments of the spinal cord, while those with paraplegia have lesions in the thoracic, lumbar, or sacral regions of the spinal cord.

Figure 3–9 depicts the neurologic level of injury at discharge from a Model System for all persons enrolled in the Database. The most common injury level at discharge is C5 (15.7%), followed by C4 (12.7%), C6 (12.6%), T12 (7.6%), C7 (6.3%), and L1 (4.8%). Overall, 52.9% of persons enrolled in the National SCI Database are classified as having tetraplegia, while 46.2% are classified as having paraplegia. The remaining 0.9% experience complete neurologic recovery by the time of discharge.

Results of population-based studies have been mixed with regard to neurologic level of injury. Consistent with the National SCI Database, the percentage of persons with tetraplegia is 55.0% in Colorado, 56.4% in Oklahoma, 57.0% in Utah, 59.5% in Virginia, 52.1% in Olmsted County, Minnesota, and 55.0% in the major trauma outcome study.[5,8,11,14,16,40] Conversely, only 44.4% of persons enrolled in the Arkansas registry, only 47.6% of persons enrolled in the Louisiana registry, and only 42.1% of the Houston-Galveston population-based sample are reported to have tetraplegia.[12,13,18] In the latter two samples, the reason for the relatively high percentage of persons with paraplegia appears to be that these samples also contain an unusually high percentage of persons whose injuries were secondary to gunshot wounds.[13,18] The reason the Arkansas population has a higher percentage of persons with paraplegia is unclear, but it does not appear to be due to an unusual etiologic distribution. Exact neurologic levels were reported only for Colorado, where the pattern is virtually identical to that of the Model Systems.[8] Therefore, the National SCI Database does not appear to be biased with respect to neurologic level of injury.

The percentage of persons enrolled in the National SCI Database who have tetraplegia peaked in the 1981–1983 time period at 55.2% and has subsequently decreased in a consistent manner to only 48.6% during the 1990–1992 time

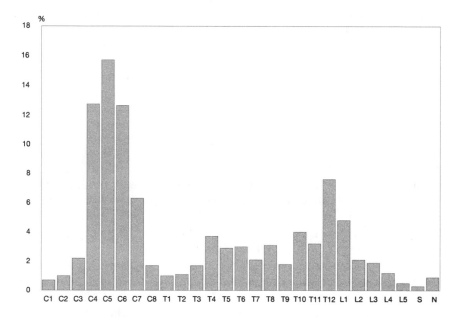

Figure 3–9 Percentages of Persons with Each Neurologic Level of Lesion at Discharge

period (Figure 3–10). This trend parallels at a reduced rate the previously discussed proportionate rise in gunshot wounds (that usually result in paraplegia) and decline in sports-related injuries (that virtually always result in tetraplegia) occurring over that same time period. The reason the trend in neurologic level of injury is not stronger given the concomitant trend in etiology is most likely due to an offsetting combination of improved emergency medical services at the scene that lead to increasing numbers of persons with tetraplegia surviving long enough to be admitted to the hospital, coupled with changing referral patterns to Model Systems such that more persons with paraplegia are being treated at other facilities than in the past.

Neurologic Extent of Injury at Discharge

There are several measures of the neurologic extent of injury that are included in the National SCI Database. The most basic of these is to categorize all injuries

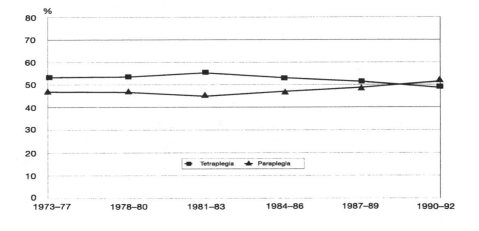

Figure 3–10 Neurologic Level of Injury at Discharge by Injury Year

neurologically as either complete or incomplete. A neurologically complete injury is defined as one in which there is no preservation of any motor and/or sensory function more than three neurologic segments below the point of damage to the spinal cord. Conversely, neurologically incomplete injuries are those in which there is preservation of either motor or sensory function more than three segments below the point of damage to the spinal cord. More detailed information on the degree of incompleteness of SCI (such as categorization by Frankel grades) is beyond the scope of this chapter, but appears in Chapter 9.

Although the recommended definitions of neurologically complete and incomplete injuries have recently changed slightly, the above definitions were in effect at the time the data were collected and were widely accepted by SCI professionals. All information on the neurologic extent of injuries that is contained in this book should be interpreted in accordance with these definitions.

Overall, 51.7% of all persons enrolled in the National SCI Database had neurologically incomplete injuries, while 48.3% had neurologically complete injuries at discharge. Interestingly, the percentage of persons with neurologically incomplete injuries increased from 44.3% between 1973 and 1977 to 56.7% between 1987 and 1989 (Figure 3–11). Once again, this can probably be attributed at least in part to improved emergency medical services at the scene of the injury. However, despite the recent advent of high-dose methylprednisolone therapy,[58] the percentage of persons with neurologically incomplete injuries at discharge decreased after 1989 to only 54.3%. Most likely, this decline in the

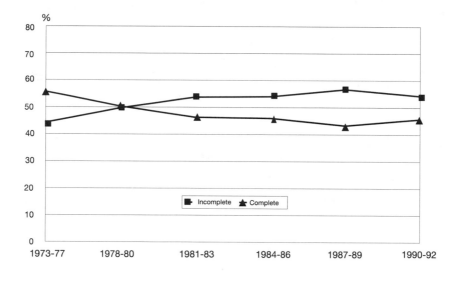

Figure 3–11 Neurologic Extent of Injury at Discharge by Injury Year

percentage of neurologically incomplete injuries during the most recent time period is due to the proportionate increase in SCIs that are secondary to gunshot wounds. As indicated previously, SCIs due to gunshot wounds are usually neurologically complete.

It has long been suspected that the National SCI Database is biased toward substantial over-representation of more severe injuries. This bias is confirmed by findings from several statewide SCI registries. In Louisiana, approximately 42% of persons with known extent of injury were reported to have neurologically complete injuries at discharge.[18] In Arkansas, only 36.4% of persons whose extent of injury was known were reported to have neurologically complete injuries at discharge.[12] The percentage of persons with neurologically complete injuries at discharge is even lower in Oklahoma (30.3%), while in Colorado it is approximately 26.5%.[8,11] Only in the Houston-Galveston sample[13] was the percentage of persons with neurologically complete injuries slightly higher (50.3%) than that seen in the National SCI Database. As is discussed in the next section, the increased percentage of neurologically complete injuries in that sample is likely due at least in part to the relatively high percentage of injuries that resulted from gunshot wounds.

Neurologic Category

Overall injury severity is usually measured by a combination of both the neurologic level and extent of injury. The standard combination involves the creation of five neurologic categories: incomplete paraplegia, complete paraplegia, incomplete tetraplegia, complete tetraplegia, and complete recovery/minimal deficit. The most common discharge neurologic category in the National SCI Database is incomplete tetraplegia (31.2%), followed by complete paraplegia (26.0%), complete tetraplegia (21.9%), incomplete paraplegia (20.0%), and complete recovery (0.9%). This pattern is very similar to that seen in Colorado, but it is strikingly different from that observed in Oklahoma and Houston-Galveston.[8,11,13] In Oklahoma, only 14.6% of persons are reported to have complete tetraplegia, while in the Houston-Galveston sample, the comparable figure is only 12.6%.[11,13] Moreover, in Louisiana, 20.4% of persons known to have thoracic or lumbosacral injuries experience complete recovery by discharge, while the comparable figure among persons with cervical level injuries is 9.5%.[18] In Utah, 11% of all persons enrolled in the registry are completely recovered by discharge.[14] Once again, taken in aggregate, these population-based data suggest that the National SCI Database is somewhat biased toward over-representation of persons with the most severe injuries.

Interestingly, the pattern of neurologic categories at discharge has changed somewhat since the Model System program began in 1973. The percentage of persons with neurologically incomplete tetraplegia and neurologically complete paraplegia has remained relatively stable over time. However, the percentage of persons with neurologically incomplete paraplegia has increased steadily from 17.0% between 1973 and 1977 to 23.1% since 1990, while the percentage of persons with neurologically complete tetraplegia has declined steadily from 26.3% to 17.5% over the same time period.

Once again, this trend can be explained at least in part by the trend in etiology of SCI discussed previously. Sports-related SCIs are the most likely to result in neurologically complete tetraplegia, yet the percentage of SCIs due to sports activities has been cut almost in half over this same time period.

The distribution of neurologic categories by grouped etiologies of SCI appears in Figure 3–12. When SCI results from a motor vehicle crash, the pattern of resulting neurologic categories is similar to that of the National SCI Database as a whole. However, other etiologies of SCI result in somewhat different neurologic outcomes. Complete paraplegia (42.1%) and incomplete paraplegia (27.5%) are the usual outcomes of SCI resulting from acts of violence. As previously mentioned, SCI secondary to sports incidents almost always results in tetraplegia, with an almost equal outcome probability of complete tetraplegia (42.5%) and

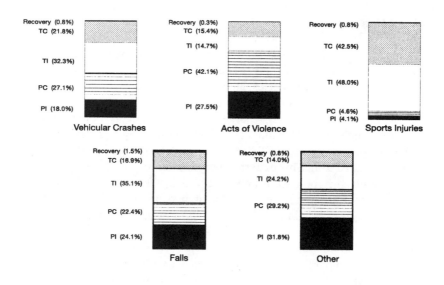

Figure 3–12 Neurologic Category at Discharge by Grouped Etiology

incomplete tetraplegia (48.0%). Falls are more likely to result in incomplete injuries, with incomplete tetraplegia being the most likely neurologic category (35.1%), followed by incomplete paraplegia (24.1%). SCI due to a fall is also the most likely to result in complete neurologic recovery (1.5%). Most SCIs due to "other" etiologies result in either neurologically incomplete or complete paraplegia.

Examination of neurologic category at discharge by age at injury is also revealing (Figure 3–13). Up to age 45, there is a relatively even distribution of neurologic categories, with slightly more persons having either incomplete tetraplegia or complete paraplegia. However, beginning at age 46, the percentage of persons with incomplete tetraplegia increases rapidly with advancing age at time of injury. Virtually all persons in the oldest age group at time of injury have tetraplegia, with 62.3% having incomplete tetraplegia and 23.5% having complete tetraplegia.

Again, this trend is due at least in part to underlying differences in etiologies of SCI across age groups that have been discussed previously. As indicated previously, SCIs among the elderly are usually the result of falls, whereas younger persons are more likely to be injured in motor vehicle crashes, acts of violence, or sports activities.[35]

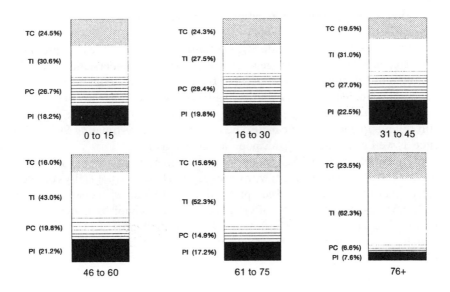

Figure 3–13 Neurologic Category at Discharge within Age Groups

CONCLUSION

In summary, current Model System statistics reveal that most persons who sustain SCIs are white males in their late teens or 20s who have graduated from high school and have never been married. These persons are most often injured in automobile crashes, with a disproportionate share of injuries occurring on the weekend and during the summer. When an SCI occurs, it is about equally likely to result from a broken neck or a broken back, and other broken bones frequently occur at the same time as the SCI.

There have been many interesting trends in the demographics and etiologies of SCIs since the inception of the Model System program in 1973. The average age at injury is increasing. Acts of violence have increased to the point that they are now the second leading cause of SCI behind only motor vehicle crashes. The percentage of persons enrolled in the Database who are African-American has also increased substantially. The proportion of neurologically incomplete injuries increased until very recently, when this trend began to reverse itself, most likely due to the increasing proportion of gunshot wounds. Each of these trends has important implications for the identification of appropriate primary prevention strategies and target populations, as well as in resource allocation among potential prevention programs to achieve the greatest cost-effectiveness.

The recent advent of statewide SCI population-based registries has provided a welcomed addition to our general knowledge and understanding of the etiologies and demographics of SCI. For the first time, it should be possible to monitor the incidence of SCI over time and thereby determine the effectiveness of various types of primary prevention programs. Eventually, those registries with follow-up components can also be of assistance in estimating SCI prevalence as well as the needs of this population as it ages.

In general, the National SCI Database appears to be representative of all new cases of SCI that occur each year with the exception that neurologically complete injuries (particularly high level complete injuries) are somewhat over-represented. Nonwhites, males, and acts of violence are also probably over-represented slightly. These potential and confirmed biases in the National SCI Database may need to be considered by readers when interpreting information contained elsewhere in this book.

REFERENCES

1. Kraus JF, Franti CE, Riggins RS, Richards D, Borhani NO. Incidence of traumatic spinal cord lesions. *J Chronic Dis* 1975;28:471–492.

2. Bracken MB, Freeman DH, Hellenbrand K. Incidence of acute traumatic hospitalized spinal cord injury in the United States, 1970–1977. *Am J Epidemiol.* 1981;113:615–622.

3. Ergas Z. Spinal cord injury in the United States: A statistical update. *Cent Nerv Syst Trauma.* 1985;2:19–30.

4. Fine PR, Kuhlemeier KV, DeVivo MJ, Stover SL. Spinal cord injury: An epidemiologic perspective. *Paraplegia.* 1979;17:237–250.

5. Griffin MR, Opitz JL, Kurland LT, Ebersold MJ, O'Fallon WM. Traumatic spinal cord injury in Olmsted County, Minnesota, 1935–1981. *Am J Epidemiol.* 1985;121:884–895.

6. Kalsbeek WD, McLaurin RL, Harris BSH, Miller JD. The national head and spinal cord injury survey: Major findings. *J Neurosurg.* 1980;53(suppl):S19–S31.

7. Relethford JH, Standfast SJ, Morse DL. Trends in traumatic spinal cord injury—New York, 1982-1988. *MMWR.* 1991;40:535–537, 543.

8. Colorado Department of Health. *1992 Annual Report of the Spinal Cord Injury Early Notification System.* Denver, Colo: Colorado Department of Transportation Printing Office; 1993.

9. Gerhart KA. Spinal cord injury outcomes in a population-based sample. *J Trauma.* 1991;31:1529–1535.

10. Injury Prevention Service. *Summary of Reportable Injuries in Oklahoma, 1988–1992.* Oklahoma City, Okla: Oklahoma State Department of Health; 1993.

11. Price C, Makintubee S, Herndon W, Istre GR. Epidemiology of traumatic spinal cord injury and acute hospitalization and rehabilitation charges for spinal cord injuries in Oklahoma, 1988–1990. *Am J Epidemiol.* 1994;139:37–47.

12. Acton PA, Farley T, Freni LW, Ilegbodu VA, Sniezek JE, Wohlleb JC. Traumatic spinal cord injury in Arkansas, 1980 to 1989. *Arch Phys Med Rehabil.* 1993;74:1035–1040.

13. Clifton GL. Spinal cord injury in the Houston-Galveston area. *Tex Med.* 1983;79:55–57.

14. Bureau of Epidemiology. *Utah Spinal Cord Injury Surveillance Summary, 1989–1991.* Salt Lake City, Utah: Utah Department of Health; 1993.

15. Georgia Central Registry. *Spinal Cord Disabilities and Traumatic Brain Injury.* Warm Springs, Ga: Roosevelt Warm Springs Institute for Rehabilitation; 1993.

16. Hickman JK. *Spinal Cord Injury in Virginia: A Statistical Fact Sheet.* Fishersville, Va: Virginia Department of Rehabilitative Services; 1993.

17. Lawrence DW, Bayakly AR, Mathison JB. *Traumatic Spinal Cord Injury in Louisiana: 1990 Annual Report.* New Orleans, La: Louisiana Office of Public Health; 1992.

18. Bayakly AR, Lawrence DW. *Spinal Cord Injury in Louisiana: 1991 Annual Report.* New Orleans, La: Louisiana Office of Public Health; 1992.

19. Harvey C, Rothschild BB, Asmann AJ, Stripling T. New estimates of traumatic SCI prevalence: A survey-based approach. *Paraplegia.* 1990;28:537–544.

20. Berkowitz M, Harvey C, Greene CG, Wilson SE. *The Economic Consequences of Traumatic Spinal Cord Injury.* Washington, DC: Paralyzed Veterans of America; 1990.

21. DeVivo MJ, Fine PR, Maetz HM, Stover SL. Prevalence of spinal cord injury: A reestimation employing life table techniques. *Arch Neurol.* 1980;37:707–708.

22. Anderson DW, Kalsbeek WD, Hartwell TD. The national head and spinal cord injury survey: Design and methodology. *J Neurosurg.* 1980;53(suppl):S11–S18.

23. Fine PR, DeVivo MJ, McEachran AB. Re: Incidence of acute traumatic hospitalized spinal cord injury in the United States, 1970–1977. *Am J Epidemiol.* 1982;115:475–477. Letter.

24. Harrison CL, Dijkers M. Spinal cord injury surveillance in the United States: An overview. *Paraplegia.* 1991;29:233–246.

25. Graitcer PL. The development of state and local injury surveillance systems. *J Saf Res.* 1987;18:191–198.

26. Cowan LS, Cannon ME, Hathcock AL Jr, Konigsberg C Jr. Fatal injury surveillance report, Delaware, 1990 head and spinal cord injuries. *Del Med J.* 1993;65:435–448.

27. Kurtzke JF. Epidemiology of spinal cord injury. *Exp Neurol.* 1975;48:163–236.

28. Gibson CJ. Overview of spinal cord injury. *Phys Med Rehabil Clin North Am.* 1992;3: 699–709.

29. Griffin MR, O'Fallon WM, Opitz JL, Kurland LT. Mortality, survival and prevalence: Traumatic spinal cord injury in Olmsted County, Minnesota, 1935-1981. *J Chronic Dis.* 1985;38:643–653.

30. Gibson CJ. Criteria for evaluating performance of the system. In: Apple DF Jr, Hudson LM, eds. *Spinal Cord Injury: The Model.* Atlanta, Ga: Georgia Regional Spinal Cord Injury Care System; 1990:45–48.

31. Granger CV, Hamilton BB. The uniform data system for medical rehabilitation: Report of first admissions for 1991. *Am J Phys Med Rehabil.* 1993;72:33–38.

32. U.S. Bureau of the Census. *Statistical Abstract of the United States: 1991.* 111th ed. Washington, DC: U.S. Department of Commerce; 1991.

33. U.S. Bureau of the Census. *Statistical Abstract of the United States: 1992.* 112th ed. Washington, DC: U.S. Department of Commerce; 1992.

34. DeVivo MJ, Rutt RD, Black KJ, Go BK, Stover SL. Trends in spinal cord injury demographics and treatment outcomes between 1973 and 1986. *Arch Phys Med Rehabil.* 1992;73:424–430.

35. DeVivo MJ, Kartus PL, Rutt RD, Stover SL, Fine PR. The influence of age at time of spinal cord injury on rehabilitation outcome. *Arch Neurol.* 1990;47:687–691.

36. DeVivo MJ, Shewchuk RM, Stover SL, Black KJ, Go BK. A cross-sectional study of the relationship between age and current health status for persons with spinal cord injuries. *Paraplegia.* 1992;30:820–827.

37. Roth EJ, Lovell L, Heinemann AW, Lee MY, Yarkony GM. The older adult with a spinal cord injury. *Paraplegia.* 1992;30:520–526.

38. Whiteneck GG, Charlifue SW, Gerhart KA, et al., eds. *Aging with Spinal Cord Injury.* New York, NY: Demos Publications; 1993.

39. Stover SL, Fine PR, eds. *Spinal Cord Injury: The Facts and Figures.* Birmingham, Ala: University of Alabama at Birmingham; 1986.

40. Burney RE, Maio RF, Maynard F, Karunas R. Incidence, characteristics, and outcome of spinal cord injury at trauma centers in North America. *Arch Surg.* 1993;128:596–599.

41. National Safety Council. *Accident Facts.* 1993 ed. Itasca, Ill: National Safety Council; 1993.

42. National Center for Health Statistics. *Vital Statistics of the United States, 1988.* Vol 2. *Mortality, Part A.* Washington, DC: U.S. Public Health Service; 1991.

43. DeVivo MJ, Richards JS, Stover SL, Go BK. Spinal cord injury: Rehabilitation adds life to years. *West J Med.* 1991;154:602–606.

44. DeVivo MJ, Rutt RD, Stover SL, Fine PR. Employment after spinal cord injury. *Arch Phys Med Rehabil.* 1987;68:494–498.

45. James M, DeVivo MJ, Richards JS. Postinjury employment outcomes among African-American and white persons with spinal cord injury. *Rehabil Psychol.* 1993;38:151–164.

46. Mawson AR, Snelling L, Winchester Y, Biundo JJ Jr. 526 spinal cord injuries: Experience of the Louisiana Rehabilitation Institute, 1965–1984. *J La State Med Soc.* 1991;143(7):31–37.

47. DeVivo MJ, Fine PR. Spinal cord injury: Its short-term impact on marital status. *Arch Phys Med Rehabil.* 1985;66:501–504.

48. DeVivo MJ, Jenkins KD, Go BK. Outcomes of post-spinal cord injury marriages. *J Am Paraplegia Soc.* 1990;13:39–40.

49. Mueller FO, Cantu RC. Catastrophic injuries and fatalities in high school and college sports, fall 1982–spring 1988. *Med Sci Sports Exerc.* 1990;22:737–741.

50. Fine PR, Stafford MA, Miller JM, Stover SL. Gunshot wounds of the spinal cord: A survey of literature and epidemiologic study of 48 lesions in Alabama. *Ala J Med Sci.* 1976;13:173–180.

51. Kraus JF, Franti CE, Riggins RS. Neurologic outcome and vehicle and crash factors in motor vehicle related spinal cord injuries. *Neuroepidemiology.* 1982;1:223–238.

52. Wigglesworth EC. Motor vehicle crashes and spinal cord injury. *Paraplegia.* 1992;30:543–549.

53. Weingarden SI, Graham PM. Falls resulting in spinal cord injury: Patterns and outcomes in an older population. *Paraplegia.* 1989;27:423–427.

54. Shrosbree RD. Spinal cord injuries as a result of motorcycle accidents. *Paraplegia.* 1978;16:102–112.

55. Rosenberg NL, Gerhart K, Whiteneck G. Occupational spinal cord injury: Demographic and etiologic differences from non-occupational injuries. *Neurology.* 1993;43:1385–1388.

56. Lawrence DW, Hooten EAG, Mathison JB, et al. Firearm-related deaths—Louisiana and Texas, 1970–1990. *MMWR.* 1992;41:213–215, 221.

57. Fine PR, Stover SL, DeVivo MJ. A methodology for predicting lengths of stay for spinal cord injury patients. *Inquiry.* 1987;24:147–156.

58. Bracken MB, Shepard MJ, Collins WF, et al. A randomized, controlled trial of methylprednisolone or naloxone in the treatment of acute spinal-cord injury. *N Engl J Med.* 1990;322:1405–1411.

4

Emergency and Acute Management of Spine Trauma

Robert L. Waters, David F. Apple, Jr., Paul R. Meyer, Jr.,
Jerome M. Cotler, and Rodney H. Adkins

INTRODUCTION

Significant progress has been made since the Egyptians labeled SCI "an ailment not to be treated."[1] The initial improvements starting in the early 1900s were in the management of paralysis. Only in the last 30 years have there been advancements in spinal column management and coordination of emergency, acute, and rehabilitation care.

Variables that can be used to assess emergency care in detail are not included in the National SCI Database. However, data on such variables are collected within the Midwest Regional Spinal Cord Injury Care System and therefore are included in this chapter.

Variables to describe the basic categories of spinal column surgery were introduced in October 1986 to the National SCI Database. Since that time, 4102 cases had been reported for data analysis. Of the total number reported, 53.7% (2204 cases) were admitted to a Model System within 24 hours, 8.3% (339 cases) between 1 day and 1 week, 24.1% (988 cases) between 1 week and 1 month, and 13.9% (571 cases) between 1 and 2 months. Information on injuries admitted to a Model System on the day of injury is gathered prospectively by trained data collectors. Furthermore, treatment decisions regarding patients admitted to a Model System on the day of injury are made by clinicians experienced in the management of SCI. For these reasons, the data presented are restricted to the 2204 cases admitted after October 1986 who were admitted to a Model System within the first 24 hours of injury.

EMERGENCY MEDICAL CARE

The primary justification for the implementation of nationwide emergency medical systems (EMS) as it relates to SCI is twofold: (1) the saving of lives and

(2) the prevention of additional progressive neurologic trauma. While the specifics of such a system are discussed later in this chapter, the final results, as demonstrated by data collected at the Midwest Regional Spinal Cord Injury Care System (MRSCICS), are dramatic.

Specifically, the time between injury and admission for the person with spine trauma has become amazingly shortened. In 1972, when data were first collected at MRSCICS, only 25% of the patients were transferred into the System in under 72 hours; for some persons, months elapsed between onset and admission. Rcently, MRSCICS reports that over 78% of the persons admitted in 1992 were transferred in under 72 hours, with a median time to admission of only 5 hours.

Commensurate with this decrease in time to admission to MRSCICS is a marked change in the overall extent of neurologic injury seen at admission. In 1972, the incidence of SCI among persons with spinal fractures or other spinal insults admitted to the MRSCICS was 81%. By 1992, this had dropped to only 57%—a 24% reduction in the occurrence of SCI.

Several factors are probably responsible for this dramatic change, including safer automotive designs, mandatory seat belt legislation, posted diving warnings at pools and at the lakeshore, and so forth. However, the influence of an "in-place" and smoothly functioning EMS (as discussed later in this chapter) within the Model System cannot be overlooked, and is most likely a strong contributor to these results.[2,3] While it is possible that this increase in the percentage of neurologically normal patients could have been due to a "shift" in patient referrals to MRSCICS, it does stand to reason that a higher percentage of persons with SCI should have been transferred to the System if that were the case, rather than the reverse.

There are two outcomes that ultimately determine the effectiveness of the acute care component of the System as a whole: duration of acute hospitalization and patient mortality. With the application of appropriate surgical and medical stabilization, as well as the total integration of patient rehabilitation into the acute care phase, the result is a length of stay for the patient with acute SCI that has been reduced from an average of 43 days in 1972 to an average of 17 days in 1992.

Several factors affecting the length of acute hospitalization can be analyzed. Multiple organ system trauma (multitrauma) frequently occurs at the time an individual sustains a spine injury. Evaluation of the MRSCICS dataset reveals that while SCI occurred singularly in 58% of the persons admitted between 1972 and 1992, injuries to other organ systems occurred in the following order: one additional system, 28%; two systems, 10%; three systems, 4%; four or more systems, 0.06%. Also, as expected using the 1972–1992 data, the incidence of multiple-system trauma has a definite impact on the average duration of acute hospitalization: spine injury alone, 21 days; one additional system, 27 days; two systems, 29 days; three systems, 36 days; four or more systems, 32 days.

Additionally, the extent of the neurologic injury has a marked impact on the average acute length of stay: no neurologic injury, 16 days; incomplete injuries, 25 days; complete injuries, 33 days.

As for patient mortality, the influence of emergency care within the System becomes immediately apparent at MRSCICS: in 1972, patient mortality during the initial hospitalization was 13%; in 1992, mortality dropped to 5%.

ACUTE SURGICAL TREATMENT

Surgical Frequency

Among all Model Systems, of 2204 patients admitted within 24 hours of injury, 45.3% did not undergo any spine surgery procedures, 49.3% underwent one procedure, 5.0% two procedures, and 0.4% three or more procedures (Table 4–1). Application of a halo is common in the treatment of cervical injuries following surgery and may be employed in cases not having surgery. Use of a halo was reported in 46.4% of patients with tetraplegia. A halo was employed in conjunction with spine surgery in 27.6% and a halo was used as the only method of spine stabilization in 18.8%.

Each injury was classified according to etiology, neurologic level of injury, motor score of the American Spinal Injury Association (ASIA), and completeness of injury. Each patient was classified according to type of surgery. If surgical decompression *was not* performed, patients were categorized in three groups depending on the type of operative procedure: spine fusion, internal spinal fixation only, and internal fixation and fusion. If surgical decompression *was*

Table 4–1 Number of Spine Surgeries*

No. of Surgeries	No. of Cases	Frequency (%)
None	990	45.3
1	1078	49.3
2	110	5.0
3	8	0.4
4	1	0.0
Total	2187	100.0

*Data from the 2204 cases admitted to a Model System within 24 hours of injury. 17 cases had incomplete data.

performed, patients were classified in the following groups whether or not fusion or internal fixation was performed: anterior decompression, posterior decompression, anterior and posterior decompression. A separate category, "other decompression," was included for less frequent types of spinal canal decompression procedures (i.e., anterolateral, posterolateral, etc.).

Procedures by Level and Completeness of Injury

Table 4–2 summarizes the percentage frequency of the different surgical categories by level and completeness of injury of the persons admitted to a Model System within 24 hours.

Table 4–2 Surgical Procedures by Level and Completeness of Injury*

Procedure	Incomplete Paraplegia	Complete Paraplegia	Incomplete Tetraplegia	Complete Tetraplegia	Total (%)
No Surgery	171	287	337	189	984 (45.4)
Fusion Only	1	7	57	42	107 (4.9)
Internal Fixation Only	16	11	8	4	39 (1.8)
Fusion and Internal Fixation Only	125	201	168	164	658 (30.4)
Anterior Decompression with or without Internal Fixation and/or Fusion	46	8	69	35	158 (7.3)
Posterior Decompression with or without Internal Fixation and/or Fusion	92	62	25	15	194 (9.0)
Anterior and Posterior Decompression	2	3	2	3	10 (0.5)
Other Decompression	10	3	3	0	16 (0.7)
Total (%)	463 (21.3)	582 (26.9)	669 (30.9)	452 (20.9)	2166 (100.0)

*Data from the 2204 cases admitted to a Model System within 24 hours of injury. 38 cases had incomplete data.

Spine fusion without internal fixation is rarely indicated in the management of acute paraplegia and accounted for 0.8% of persons with paraplegia. Fusion without fixation may be employed in chronic injuries when correction of deformity or spinal realignment is not desirable and acute instability is not present. Similarly, internal fixation without fusion is rarely indicated and was performed in only 2.6% of persons with paraplegia. Properly performed combined internal fixation and fusion enables restoration of spinal alignment, diminishes the chance of pseudoarthrosis, and provides spine stability. For these reasons, combined internal fixation and fusion is the most commonly performed surgical procedure and was performed in 31.2% of persons with paraplegia.

A similar trend was observed among persons with tetraplegia. Internal fixation with fusion was the most common surgical procedure, accounting for 29.6% of persons with tetraplegia. Internal fixation alone was rare, accounting for only 1.1% of persons with tetraplegia. Fusion without internal fixation was performed in 8.8% of persons with tetraplegia. The higher incidence of fusion without internal fixation among persons with tetraplegia versus those with paraplegia probably reflects a lag in the development of internal fixation systems for the cervical region as compared with the thoracic and lumbar regions. In the past, the most common technique available for internal fixation, posterior wiring, was judged inadequate in certain situations such as the presence of multiple fractures of the posterior lamina. However, various internal fixation systems employing specially designed hooks, screws, and plates have been developed recently and now provide a reliable means of obtaining secure internal fixation of most fractures when fusion is performed.

Among persons with tetraplegia, those with complete injuries were more likely to undergo operative intervention (58.2%) than those with incomplete injuries (49.6%). The opposite was true in paraplegia: surgery was performed in 50.7% of persons with complete paraplegia and in 63.1% of persons with incomplete paraplegia.

Among persons with paraplegia, posterior decompression was performed approximately three times more frequently than anterior decompression. Among persons with tetraplegia the opposite was true: anterior decompression was performed approximately two and one-half times more frequently.

Procedures by Etiology

As can be seen in Table 4–3, the etiology of injury influenced the frequency of surgery. Among patients admitted to a Model System within 24 hours of injury, surgical intervention was performed with approximately the same frequency in patients sustaining nonpenetrating injuries from motor vehicle crashes (66.4%), motorcycle crashes (70.3%), diving (72.5%), and falls (65.0%). On the other

Table 4-3 Surgical Procedures by Etiology*

Procedure	Motor Vehicle Crash	Motorcycle Crash	Other Vehicular	Gunshot Wound	Other Penetrating Wound	Other Violent	Diving	Other Sport	Fall	Other	Total
No Surgery	228	33	20	359	36	17	39	15	174	67	988
Fusion Only	45	6	3	0	0	1	17	7	24	4	107
Internal Fixation Only	15	5	2	0	0	0	2	2	11	4	41
Fusion and Internal Fixation Only	275	45	19	3	3	8	53	29	172	53	660
Anterior Decompression	43	10	5	2	0	4	23	6	50	16	159
Posterior Decompression	66	10	4	27	3	3	6	3	56	17	195
Anterior and Posterior Decompression	1	1	0	0	0	2	2	0	3	1	10
Other Decompression	5	1	0	1	0	0	0	2	7	1	17
Total	678	111	53	392	42	35	142	64	497	163	2177
(%)	(31.2)	(5.1)	(2.5)	(18.0)	(1.9)	(1.6)	(6.5)	(2.9)	(22.8)	(7.5)	(100.0)

*Data from the 2204 cases admitted to a Model System within 24 hours of injury. 27 cases had incomplete data.

hand, surgery was infrequently performed in patients with penetrating injuries caused by gunshot (8.4%) and other penetrating (stab) injuries (14.3%).

The more common performance of surgery following nonpenetrating injury is consistent with the fact that these injuries more likely result in spine instability when associated with SCI and the need for internal fixation and fusion, in contrast to penetrating injuries, which are generally stable. Moreover, patients with injuries resulting from high-energy trauma, in addition to being unstable, are more likely to have bone fragments in the spinal canal, which are considered by some surgeons to be an indication for decompression.

Procedures by Age

Age was not a factor in the use of surgical treatment among persons who were 60 years of age or younger and were admitted to a Model System within 24 hours of injury. The incidence of surgery within the age intervals 0 to 15 years was 56.9%; 16 to 30 years, 60.0%; 31 to 45 years, 60.2%; 46 to 60 years, 50.9%. Among individuals more than 60 years of age, 37.0% underwent surgery.

Procedures by Sex

Of patients admitted to a Model System within 24 hours of injury, 17.4% were female and 82.6% were male (Table 4-4). Males were less likely to undergo a spine surgery than females (46.9% of males received nonoperative treatment versus 38.0% of females). One explanation for this difference is the higher incidence of penetrating injuries due to violence (gunshot wounds and stabs) in males compared with females (19.3% versus 11.5%). Since penetrating injuries are generally stable injuries, they are less likely to require surgical stabilization. Ninety-one percent of patients injured by gunshot wound received nonoperative treatment.

COMPLICATIONS DIRECTLY ASSOCIATED WITH SPINE SURGERY

Revision Surgery

Failure of instrumentation to stabilize the spine adequately was rare, judging by the low incidence of reoperation to revise or remove hardware during hospitalization. Of the 1256 patients undergoing at least one surgical procedure,

Table 4–4 Etiology by Gender*

Etiology	Male		Female	
	n	*(%)*	*n*	*(%)*
Motor Vehicle Crash	502	(73.1)	185	(26.9)
Motorcycle Crash	109	(95.6)	5	(4.4)
Other Vehicular	50	(92.6)	4	(7.4)
Gunshot Wound	352	(88.9)	44	(11.1)
Other Penetrating Wound	36	(85.7)	6	(14.3)
Other Violent Trauma	28	(80.0)	7	(20.0)
Diving	133	(92.4)	11	(7.6)
Other Sport	52	(81.2)	12	(18.8)
Fall	413	(82.4)	88	(17.6)
Other	144	(87.8)	20	(17.4)
Total	1819	(82.6)	382	(17.4)

*Data from the 2204 cases admitted to a Model System within 24 hours of injury. 3 cases had incomplete data.

reoperation to repair internal fixation was performed on 0.9% of patients, and an additional 0.9% had fixation removed.

Wound Infection

It is reasonable to assume that persons who are in the acute phase of SCI are at greater risk for infection following surgery than the general population. Bowel and bladder incontinence, pathophysiologic changes in insensate skin, and pressure ulcers increase the concentration of skin bacteria. Extensive dissection needed for spine exposure and bleeding from bone surfaces creates a large wound surface with a potential for hematoma formation. These reasons may in whole or part account for the relatively high overall postoperative infection rate of 4.4% (Table 4–5).

Motor Loss and Recovery

Further motor loss after the initial SCI is one of the most devastating complications a person with SCI can sustain. Within the National SCI Database, motor loss and recovery are documented by use of a muscle-scoring system and

Table 4–5 Postoperative Wound Infection by Surgical Procedure*

Procedure	No Infection	Infection	No. of Cases	% Frequency
Fusion Only	103	2	105	1.9
Internal Fixation Only	38	3	41	7.1
Fusion and Internal Fixation Only	626	30	656	4.8
Anterior Decompression	155	4	159	2.6
Posterior Decompression	185	10	195	5.1
Anterior and Posterior Decompression	9	1	10	10.0
Other Decompression	15	2	17	11.8
Total	1131	52	1183	4.4

*Data from the 2204 cases admitted to a Model System within 24 hours of injury. 31 cases had incomplete data.

recorded according to the following categories: (1) no motor loss; (2) motor loss following spinal surgery, with recovery to the preoperative level prior to discharge (transient motor loss); (3) motor loss following spinal surgery, with no recovery prior to discharge (extended motor loss); (4) motor loss not following spinal surgery, with recovery prior to discharge; and (5) motor loss not following spinal surgery, with no recovery prior to discharge. Among those persons not undergoing surgery, the incidence of transient motor loss that recovered by the time of rehabilitation discharge was 1.1% and the incidence of motor loss that did not resolve by the time of hospital discharge was 1.2%. The incidence of transient motor loss after surgery that resolved by the time of discharge from rehabilitation was 0.7% and the incidence of motor loss that did not recover by the time of discharge was 0.5% (Table 4–6).

OTHER COMPLICATIONS

The development of the various complications discussed below may or may not be influenced by spine surgery or influence decisions regarding spine surgery. Because data specifying the sequence of events are not maintained within the National SCI Database, strong conclusions cannot be drawn regarding associations between surgery and the occurrence of a particular complication. For example, a person may undergo surgery within the first week of System admission and develop pneumonia within the next 3 days, another patient may undergo similar surgery within a similar time frame and develop pneumonia 2 months later, and still another may develop pneumonia within the first week and

Table 4–6 Motor Loss and Recovery by Surgical Procedure*

Procedure	No Motor Loss	Transient Motor Loss[†] after Spinal Surgery	Extended Motor Loss[‡] after Spinal Surgery	Transient Motor Loss[†] Not following Surgery	Extended Motor Loss[‡] Not following Surgery	Total
No Surgery	947	N/A	N/A	14	19	980
Fusion Only	104	1	1	0	0	106
Internal Fixation Only	40	0	1	0	0	41
Fusion and Internal Fixation Only	641	4	6	5	2	658
Anterior Decompression	151	3	1	3	1	159
Posterior Decompression	182	2	3	5	4	196
Anterior and Posterior Decompression	10	0	0	0	0	10
Other Decompression	16	1	0	0	0	17
Total	2091	11	12	27	26	2167
(%)	(96.5)	(0.5)	(0.6)	(1.2)	(1.2)	(100.0)

*Data from the 2204 cases admitted to a Model System within 24 hours of injury. 37 cases had incomplete data.
†Motor loss with recovery to preoperative level prior to discharge.
‡Motor loss with no recovery prior to discharge.

surgery may be delayed for several weeks until the complication is resolved. However, all three of these hypothetical cases would be documented identically within the National SCI Database. The data would show that each had a particular type of spine surgery and had developed pneumonia during treatment within a System and no more. Thus, although the coinciding incidence of certain events can be established using the National SCI Database, cause-and-effect links cannot.

In the following sections addressing the incidence of pressure ulcers, deep venous thrombosis, pulmonary embolism, pneumonia, and death, data from the 2204 patients admitted to a Model System within 24 hours of injury were analyzed.

Pressure Ulcers

Pressure ulcers were graded on a four-point classification system: grade 1 ulcers are limited to the superficial epidermal and dermal layers, grade 2 ulcers involve the epidermal and dermal layers and extend into the adipose tissue, grade 3 ulcers extend through superficial structures and adipose tissue down to and including muscle, and grade 4 ulcers destroy all soft tissue structures and communication with bone or joint structures. Each patient was categorized according to the highest-pressure-ulcer grade recorded during hospitalization. The overall incidence of pressure ulcers was 30% for those persons treated nonoperatively and 31% for those who underwent spine surgery (Table 4–7).

Grade 1 and grade 2 pressure ulcers customarily heal if pressure is removed from the affected area. Grade 3 and grade 4 pressure ulcers generally require surgery or prolonged bed rest and delay rehabilitation if they are located over the sacrum or ischium. The incidence of grade 3 and grade 4 pressure ulcers was 5% for those persons not undergoing surgery and 4% for those having surgery.

Deep Venous Thrombosis

Deep venous thrombosis (DVT) is a frequent complication following SCI. Bed rest, hypercoaguability, and paralysis predispose those with SCI to DVT.

Table 4–7 Most Severe Pressure Ulcer Grade by Surgical Procedure*

Procedure	None	Grade 1	Grade 2	Grade 3	Grade 4	Total
No Surgery	686	119	121	39	12	977
Fusion Only	72	11	12	8	0	103
Internal Fixation Only	30	2	3	3	2	40
Fusion and Internal Fixation Only	442	86	92	20	6	646
Anterior Decompression	101	26	26	2	0	155
Posterior Decompression	141	28	20	3	2	194
Anterior and Posterior Decompression	8	1	1	0	0	10
Other Decompression	10	4	2	1	0	17
Total	1490	277	277	76	22	2142
(%)	(69.6)	(12.9)	(12.9)	(3.6)	(1.0)	(100.0)

*Data from the 2204 cases admitted to a Model System within 24 hours of injury. 62 cases had incomplete data.

A diagnosis of DVT was made in 13.8% of persons admitted to a System within 24 hours (Table 4–8). DVT was confirmed by fibrinogen uptake, impedance plethysmography, Doppler ultrasound, or venography studies. The incidence of DVT was 10.6% for persons treated nonoperatively and 14.0% for persons undergoing surgery.

The diagnosis of DVT may be underestimated in a clinical population if confirmatory studies are performed only on persons having clinical symptoms. Because different studies were utilized in the various Model Systems and because these studies were not conducted prospectively, the incidences of DVT reported above may underestimate the true incidence.

Pulmonary Embolism

The data on the incidence of pulmonary embolism gathered from the National SCI Database probably underestimate the actual incidence for the same reasons as those associated with DVT. The reported incidence of pulmonary embolism based on ventilation-perfusion lung scan, pulmonary angiography, or ventilation-perfusion lung scan and angiography was 4.0% in persons not undergoing surgery (Table 4–9). Using the same techniques, the incidence was 2.5% for those persons who had surgery.

Pneumonia

The overall incidence of pneumonia was 18.5% (Table 4–10). The incidence for the group of patients having no surgery, 18.8%, was similar to that of the group having surgery, 18.2%. As would be expected, the incidence of pneumonia for those individuals with tetraplegia was higher than that for those with paraplegia, 25.6% versus 11.3%. For those with paraplegia who also underwent spine surgery, the incidence was 9.5% compared with 13.7% for those who did not have surgery. For those with tetraplegia who also underwent spine surgery, the incidence was 27.4% compared with 23.5% for those who did not have surgery.

Death

The death rate during initial hospitalization for those patients who did not have spine surgery was much higher than that for those who had spine surgery, 7% compared with 1.9%. The highest death rate was for those with complete tetraplegia who did not have surgery, 21%. Death rates among other groups were

Table 4-8 Occurrence of Deep Venous Thrombosis (DVT) by Surgical Procedure and Diagnostic Confirmation Procedure*

Procedure	No DVT	Confirmed by Fibrinogen Uptake	Confirmed by Impedance Plethysmography	Confirmed by Doppler	Confirmed by Venography	Confirmed by Other Procedure	Unconfirmed Diagnostic Procedure	Total
No Surgery	859	5	17	36	46	7	8	978
Fusion Only	95	0	4	2	5	1	0	107
Internal Fixation Only	36	0	1	2	1	1	0	41
Fusion and Internal Fixation Only	549	5	15	32	52	4	2	659
Anterior Decompression	135	0	7	5	10	1	1	159
Posterior Decompression	168	0	2	9	13	1	3	196
Anterior and Posterior Decompression	9	0	0	0	1	0	0	10
Other Decompression	16	0	0	0	1	0	0	17
Total	1867	10	46	86	129	15	14	2167
(%)	(86.1)	(0.5)	(2.1)	(4.0)	(6.0)	(0.7)	(0.6)	(100.0)

*Data from the 2204 cases admitted to a Model System within 24 hours of injury. 37 cases had incomplete data.

Table 4–9 Occurrence of Pulmonary Embolism by Surgical Procedure and Diagnostic Confirmation Procedure*

Procedure	No Pulmonary Embolism	Confirmed by Vent-Perfusion Lung Scan	Confirmed by Pulmonary Angiography	Confirmed by Vent-Perfusion Lung Scan and Pulmonary Angiography	Confirmed by Other Procedure	Unconfirmed Diagnostic Procedure	Total
No Surgery	931	29	8	2	3	8	981
Fusion Only	106	0	0	0	0	1	107
Internal Fixation Only	40	1	0	0	0	0	41
Fusion and Internal Fixation Only	642	13	1	2	0	0	658
Anterior Decompression	154	2	1	1	1	0	159
Posterior Decompression	187	4	1	3	0	1	196
Anterior and Posterior Decompression	9	0	0	0	0	1	10
Other Decompression	16	1	0	0	0	0	17
Total	2085	50	11	8	4	11	2169
(%)	(96.1)	(2.3)	(0.5)	(0.4)	(0.2)	(0.5)	(100.0)

*Data from the 2204 cases admitted to a Model System within 24 hours of injury. 35 cases had incomplete data.

Table 4–10 Number of Cases and Percentage Frequency of Pneumonia by Surgical Procedure*

Procedure	Total No. of Cases	No. of Cases with Pneumonia	% Frequency
No Surgery	977	184	18.8
Fusion Only	107	23	21.5
Internal Fixation Only	41	5	12.2
Fusion and Internal Fixation Only	656	134	20.4
Anterior Decompression	158	30	19.0
Posterior Decompression	195	21	10.8
Anterior and Posterior Decompression	10	1	10.0
Other Decompression	17	1	5.9
Total	2161	399	18.5

*Data from the 2204 cases admitted to a Model System within 24 hours of injury. 43 cases had incomplete data.

---

as follows: incomplete tetraplegia, no surgery—5.7%; complete tetraplegia, surgery—3.7%; complete paraplegia, no surgery—3%; incomplete tetraplegia, surgery—2.7%; incomplete paraplegia, no surgery—2.2%; incomplete paraplegia, surgery—1%; and complete paraplegia, surgery—0.4%. It should be reiterated, however, that information regarding the sequence of events is not provided in the National SCI Database, and therefore no significant correlations can be confirmed. Nevertheless, it is highly likely that the medical stability of many of those patients who died and had no surgery strongly influenced decisions not to perform surgery.

COLLABORATIVE STUDIES

Although surgery is performed to realign the spine, correct deformity, provide spine stability, and alleviate spinal cord compression, the National SCI Database does not classify cases according to the type of fracture. Without a fracture classification to describe the type and extent of injury, it is not possible to evaluate the effectiveness of different surgical procedures or nonoperative methods and control for type of injury.

The fracture classification systems most commonly used in clinical practice are the Allen et al. system[4] for the lower cervical spine and the Denis system[5] for the thoracolumbar spine. The Allen et al. system groups fractures into various phylogenies based on mechanism of injury as described by the force of injury and the position of the spine at the time of injury. The common fracture and dislocation classifications are compressive flexion, distractive flexion, lateral flexion, vertical compression, compressive extension, and distractive extension. This system, however, was devised prior to the widespread use of computed tomography (CT) scans in evaluating spine fractures and relies only on the roentgenographic appearance of fractures for classification. The Denis system proposes a "three-column" model for fracture classification. The fracture types in this classification system are compression fracture, burst fracture, seat belt–type fracture, and fracture dislocation. In both the Allen et al. system and the Denis system, the authors state that there is a correlation between the fracture type and the neurologic deficit. In neither of the systems, however, is the neurologic deficit described in a detailed manner, nor is the issue of recovery addressed. Additionally, neither of these two commonly used fracture classification systems has been evaluated for intertester or intratester reliability.

Detailed studies characterizing specific types of injury conducted in a prospective manner are necessary. An example of such a study is described below.

Bullet Removal from the Spinal Canal

Gunshot injuries account for 14.6% of all admissions to the Model Systems. Most of these result from low-velocity bullets fired from handguns. In approximately one-third of cases the bullet does not enter the spinal canal, and injury is sustained as a result of concussive impact analogous to closed head trauma. In one-third of patients the bullet traverses the spinal canal. In one-third of cases the bullet or the major bullet fragment becomes lodged inside the spinal canal.[6]

To address the surgical question regarding whether or not bullets should be removed from the spinal canal, a collaborative investigation[7] among the Model Systems was conducted using the ASIA *International Standards for Neurological and Functional Classification of Spinal Cord Injury.*[8] Serial motor and sensory examinations were performed prospectively on 66 patients with bullet fragments lodged in the spinal canal. The majority had bullets lodged in the thoracic region (59.1%), followed by the cervical region (21.2%) and the lumbar region (19.7%).

Multivariate analysis of variance was used to assess the effects of bullet removal on changes in ASIA motor index score and sharp/dull and light touch sensation scores between the initial and annual examinations. These analyses revealed an overall significant difference ($P < 0.035$) between those who had bullets removed and those who did not. There was, however, general improvement in all three scores at annual follow-up regardless of whether or not bullets were removed.

Subsequent univariate analysis of variance demonstrated that the difference between those who had bullets removed and those who did not was due exclusively to changes in ASIA motor scores. The change in ASIA motor score for those with bullet removal was 10.4 ± 7.8 points, while those individuals who did not have bullet removal improved an average of 4.4 ± 8.0 points ($P < 0.004$).

Since a larger proportion of the cases with bullets located at lower vertebral levels had bullets removed, data were partitioned according to the vertebral location of the bullet. Subjects were divided into three groups: cervical, C1 to C7 (n = 14); thoracic, T1 to T11 (n = 32); and lumbar, T12 to L5 (n = 20).

In the cervical and thoracic regions there was no statistically significant difference in ASIA motor scores between those who had bullet removal and those who did not (Table 4–11). ASIA motor scores for persons with bullet removal from the lumbar region increased an average of 12.9 ± 6.1 points, while scores for those without bullet removal increased 3.3 ± 3.6 points ($P < 0.001$).

Ankylosing Spondylitis

Ankylosing spondylitis is an inflammatory condition affecting the spine, the sacroiliac joints, and the hips. The average age at onset of this disease is 28 years, with males predominating 10:1. From 1985 to 1989, a collaborative study among the Model Systems identified 59 persons with paralysis associated with spine trauma and ankylosing spondylitis.[9] Twenty-two of these were managed operatively and 37 nonoperatively. The spinal management of both groups of persons attempted to place the spine in the premorbid condition while healing took place. Analysis revealed no statistical difference between the two groups in regard to neurologic loss or improvement or number of complications. However, there was a statistically significant increase in the length of stay for persons in the operative group. All but two of the persons in this group underwent some period of time

---

Table 4–11 Motor and Sensory Changes from Initial Hospitalization to Annual Follow-Up*

	Bullet Removed	Bullet Not Removed
Motor (All Levels)	10.4 ± 7.8	4.4 ± 8.0
T1 to T11	8.8 ± 9.2	3.8 ± 8.1
T12 to L5	12.9 ± 6.1†	3.3 ± 3.6
Sharp/Dull Sensory	4.5 ± 11.6	3.9 ± 12.1
Light Touch Sensory	4.4 ± 8.4	6.4 ± 20.1

*Data from Model Systems' collaborative study.
†$P < 0.05$.

in traction before surgery was attempted, and this may account for the increased length of stay. The conclusion was that nonoperative management by placing the patient in traction to duplicate the premorbid spine position with conversion to a halo was the safest and most appropriate method of treatment. However, during the course of this study, newer methods of internal fixation of the spine were developed. With better methods of internal fixation, managing the long lever arm of a spondylytic spine operatively may become easier and safer.

EMERGENCY MEDICAL SYSTEMS DEVELOPMENT AND SPINE TRAUMA MANAGEMENT

With serendipity, the year 1971 saw the initiation of a move toward the development of an EMS system and a system of federally sponsored and supported SCI Model Systems. Neither was in response to the other; rather, both were in response to their absence in society. This awareness was heightened by the 1966 publication of the National Academy of Sciences, National Research Council's document, *Accidental Death and Disability: The Neglected Disease of Modern Society.*[10]

Additional emphasis on the need for the development of "trauma" health care delivery systems arose historically from the lack of war casualty management schemes dating back to the Civil War.[11] Disastrous consequences followed the Union army's battle at Bull Run on July 21, 1861. With no prior plans for the management of an unanticipated mass of war wounded, the result was a blood bath. With each successive war, improvement in casualty care began to evolve. Battle casualty death rates fell from 8% (100% of persons with SCI within 1 year) following World War I, to 4.5% in World War II (with persons with SCI now surviving 10 years), to 2.5% in Korea, and mortality rates of less than 2% in Vietnam.[11] These changes were brought about as a result of intensive planning and implementation of innovative programs by leaders in military medicine. It became apparent that the same issues needed to be addressed in the civilian society.

These impressive reduced mortality-increased survival statistics were responsible for influencing President Lyndon Johnson to establish the Highway Safety Act in 1966.[12] Concurrent with the focus of attention on emergency medical care came the initiation of two new classes of ambulance attendants: emergency medical technicians (EMTs)[13] and paramedics.[14] Prior to the 1970s, neither existed. Accompanying their arrival came ambulances of new design, with new workspace and communication capabilities between ambulance and hospital. For the first time, trained paraprofessionals were able to provide in-transit emergency patient resuscitation and drug administration. The result was a dramatic improvement in patient survival.

The 1966 encyclical on trauma[10] and the EMS Act of 1973,[15-17] along with the Rehabilitation Services Administration's first Model SCI System demonstration grant award in Phoenix in 1970, focused attention on both trauma and SCI. Federal demonstration grants in both areas soon led to the purposeful integration of these activities into a highly effective and efficient emergency health care delivery system.

Trauma Network Structure

The underlying concept of a trauma network or system, regardless of the trauma etiology and irrespective of the site or location of injury, is that the injured person shall always have access to immediate medical attention. Then, depending on the nature and severity of injury, the patient is transported, whether by ground or air (fixed or rotary), to a designated trauma center capable of delivering the level of care commensurate with the existing injury.

Key to the success of any trauma system are four components: (1) access to the system, (2) immediate attention, (3) transport and resuscitation, and finally (4) the delivery of the level of medical care required to meet the needs of the patient's injury.[18] To achieve this end, every component of the trauma system must be airtight and thoroughly integrated. A prerequisite to success is the uniform availability of emergency and rescue services personnel, appropriately dispersed across rural, suburban, and urban America. This implies the presence of, and a careful integration of city, state, and federal emergency medical services, with participation by both municipality fire or police departments and private ambulance companies. Access must be via a universally available emergency telephone access number (911), which in turn becomes the dispenser of the responding service. As noted, a trauma system must exist within every community, whether urban or rural.

Included within an organized trauma network system are levels or categories of sophisticated care. It is obvious that not every community having a designated trauma center will have the capability of either manning or supporting the highest (center) level of care required. While that may be the case, every center should have the availability of immediate access to a Level I trauma center capable of managing neurologic injuries (such as SCI) or burns. A Level II trauma center, usually a suburban hospital, is a care facility with slightly less sophistication or availability of staff and equipment. The least sophisticated trauma care facility, and probably the busiest, is the Level III trauma center. While its primary function is to provide emergency care when required, it has access to Level I and Level II facilities, depending on the demands of the patient's injury.

SCI Trauma Centers

Just as there are organizational levels throughout the trauma network system, there are components within the SCI Model System. Included are (1) prevention; (2) emergency care, resuscitation, retrieval, and transport; (3) acute care; (4) rehabilitation care; and (5) follow-up. While each section stands alone, collectively (from a System standpoint) they are highly integrated and interdependent. Looking across the broad field of trauma, and specifically SCI trauma, it is incumbent on the reader to appreciate the effort that has been expended across the United States to develop simultaneously, with assistance from the federal government, two very critical systems in the chain of trauma health delivery: that of a nationwide network of trauma centers and the initiation of the development of a nationwide system of SCI centers (located either within, or as a function of, a Level I trauma center environment). An additional prerequisite has been the incorporation of rehabilitation centers within the trauma system concept. The union of these latter three systems has come to serve as the model of "specific entity" (trauma–SCI–rehabilitation) health care delivery systems for the future.

SPINE FRACTURES

The goals of the surgeon taking care of persons with traumatic SCI should be to restore spinal alignment, establish spinal stability, prevent further neurologic deterioration, and perhaps enhance neurologic recovery. The advent of better diagnostic capabilities has significantly affected the management of the spinal column and spinal cord in recent years.

Until the mid-1970s, the primary diagnostic tools were routine roentgenograms and myelograms. The use of the myelogram in the evaluation demonstrated many complete blocks, which led to the employment of laminectomy as a routine procedure in the management of SCI. As the failure of this method to improve neurologic function has been documented, and with the advent of the newer modalities, laminectomy is seldom indicated. Use of CT either alone or augmented with less toxic radio-opaque fluids, improved the surgeon's capability of delineating bone as well as disc components.[19]

The use of wires in the cervical spine and rod and hook techniques in the thoracic and lumbar spine improved the surgeon's ability to realign the spine as well as provide effective stabilization. However, the limitations of these techniques soon became evident. In the last 10 years and certainly in the last 5 years, more exacting techniques and new generations of stabilizing implantable devices have added to the armamentarium. Now anterior and posterior plating with screws and more rigid rodding supplemented by screw fixation have become available. These devices now provide an appropriately trained spine surgeon with the instrumentation to stabilize reliably nearly all unstable acute injuries.

With the improved ability to restore spinal alignment and thus reduce fracture fragments has come the question of what to do with bone that remains in the spinal canal. One group proposes to remove bone in the canal,[20–22] restoring the canal to near anatomic capacity. Another group feels that with realigning the spine,[23] and stabilizing it, sufficient decompression occurs to allow any neurologic recovery to take place that would normally take place. There is gathering evidence that bone left in the canal remodels over a period of time.[24] However, there is general agreement that restoration of spinal alignment as quickly as possible enhances neurologic recovery.[25]

During the course of the 5 years corresponding to the data analyzed for this report, the use of high doses of methylprednisolone was introduced. Other studies are now taking place advocating the use of gangliosides such as GM_1 with and without methylprednisolone. While continued collection of data on a large number of persons with SCI will continue to delineate the efficacy of treatment efforts such as these and surgical treatment as discussed above, the National SCI Database was not designed to address such issues in the details required. The Database provides a broad picture of SCI and the influence of systematic care provision, and serves to foster in-depth, focused research that can be conducted appropriately in single-site or collaborative studies among various Systems.

CONCLUSION

Improved techniques for internal fixation of unstable spine fractures during the past several decades now provide reliable methods of stabilizing acutely unstable spine fractures, permitting rapid mobilization and full participation in the rehabilitation program soon after injury. New imaging techniques permit visualization of spine and spinal cord pathology to assess the need for surgical decompression more accurately.

Because of the low incidence of SCI in the general population, it is difficult for a single System to accumulate prospectively a sufficient number of cases to determine whether surgery improves neurologic outcome by comparison with control subjects. Collaborative studies between Systems are necessary to accumulate a statistically sufficient number of cases in a reasonable time frame. Collaborative studies necessitate common methods of classifying the type of fracture and assessing neurologic function.

ASIA's *International Standards for Neurological and Functional Classification of Spinal Cord Injury*[8] has become the standard means of measuring neurologic function. At the present time there is no fracture classification system to categorize different types of injuries. Such a classification system is needed to permit evaluation of the effectiveness of surgery in promoting neurologic recovery.

Information from the National SCI Database indicates the incidence of certain types of surgical complications. The overall incidence of infection was 4.4% and the incidence for reoperation to revise or remove instrumentation was 1.8%. While no cause-and-effect connections can be verified within the Database regarding pressure ulcers, DVT, pulmonary embolism, or pneumonia, the overall incidence of each complication was similar in persons undergoing spine surgery when compared with those treated nonoperatively.

REFERENCES

1. Smith E. T*he Edwin Smith Surgical Papyrus* (Breasted JH, trans from the hieroglyphics). Chicago: University of Chicago Press; 1930:1,323–332.

2. Green E, Eismont FJ, O'Heir JT. Pre-hospital management of spinal cord injuries. *Paraplegia.* 1987;25:229–238.

3. Garfin SR, Shakford SR, Marshall LF, Drummond JC. Care of the multiply injured patient with cervical spine injury. *Clin Orthop.* 1989;239:19–29.

4. Allen BL, Ferguson RL, Lehmann TR, O'Brien RP. A mechanistic classification of closed indirect fractures and dislocation of the lower cervical spine. *Spine.* 1982;7:1–27.

5. Denis F. The three column spine and its significance in the classification of acute thoracolumbar spinal injuries. *Spine.* 1983;8:817–831.

6. Waters RL, Adkins RH, Yakura J, Sie I. Profiles of spinal cord injury and recovery after gunshot injury. *Clin Orthop.* 1991;267:14–21.

7. Waters RL, Adkins RH. The effects of removal of bullet fragments retained in the spinal canal. A collaborative study by the National Spinal Cord Injury Model Systems. *Spine.* 1991;16:934–939.

8. *International Standards for Neurological and Functional Classification of Spinal Cord Injury.* Rev. 1992. Chicago: American Spinal Injury Association/International Medical Society of Paraplegia/American Paraplegia Association; 1992;1–26.

9. Apple DF Jr, et al. Spinal cord injury occurring in patients with ankylosing spondylitis: A multi-center study. *Orthopedics.* In press.

10. Division of Medical Sciences, National Academy of Sciences. *Accidental Death and Disability: The Neglected Disease of Modern Society.* Washington, DC: National Research Council; September 1966.

11. Adams GW. *Doctors in Blue.* New York: Collier Books; 1961.

12. Law of the 89th Congress. Highway Safety Act of 1966, Washington, DC; 1966.

13. Committee on Emergency Medical Services and Subcommittee on Ambulance Services. National Academy of Sciences, National Highway Traffic Safety Administration. *Emergency Medical Technician.* Advanced Training Program. U.S. Department of Transportation, Washington, DC; November 1973.

14. Boyd DR. Emergency medical services systems development: A national initiative. IEEE *Trans Vehic Technol.* November 1976; VT-25(4).

15. Law of the 93rd Congress. Emergency Medical Services Systems Act of 1973. Pub L 93–154. Washington, DC; 1973.

16. Law of the 94th Congress. Emergency Medical Services Amendments of 1976. Pub L 94–173. Washington, DC; 1976.

17. Law of the 96th Congress. Emergency Medical Services Amendments of 1979. Pub L 96–142. Washington, DC; 1979.

18. Meyer PR. Acute injury retrieval and splinting techniques: On-site care. In: *Surgery of Spine Trauma*. New York: Churchill-Livingstone; 1989:1–21.

19. Rizzolo SJ, Piazza MR, Cotler JM, Balderston RA, Schaefer D, Flanders A. Intervertebral disc injury complicating cervical spine trauma. *Spine.* 1991;16(6 suppl):S187–S189.

20. Riska EB, Myllynen P, Brostman O. Anterolateral decompression for neural involvement in thoracolumbar fractures: A review of 78 cases. *J Bone Joint Surg [Br].* 1982;69:704–708.

21. Anderson PA, Bohlman HH. Anterior decompression and arthrodesis of the cervical spine: Long term motor improvement. Part I: Improvement in incomplete traumatic quadriplegia. *J Bone Joint Surg [Am].* 1992;74:671–682.

22. Anderson PA, Bohlman HH. Anterior decompression and arthrodesis of the cervical spine: Long term motor improvement. Part II: Improvement in complete traumatic quadriplegia. *J Bone Joint Surgery [Am].* 1992;74:683–699.

23. Crutcher JP Jr, Anderson PA, King HA, Montesana PX. Indirect spinal canal decompression in patients with thoracolumbar burst fractures treated by posterior distraction rods. *J Spinal Dis.* 1991;4:39–48.

24. Mumford J, Weinstein JN, Spratt KF, Goel VK. Thoracolumbar burst fractures: The clinical efficacy and outcome of nonoperative management. *Spine.* 1993;18:955–970.

25. Cotler JM, Herbison GJ, Nasuti JF, Ditunno JF Jr, An H, Wolff BE. Closed reduction of traumatic cervical spine dislocation using traction weights up to 140 pounds. *Spine.* 1993;18:386–390.

5

Management of Pulmonary, Cardiovascular, and Metabolic Conditions after Spinal Cord Injury

Kristjan T. Ragnarsson, Karyl M. Hall,
Conal B. Wilmot, and R. Edward Carter

INTRODUCTION

Pulmonary and cardiovascular conditions after SCI are a frequent source of morbidity. In fact, pulmonary complications are the most common cause of death, during both the acute and chronic phases after injury. These two conditions, therefore, have received much attention in the National SCI Database. Metabolic conditions related to SCI are quite varied, and although these may also be a source of morbidity, they rarely result in death. Limited data on metabolic conditions were collected by all Model Systems. These data, which addressed mainly osteoporosis, fractures, and heterotopic ossification, are presented in Chapter 8.

In this chapter, data on pulmonary and cardiovascular conditions collected by the SCI Model Systems since October 1986 are presented and discussed. First, the reader should note that information on individuals with SCI relating to events that occurred prior to their admission to a Model System was collected retrospectively. These data included their status before and after the SCI occurred, but before they were admitted to a Model System acute care or rehabilitation service. In general, it was very difficult to obtain reliable information from the referring hospitals on the various pulmonary and cardiovascular conditions that occurred prior to System admission. These pre-System data could not be analyzed and interpreted in a meaningful way and therefore are not presented in this chapter. The data that are presented are restricted to cardiovascular conditions that were documented: (1) during inpatient acute care and rehabilitation within a Model System and (2) during annual follow-up.

Second, the data presented here on pulmonary and cardiovascular complications during inpatient System stay are restricted to persons admitted to a System within 24 hours of injury, whereas the data collected annually during follow-up were obtained from the entire sample (i.e., not only from those who entered a System within 24 hours of injury, but also from those who were admitted up to 60 days after injury).

Third, data were collected on System admission and at definitive discharge following inpatient rehabilitation. Data were also collected annually by clinic visit or by telephone, and are reported here for 6 years after injury. The data were analyzed by age, gender, neurologic categories, and/or Frankel grade.

PULMONARY CONDITIONS

The National SCI Database provides the opportunity to investigate the long-term pulmonary status of individuals with SCI. This information is particularly relevant to the well-being of those with SCI, as pulmonary conditions are the leading cause of mortality for both tetraplegia and paraplegia.[1] Histories of aspiration, atelectasis, pneumonia, and ventilatory failure were documented. The definitions used for each of these conditions can be found in Appendix A.

Pulmonary Conditions during System Stay

Occurrences of aspiration, atelectasis, pneumonia, and ventilatory failure during System stay were documented by age group, gender, neurologic category (complete paraplegia, incomplete paraplegia, complete tetraplegia, incomplete tetraplegia) and Frankel grade. The number of persons on whom data were collected during System stay ranges from 2089 to 2196. Percentages in tables reflect the percentages of persons with SCI who had the condition, calculated from the total number in that neurologic category or Frankel grade. The use of χ^2 analyses determined the statistical significance of association between pulmonary conditions and other factors. A value of $P < 0.05$ was required to be considered statistically significant.

Aspiration

Aspiration occurred in 4.3% of persons by System discharge. There was a significant association between age and aspiration, with older age groups showing higher incidence. The incidence increases from a range of 3% to 5% in age groups up to 60 years to a range of 12% to 13% in the group of persons older than 60 years.

No statistically significant gender differences were found for incidence of aspiration. Neurologic category at admission to the System was significantly related to episodes of aspiration (Table 5–1). Only 1.3% of those with incomplete paraplegia aspirated during System stay, whereas 11.4% of those with complete tetraplegia aspirated. No occurrences of aspiration were recorded for those with minimal disability.

Likewise, there was a significant association between Frankel grade at System admission and aspiration (Table 5–2). Three percent of individuals with incomplete injuries aspirated, whereas 5.8% of individuals with Frankel grade A (complete injuries) aspirated.

Atelectasis

Atelectasis occurred in 23.6% of persons by definitive System discharge. Neither age nor gender was associated with atelectasis during System stay. There was, however, a significant association between neurologic category and atelectasis (Table 5–1). Note that very little difference in incidence existed between individuals with incomplete paraplegia and incomplete tetraplegia. The large differences were seen between those with incomplete and complete injuries and between persons with paraplegia complete injuries and tetraplegia complete injuries. Also, those with complete injuries had a significantly higher incidence of atelectasis (Table 5–2).

Pneumonia

Pneumonia occurred in 18.4% of persons. There was a significant association between age and occurrences of pneumonia during System stay (Table 5–3). The greatest incidence of pneumonia was seen in the age categories beyond 60 years.

Table 5–1 Percentage Occurrence of Selected Pulmonary Conditions during System Stay by Neurologic Category

Neurologic Category*	Aspiration	Atelectasis	Pneumonia	Ventilatory Failure
Paraplegia, Incomplete	1.3	13.2	6.0	4.4
Paraplegia, Complete	1.5	28.3	15.2	9.2
Tetraplegia, Incomplete	4.3	16.3	13.6	11.5
Tetraplegia, Complete	11.4	39.3	37.8	37.1

*n = 2106 to 2156.

Table 5–2 Percentage Occurrence of Selected Pulmonary Conditions during System Stay by Frankel Grade

Frankel Grade*	Aspiration	Atelectasis	Pneumonia	Ventilatory Failure
A	5.8	33.1	26.6	21.4
B	5.4	23.3	16.9	12.7
C	2.7	15.5	12.8	8.5
D	1.7	9.5	5.7	5.9

*n = 2089 to 2196.

There were no statistically significant gender differences in incidence of pneumonia. Neurologic category was significantly related to pneumonia: the higher and more complete the injury, the greater the number of persons who developed pneumonia (Table 5–1). There were no reported cases of pneumonia for those with minimal neurologic deficits. Likewise, those with complete injuries had a higher incidence of pneumonia (Table 5–2).

Ventilatory Failure

Ventilatory failure occurred in 14.7% of persons by System discharge. Age and ventilatory failure were significantly related during System stay. Incidence was approximately 12% in persons under age of 30, 15% to 17% in persons aged 31 to 60, and 22% to 23% in persons over age 60. This association between age and ventilatory failure was statistically significant.

No statistically significant difference was seen in the occurrence of ventilatory failure by gender. Both neurologic category (Table 5–1) and Frankel grade (Table 5–2), however, were significantly related to the occurrence of this

Table 5–3 Percentage Occurrence of Pneumonia during System Stay by Age Group*

Age	%
0–15	9.8
16–30	15.7
31–45	21.5
46–60	17.4
61–75	27.8
76+	34.0

*n = 2178.

condition during System stay. It is evident that individuals with complete tetraplegia are at greatest risk, as expected.

Pulmonary Conditions at Annual Follow-Up

The number of persons on which follow-up data were collected ranged from 2743 to 2891 for year 1 to 1487 to 1539 for year 6. Occurrences of aspiration, atelectasis, pneumonia, and ventilatory failure were documented. Findings are classified by neurologic category.

Aspiration

Neurologic category and incidence of aspiration were significantly associated for follow-up years 1, 2, and 6 only, with fewer episodes of aspiration occurring in those with paraplegia than in those with tetraplegia, as expected. The overall incidence of aspiration at all neurologic levels during follow-up was very low, less than 1%.

Atelectasis

There was a significant association between neurologic category and incidence of atelectasis in follow-up years 1 through 5, with fewer episodes in persons with paraplegia than in those with tetraplegia. For persons with paraplegia, completeness of injury was not a factor in incidence of atelectasis (the incidence was less than 0.4% for those with paraplegia). As expected, the incidence of atelectasis was significantly reduced during follow-up years after injury, compared with during System stay. Atelectasis averaged 1.3% per year for individuals with incomplete tetraplegia, but even for persons with complete tetraplegia, the annual incidence averaged only 2.6%. No trends in frequency were evident across the 6 follow-up years, with the annual incidence of atelectasis remaining fairly stable.

Pneumonia

Neurologic category and incidence of pneumonia were significantly associated in follow-up years 1 through 4, with a strong trend in follow-up years 5 and 6. Generally, the lowest incidence of pneumonia was observed for those with incomplete paraplegia, as expected. Even those with complete paraplegia had only a 1% incidence of pneumonia, on the average, in any given year postinjury. Individuals with incomplete tetraplegia averaged only a 2.2% incidence per year, and those with complete tetraplegia, 4.7% per year. In this last group, the average incidence decreased generally through each year of follow-up, being highest during the first and second years (6.3% and 6.4%) and lowest during the sixth year (3.0%).

Ventilatory Failure

There was a significant association between neurologic category and incidence of ventilatory failure in follow-up years 1, 2, 4, and 5 only, with the least number of episodes for persons with paraplegia, as expected. Results for those with incomplete tetraplegia yielded less than 1% incidence per year. Incidence of ventilatory failure for individuals with complete tetraplegia ranged from 0.5% to 2.3%, with no trend evident over time.

Findings of the National SCI Database

During System stay, it was found that age was significantly related to the occurrence of aspiration, pneumonia, and ventilatory failure. That is, the older the individual, the more likely these complications were to occur, findings in accord with previous work.[2] Neurologic level and Frankel grade were also consistently related to all the complications. The higher the level of neurologic lesion and the more complete the injury, the higher was the incidence of these conditions. No statistically significant gender differences were found for any of these conditions.

Incidence of aspiration during System stay was infrequent (4.3%) on the average, but was more common for those over the age of 60 (11.9%) and for individuals with complete tetraplegia (11.4%). Atelectasis was fairly common across all age groups during System stay, with a somewhat higher risk noted for increasing age (16% to 30%). Persons with complete injuries were at higher risk than those with incomplete injuries, and individuals with complete tetraplegia had the highest incidence of atelectasis during System stay (39.3%). Pneumonia was much more prevalent among older individuals, but was present in all age groups (10% to 34%).

Individuals with complete tetraplegia were also at greatest risk of developing pneumonia during System stay (37.8%). Incidence of ventilatory failure was most frequent for those with complete tetraplegia (37.1%) and for those over the age of 60, as expected.

In a study of 2619 individuals who sustained SCI between the years 1959 and 1985, 68% were reported to have marked respiratory problems.[3] Atelectasis and pneumonia were found to be the most common respiratory complications[2] within the first month after injury. In a sample of 261 persons with SCI admitted to 5 Model Systems within 48 hours of injury, with a neurologic level of C1 to T12 and Frankel grade A, B, or C, 36% were reported to have had atelectasis, followed by pneumonia (31%) and ventilatory failure (23%).[4] In that study, atelectasis was diagnosed an average of 18 days following injury, pneumonia was diagnosed an average of 25 days following injury, and ventilatory failure was diagnosed 4.5 days following injury.

During the first 6 follow-up years, the incidence of aspiration was quite low. Atelectasis was a significant concern only for those with tetraplegia. Pneumonia and ventilatory failure were significantly related to neurologic level in the expected direction during all 6 years. However, the occurrence of these conditions was very low. The respiratory condition with the highest incidence was pneumonia, which occurred at an annual average in 4.7% of individuals with complete tetraplegia. Pneumonia was most common during follow-up years 1 and 2 (6%), but its incidence dropped thereafter for this group.

Pulmonary Mortality

In 1968, Silver and Gibbon[5] proposed that respiratory complications might account for as many as half of the deaths in those with complete tetraplegia. Bellany et al.[6] reported 40% mortality within 1 year of cervical injury, confirming with autopsy that pulmonary complications were related to most deaths. Reines and Harris[2] found a mortality rate of 30% for persons with tetraplegia, and an overall mortality rate of 11% for all persons with SCI due to pulmonary complications alone within the first month after injury.

A recent study of mortality during the first 12 years after SCI in a sample of 9135 individuals, of whom 854 had died, reported the leading primary cause of death as pneumonia.[1] Pneumonia was the leading cause of death of every age group through these 12 years after injury. It was the primary cause of death for persons with both complete and incomplete injuries, although it was much less common for persons with incomplete lesions. The deaths occurred most often relatively early after injury, contributing substantially to a reduced life expectancy for these persons.

Once an individual has completed inpatient rehabilitation and has stable respiration, mortality rates can approach those of the normal population. However, this may not be the case when complicating factors are present, such as intrinsic lung or heart disease, open tracheostomy, or the need for ventilator support. Neurologic level, completeness of cord lesion, and advancing age significantly affect survival statistics. For example, those who sustain SCI after age 50 have a survival rate of 43.4%[3,7] 6 years postinjury. For a review of mortality findings based on the current National SCI Database, see Chapter 14.

Pulmonary Morbidity

Even when the innervation of the phrenic nerve is intact, individuals with tetraplegia and high-level paraplegia will have reduced effective maximum respiratory vital capacity and tidal volume.[8] If, for example, an individual's vital capacity is 5 liters prior to injury, this lung capacity may be reduced to 1.3 liters following SCI with a complete C6 neurologic lesion.

Following acute SCI, while the person is in spinal shock, oxygen diffusion capacity may be impaired.[9] Overhydration can make cord edema worse while this condition exists. Further fluid overload reduces the effective gaseous exchange of O_2 and CO_2, therefore reducing vital capacity.[10] If not adequately managed, this condition may cause mucous plugs to develop within the respiratory tract, and atelectasis of the lung, further reducing the gaseous exchange area. If the lung becomes infected, pneumonia will result. This condition is more serious the higher the neurologic lesion, because individuals with tetraplegia and high paraplegia (i.e., those with neurologic lesions above T8) have a markedly diminished cough and reduced vital capacity. Because of the progressive pathologic changes within the spinal cord during the first days after injury, the neurologic level may rise at least temporarily, causing further impairment of respiratory functions. This phenomenon can be very significant for persons with tetraplegia, for whom the vital capacity is already severely compromised. Physical fatigue, including fatigue of the partially innervated diaphragm in persons with SCI who are barely able to breathe spontaneously, is also a factor that can reduce respiratory capacity and increase the risk of pulmonary complications.[7]

Prophylaxis

Comprehensive respiratory management has been shown to reduce considerably the mortality from respiratory failure.[11] A very active prophylactic respiratory therapy program has therefore been recommended, starting immediately following injury.[9,12] The basic elements of such a program would include the following:[13]

- postural drainage, Trendelenburg and reverse Trendelenburg
- assisted coughing
- intermittent positive-pressure breathing with saline and/or $NaHCO_3$ bronchodilators
- active program to increase strength and excursion of diaphragm and other innervated accessory muscles of respiration, such as the sternocleidomastoid and trapezius muscles
- vital capacity assessment

- arterial blood gas assessment as needed
- chest X-rays as needed
- oxygen saturation monitoring

The general treatment goal for persons with SCI is to achieve approximately 60% of predicted vital capacity, but the specific therapeutic procedures vary from System to System.[14] It has been recommended that intubation or tracheostomy be done and mechanical respiration initiated if vital capacity decreases to 1000 mL or less, if arterial blood gases become increasingly abnormal (increased Pco_2 and decreased Po_2), if atelectasis becomes frequent, or if the chest X-ray shows consolidation.[15] This will allow the individual to be ventilated properly and to receive adequate pulmonary toilet.

Tidal volumes for patients on a ventilator should be higher than normal breathing, that is, at least 20 mL/kg[15,16] rather than the 10 mL/kg recommended for the able-bodied person. The larger volume has been found to reduce complications and shorten the time the person with SCI is required to be on the ventilator. These volumes have reduced the use of the positive end-expiratory pressure technique, which can cause pneumothorax.

Once the respiratory status has stabilized, the patient can be weaned from the ventilator. The subsequent respiratory care program should continue to stress pulmonary toilet and strengthening of the respiratory muscles. As the respiratory status improves, the oxygen needs are reduced, the arterial blood gases normalized, and the vital capacity increased.[9] Weaning of the patient from the ventilator may be best accomplished by progressively increasing the time off the ventilator rather than reducing the intermittent mandatory volume. Plugging of the tracheostomy tube is stopped if the vital capacity drops 25% below the ventilated status. Serial arterial blood gases are monitored regularly during weaning. When the patient tolerates plugging of the tracheostomy tube for 24 hours with adequate volumes and satisfactory arterial blood gases, the tube can be removed. The specifics of different weaning techniques must be investigated further in order to establish their comparative effectiveness.[8]

The risk of developing atelectasis can be increased if the prophylactic interventions are not vigorous or are infrequent, or if the person is not monitored adequately, making it necessary to perform tracheostomy and/or intubation.[12] Pneumonia frequently develops as a consequence of an untreated atelectasis or small pulmonary emboli. It may also result from a blood-borne spread from another site of infection. Because of the reduction of ventilated lung tissue caused by pneumonia, there may be a critical deterioration in pulmonary function. The treatment of pneumonia involves administering appropriate antibiotics, providing supportive measures, and continuing a vigorous program of pulmonary toilet.

The Ventilator-Dependent Patient

While in bed, the ventilator-dependent patient will use a large static ventilator. As mobilization out of bed is begun, the large ventilator can be exchanged for a portable ventilator if the lungs are clear by clinical or radiologic assessment. The portable ventilator can be built onto the electric wheelchair to permit greater mobility.

Another device to assist breathing is the pneumobelt, an external compression device that is used with the portable ventilator when the person with respiratory impairment is sitting upright in the chair.[17] This device allows the tracheostomy to be plugged and permits use of a fenestrated tracheostomy tube, which enables the individual to communicate verbally. The relative contraindications to pneumobelt use are obesity and spasticity.

If the neurologic lesion is complete and transverse at the C1 and C2 levels, the person with tetraplegia may be a candidate for a phrenic nerve stimulator (PNS).[18] Since the C3, C4, and C5 segments are intact, the functional phrenic nerve can be stimulated by an external electrical device. With appropriate conditioning of the diaphragm postoperatively, the PNS can produce tidal volumes up to 1000 mL per stimulation when the bilateral stimulation is performed simultaneously. The individual may alternate the use of PNS, pneumobelt, and ventilator for respiration by the time of discharge and, with increasing confidence, can gradually attain complete independence from the ventilator. This achievement obviously would increase the quality of life and reduce the need for acute medical attention.[19]

Long-Term Pulmonary Care

As persons with SCI live longer, clinical conditions related to the aging of the respiratory system have become more common.[20] Many factors contribute to this increased survival rate, such as a better understanding of the pathophysiology of SCI and the adoption of a healthier lifestyle, including reduction in smoking, maintenance of optimal weight, and regular exercise. Additional factors include pharmacologic advances, systematic follow-up, and prompt medical management of clinical conditions such as chronic and acute respiratory problems.

The inevitable deterioration that occurs with age is predicted, in part, on a person's genetic structure. However, other preventable risk factors can be identified that cause damage to the respiratory system, including air pollution, smoking, respiratory infections, obesity, and loss of physical fitness. Additional risk factors to be considered specifically for persons with SCI are higher levels and greater completeness of the cord injury, skeletal deformities of the spine and chest, and spasticity of the chest and abdominal walls, all of which affect respiratory excursion and the ability to cough.[20]

The impact of these risk factors can be reduced through education, cessation of smoking, vaccination against influenza and pneumococcal infections, and application of prophylactic treatment principles. Some individuals with severely diminished respiratory capacity can be taught new breathing techniques, such as accessory muscle respiration, or be provided with noninvasive intermittent positive-pressure ventilation.[21] These persons must have effective clearance of secretions from the respiratory tract by assisted coughing, suctioning, and postural drainage.[21] Respiratory infections and other conditions that affect breathing capacity must be treated vigorously.

CARDIOVASCULAR CONDITIONS

Cardiovascular conditions during the acute and chronic phases of SCI are major causes of morbidity and mortality. Deep venous thrombosis, pulmonary embolism, and autonomic dysreflexia have been well recognized for decades and received much interest, as is evident by the numerous scientific publications that address these conditions. Myocardial infarction following SCI is generally considered to be a rare event, but cardiopulmonary arrest, due to any of several underlying causes, is often associated with death. The relationship between these conditions and cardiovascular conditions that existed prior to the SCI is unclear.

Definitions of the cardiovascular conditions for which data were collected can be found in Appendix A.

Cardiovascular Conditions during System Stay

The number of persons on whom data on cardiovascular conditions were collected during System stay ranged from 2185 to 2204.

Autonomic Dysreflexia

Autonomic dysreflexia (AD) occurred in 8.9% of all persons during System stay (Table 5–4). All age groups are prone to develop AD, although the occurrence of this condition appears to be slightly more common among younger adults.

When analyzed by gender it was noted that AD occurred slightly, but still significantly, more often in males (9.2%) than in females (7.4%). One possible explanation could be the gender difference in the anatomy of the lower urinary tract, males having a greater tendency for bladder outlet obstruction.

Table 5–4 Percentage Occurrence of Cardiovascular Conditions during System Stay by Age Group*

Age Group	Autonomic Dysreflexia	Deep Venous Thrombosis	Pulmonary Embolism	Myocardial Infarction	Cardiopulmonary Arrest
0–15	12.7	7.9	1.6	0.0	3.2
16–30	10.2	12.6	3.1	0.5	3.6
31–45	7.7	17.5	4.5	0.2	3.6
46–60	7.8	15.1	3.5	0.4	6.3
61–75	4.6	15.2	8.8	2.2	11.8
76+	3.7	1.9	3.8	5.9	25.9
Average (All Age Groups)	8.9	13.6	3.8	0.6	4.9

*n = 2186.

Autonomic dysreflexia was found in 15.4% of persons with cervical cord lesions and in 2.6% of those with thoracic cord lesions. In persons with tetraplegia, AD was more common in those with complete neurologic lesions (Table 5–5). It was found to occur in 22.7% of those with complete lesions, compared with 12.2% of those with incomplete lesions.

It is of some interest that the incidence of AD was not higher than 15.4% during System stay in patients with cervical cord lesions, since other studies have revealed a much higher frequency (30% to 85% of persons at risk,[22] that is, those with severe cord lesions above the T5 neurologic segment). The low incidence of AD for System patients may be attributed in part to anticipation, good diagnostic work-up, and appropriate and timely interventions. However, there may be other explanations. Model System data include only AD that required intervention, not transient symptoms that resolved spontaneously. Also, AD generally does not appear during the period of spinal shock, (i.e., while areflexia is present), a condition that may last for many weeks after the onset of SCI. As inpatient length of stay has been reduced in recent years, it is also possible that a relatively short hospital stay may account for the relatively low frequency of AD reported here. The higher frequency of AD reported elsewhere may not refer directly to its incidence during inpatient stay, but rather to the prevalence of the condition over a lengthy period of time, that is, how many persons with tetraplegia have experienced the condition.

Deep Venous Thrombosis

Deep venous thrombosis (DVT) during System stay occurred in 13.6% of persons (Table 5–4). Specific diagnostic studies confirmed the presence of DVT

Table 5–5 Percentage Occurrence of Cardiovascular Conditions during System Stay by Neurologic Category

Neurologic Category	Autonomic Dysreflexia	Deep Venous Thrombosis	Pulmonary Embolism	Myocardial Infarction	Cardiopulmonary Arrest
Paraplegia, Minimal Deficit	0.0	4.4	0.0	0.0	1.5
Paraplegia, Incomplete	1.8	13.2	3.5	0.2	1.2
Paraplegia, Complete	3.0	19.3	4.3	0.2	1.4
Tetraplegia, Minimal Deficit	1.6	7.9	1.6	1.6	1.1
Tetraplegia, Incomplete	12.2	11.6	4.5	0.9	3.9
Tetraplegia, Complete	22.7	12.8	3.3	1.3	8.7
Average (All Categories)	8.8	13.7	3.8	0.6	3.5

*n = 2204.

in 94.6% of all those reported as having DVT. The diagnostic techniques most frequently used to confirm DVT were venography (42.6%) and Doppler ultrasound (28.7%), followed by impedance plethysmography (15.2%) and ^{125}I-labeled fibrinogen uptake (3.3%).

The DVT incidence of 13.6% during inpatient stay at a Model System is considerably lower than that reported previously by other investigators,[23–26] who have found the incidence of DVT to vary between 31% and 61%, depending on the diagnostic methods used and the prophylactic treatment. Not all Systems screen all their patients for DVT regularly during System stay, which may explain in part the low incidence of DVT reported here. This low incidence, however, can hardly be due to low level of suspicion or lack of diagnostic procedures at the Model Systems and may therefore also be interpreted as a result of effective prophylaxis.

When analyzed by age, the incidence of DVT was found to be similar in those between the ages of 16 and 75, but appeared to be lower at each end of the age spectrum (Table 5–4). When analyzed by gender, it was noted that DVT occurred more commonly in males (14.9%) than in females (9.0%). When examined by category of neurologic impairment (Table 5–5), DVT during System stay was found to occur slightly more often in persons with paraplegia (16.0%) than in those with tetraplegia (11.9%). DVT was more common in those with complete cord lesions (16.6%) than in those with incomplete lesions (12.5%) and, as expected, was least common in those with minimal deficit (6.4%).

A second episode of DVT occurred during System stay in 2.2% of persons. Those persons 31 to 45 years of age had more second occurrences of DVT (2.9%), followed by 2.7% of persons 16 to 30 years of age and 2.1% of those 45 to 60 years of age. A third or a fourth episode of DVT was exceedingly rare (< 1%).

Pulmonary Embolism

The incidence of pulmonary embolism (PE) during System stay was 3.8% (Table 5–4). PE was found least often in those 0 to 15 years of age and most often in those 60 to 75 years of age, but incidence did not vary greatly among age groups. In the 76 years plus age group, the percentage of PE was greater than the percentage of DVT, probably due to the small sample size and methods of diagnostic testing used to confirm the diagnosis.

The clinical diagnosis of PE was confirmed by ventilation perfusion lung scan (59.5%), pulmonary angiogram (13.0%), by both techniques (9.5%), and by other techniques (4.8%). It was not confirmed by any specific diagnostic technique in 13.0% of cases reported.

PE during System stay occurred in 2.6% of females and 4.1% of males, a statistically significant difference. PE occurs very rarely in those with minimal neurologic deficit (Table 5–5), but with almost equal frequency in persons with paraplegia (3.8%) and tetraplegia (3.9%), both in those who have incomplete (4.1%) and complete (3.9%) lesions.

Myocardial Infarction

Myocardial infarction (MI) occurred in only 0.6% of persons during System stay (Table 5–4). As might be expected, MI occurred most frequently in those over the age of 60. MI was diagnosed in 2.2% of those 61 to 75 years of age and in 5.9% of those over 75 years of age (Table 5–4). MI was found to occur with almost the same frequency in females (0.5%) and in males (0.6%). Examined by category of neurologic impairment (Table 5–5), MI was found to occur more commonly in persons with tetraplegia, both in those with complete and incomplete lesions, compared with those with paraplegia (1.1% vs. 0.2%).

Cardiopulmonary Arrest

Cardiopulmonary arrest occurred in 4.9% of persons during System stay. The incidence of cardiopulmonary arrest was similar in persons under the age of 45, but rose with increasing age and was by far the highest in persons over 75 years of age (Table 5–4).

Cardiopulmonary arrest was found to be significantly more common in persons with tetraplegia than in those with paraplegia, especially in those with tetraplegia and complete neurologic lesion (Table 5–5).

Cardiovascular Conditions during Follow-Up

The number of persons on whom data on cardiovascular conditions were collected on annual follow-up ranged from 2719 for year 1 to 45 for year 6, providing a sample of more than 6900 follow-up records.

Autonomic Dysreflexia

Reported frequency of AD was similar during each follow-up year, with an average incidence of 10.3% during the 6-year period.

Deep Venous Thrombosis

During 6 follow-up years, 77 episodes of DVT were diagnosed from a total of 6938 annual visits (1.1%), indicating that DVT is indeed a rare condition during the chronic phase of SCI. DVT occurs most commonly during the first follow-up year but thereafter remains a rare event, with less than 1% incidence per year.

Pulmonary Embolism

PE during follow-up was diagnosed in only 21 of 6953 visits (0.3%), indicating the rarity of this condition during the chronic phase of SCI.

Myocardial Infarction

MI was diagnosed in only 6 persons during the 6 years of follow-up from a total of 6962 entries (0.1%).

Cardiopulmonary Arrest

Cardiopulmonary arrest was documented in 22 of 6967 persons (0.3%) during the 6 years of follow-up. Of these 22, all had at least one episode of cardiopulmonary arrest, and 8 (0.1%) had an unknown number of such arrests. The frequency of cardiopulmonary arrest is similar during each of the follow-up years.

Discussion of Cardiovascular Conditions

The cardiovascular conditions associated with SCI that have received the most attention are DVT, PE, and AD. Orthostatic hypotension and dependent edema are also frequent symptoms of cardiovascular dysfunction, although usually of less clinical significance. In recent years there has been a growing interest in the effects of sympathetic dysfunction and unopposed vagal action on the heart in persons with tetraplegia.

DVT still occurs frequently during the acute phase of SCI despite prophylactic measures, and PE remains a serious complication that may result in death. Early and accurate diagnosis and aggressive management of these conditions can do much to reduce morbidity and mortality. AD may occur in virtually all persons with a level of neurologic dysfunction above T5, that is, above the major splanchnic sympathetic outflow. AD usually occurs as a response to a noxious stimulus below the level of neurologic dysfunction. Unrecognized and untreated, AD may have serious consequences, whereas removal of the offending stimulus and effective medical management may promptly suppress the symptoms. Bradycardia due to unopposed vagal influence on the heart is most likely to occur during the acute phase of high-level SCI. When this condition is profound and sustained, a cardiac pacemaker may be required to regulate the heart rate. Although cardiac function in those with high-level SCI is impaired during strenuous physical exercise (i.e., heart rate, stroke volume, and cardiac output are reduced compared to normal), this dysfunction does not appear to influence significantly the health and life expectancy of persons with SCI. It is still not known whether persons with SCI are more prone to develop coronary artery disease than able-bodied individuals, but there is speculation that the presence of several risk factors, including sedentary lifestyle, reduced lean body mass, diminished high-density lipoprotein, and abnormal glucose tolerance test, may predispose persons with SCI to cardiovascular disease.[27]

In principle, management of AD focuses on swift identification and elimination of noxious stimuli that may cause the symptoms, prompt suppression of elevated blood pressure, and prevention of recurrent episodes. Numerous noxious stimuli capable of provoking AD have been identified,[22] and these should be removed promptly whenever possible. It is particularly important to assess the condition of the bladder and rectum and ensure their evacuation. If blood pressure is still elevated, it should be lowered, first by bringing the patient to sitting or to the head-up tilt position; but if still sustained, pharmacologic treatment must be considered with a variety of neuroactive medications[22] that may include amyl nitrate, phenoxybenzamine, mecamylamine, guanethidine, and prazosin.

Orthostatic hypotension is primarily associated with high cord lesions and is most often noted transiently following periods of prolonged recumbency. It is caused by pooling of blood in the dependent body parts, decreased venous return to the heart, and reduced cardiac output, which in turn are related to impaired reflex vasoconstriction and absence of compressive muscle forces. Immediate treatment usually consists of placing the patient in the recumbent position and elevating the legs. Preventive measures include elastic stockings, abdominal binders, persistent elevation of the legs, increased salt intake, and medications such as ephedrine sulfate or fluorinated corticosteroids.

Dependent edema is commonly observed. It tends to be bilateral and symmetric. It is usually associated with the dependent position of the paralyzed limbs and impaired compressive muscle forces. Occasionally edema may be aggravated by hypoproteinemia or by fluid and electrolyte imbalance with overhydration. Unilateral edema often indicates the presence of DVT and warrants that appropriate diagnostic tests be ordered. Dependent edema is best managed with elevation and compression with elastic stockings, but diuretics are generally not indicated.

PE is a relatively frequent complication and a leading cause of death in persons with acute SCI.[25] It usually originates from thrombi that develop in the deep veins of the lower extremities,[28] apparently due to increased coagulability of blood and decreased venous return.[29,30] Prevention of DVT is superior to treatment and is considered to be of great importance in the management of acute SCI. If no contraindications exist, prophylactic treatment should begin as early as clinically possible after the injury, and generally within 14 days, when the risk of DVT is felt to be highest.[25]

Administration of low-dose subcutaneous heparin, usually in fixed doses of 5000 U every 12 hours, and external compression of the legs with elastic bandages, stockings, or pneumatic pumps are the most frequently recommended prophylactic interventions. Other prophylactic treatment has also been advocated: administration of heparin in doses that are adjusted to prolong activated partial thromboplastin time (APTT),[23] electrical stimulation of the calf muscles,[25] or administration of drugs with anticoagulant effects (aspirin and dipyridamole).[24]

Recent studies have shown that subcutaneous administration of low-molecular-weight heparin in doses of 3500 anti-Xa units once daily is safe and effective in the prevention of thromboembolism in selected patients with SCI and complete motor paralysis and is superior to standard heparin in fixed doses of 5000 U three times a day.[23,31] Currently, no single treatment guarantees that DVT or PE will not occur. Prophylactic treatment is usually continued for several weeks or even months after SCI while flaccid paralysis of the legs predominates. Development of DVT in the legs may be detected by clinical inspection or by performing specific diagnostic tests such as impedance plethysmography, ^{125}I-labeled fibrinogen uptake, Doppler ultrasound, or venography. PE may occur without clinical evidence of DVT and is accompanied by well-described clinical symptoms. PE is optimally confirmed by ventilation perfusion lung scan, pulmonary angiography, or both.

Once DVT or PE has been diagnosed, full anticoagulation is generally recommended, starting with intravenous heparin and adjusting doses daily according to the APTT. Sodium warfarin administration is started within a few days, and the heparin can usually be discontinued in 7 to 10 days, when the prothrombin time has reached a level 1.5 or 2.0 times the control value or an international normalized ratio of 2.0 to 3.0.[32] Anticoagulation treatment for DVT without PE is usually continued for 3 months, but for 6 months if PE did occur. In the chronic phase of SCI, DVT and PE are rare, and prophylactic treatment is therefore not recommended. However, should a new episode of DVT or PE develop, full anticoagulation is recommended for the same length of time as indicated above.

METABOLIC CONDITIONS

Persons with SCI may experience a wide range of metabolic dysfunctions as a result of altered endocrine function, sedentary lifestyle, and impaired neurogenic influence. Several conditions that are related to dysfunction of bone mineral metabolism[33] are discussed in Chapter 8, including heterotopic ossification, osteoporosis, pathologic bone fractures, and immobilization hypercalcemia. AD, which is associated with altered secretion of catecholamines (norepinephrine, epinephrine, and dopamine) has been discussed in this chapter. Several other metabolic conditions common to persons with SCI deserve to be noted.

The clinical findings of testicular atrophy and gynecomastia in men, and amenorrhea in women, along with reduction of serum levels of the sex hormones testosterone, luteinizing hormone, and follicle-stimulating hormone for several weeks after SCI, indicate dysfunction of the hypothalamic-pituitary-gonadal axis.[34] Similarly, it has been shown that the hypothalamic-pituitary-adrenal axis is altered during the acute phase of SCI[35] and that during the chronic phase of SCI, many hormones such as adrenocorticotropic hormone,[35] cortisol, and β-endorphins[36] are not secreted according to the normal circadian rhythm.

Persons with chronic SCI have been shown to have increased incidence of abnormal carbohydrate metabolism,[37,38] with the majority having an abnormal or diabetic oral glucose tolerance test and the majority of those with abnormal tests demonstrating hyperinsulinemia and insulin resistance.

During the acute phase of SCI, significant weight loss usually occurs, particularly in persons with tetraplegia, due to increased metabolic demands, muscle atrophy, and negative nitrogen and calcium balance. Hypoproteinemia is common and increased by secondary complications, such as pressure ulcers and infections. In contrast, during the chronic phase of SCI, energy expenditure is usually reduced and many individuals become clinically obese. Even in those persons who appear thin, body composition studies have shown that the lean body mass is reduced and the body fat is proportionally increased.[39] Other studies have shown that an inverse relationship appears to exist between the level of neurologic dysfunction and the daily total energy expenditure: the lower the cord lesion the higher the energy expenditure.[40]

Several studies have shown that persons with SCI have low levels of high-density lipoproteins,[41–43] which seems to place them at a higher risk for developing coronary artery disease. These findings have recently been disputed,[44] as well as their interpretation.[45]

There is speculation that many of the metabolic and endocrine changes following SCI are related to a sedentary lifestyle rather than to the actual neurologic deficit.[27] It would follow that prevention and management of some of these conditions should include regular physical exercise.

It has been suggested that clinical pharmacokinetics such as absorption, distribution, effectiveness, and metabolism may be altered for many drugs in persons with SCI.[46] It has been shown that volume distribution of gentamicin and its total body clearance was greater in persons with SCI than in controls.[47] This may be related to high distribution in the extracellular fluid space and minimal biotransformation of this drug and perhaps other drugs with similar qualities. Impaired gastrointestinal absorption of drugs that are passively absorbed and require intact postprandial gastric emptying also seems to be reduced proportionally to the impaired gastric emptying and the neurologic level of cord injury.[46] Absorption of drugs injected into paralyzed muscles also may be reduced, thus reducing their therapeutic efficacy.

REFERENCES

1. DeVivo MJ, Black KJ, Stover SL: Causes of death during the first 12 years after spinal cord injury. *Arch Phys Med Rehabil.* 1993;74:248–254.

2. Reines HD, Harris RC. Pulmonary complications of acute spinal cord injuries. *Neurosurgery.* 1987;21:193–196.

3. Carter RE. Respiratory aspects of spinal cord injury management. *Paraplegia.* 1987;25:262–266.

4. Jackson AB, Groomes TE: Incidence of respiratory complications following spinal cord injury. *Arch Phys Med Rehabil.* 1994;75:270–275.

5. Silver JR, Gibbon NOK. Prognosis in tetraplegia. *Br Med J.* 1968;4:79–83.

6. Bellany R, Pitts FW, Stauffer ES. Respiratory complications in traumatic quadriplegia: Analysis of 20 years experience. *J Neurosurg.* 1973;39:596–600.

7. DeVivo MJ, Kartus PL, Stover SL, Rutt RD, Fine PR. Seven-year survival following SCI. *Arch Neurol.* 1987;44:872–875.

8. Mansel JK, Norman JR. Respiratory complications and management of spinal cord injuries. *Chest.* 1990;97:1446–1452.

9. Ledsome JR, Sharp JM. Pulmonary function in acute cervical cord injury. *Am Rev Respir Dis*. 1981;124:41–44.

10. Poe RH, Reisman JL, Rodenhouse TG. Pulmonary edema in cervical spinal cord injury. *J Trauma*. 1978;18:71–73.

11. Cheshire DJE: Respiratory management in acute traumatic tetraplegia. *Paraplegia*. 1964;1:252–261.

12. McMichan JC, Michel L, Westbrook PR. Pulmonary dysfunction following traumatic quadriplegia. *JAMA*. 1980;243:528–531.

13. Wood M. Respiratory therapy. In: Whiteneck G, et al, eds. *The Management of High Quadriplegia*. New York: Demos Publications, Inc; 1989:51–60.

14. Wicks AB: Ventilator weaning. In: Whiteneck G, et al, eds. *The Management of High Quadriplegia*. New York: Demos Publications, Inc; 1989:141–147.

15. Peterson P. Pulmonary physiology and medical management, In: Whiteneck G, et al, eds. *The Management of High Quadriplegia*. New York: Demos Publications, Inc; 1989:35–50.

16. Massaro GD, Massaro D. Morphologic evidence that large inflations of the lung stimulate secretion of surfactant. *Am Rev Respir Dis*. 1983;127:235–236.

17. Miller HJ, Thomas E, Wilmot CB: Pneumobelt use among the high quadriplegia population. *Arch Phys Med Rehabil*. 1988;69:369–372.

18. Carter RE, Menter R, Wood M, Wilmot CB, Hall KM: Available respiratory options. In: Whiteneck G, et al, eds. *The Management of High Quadriplegia*. New York: Demos Publications, Inc; 1989:149–172.

19. Whiteneck GG, Carter RE, Charliefue SW, et al. A collaborative study of high quadriplegia. *ASIA Bull*. 1986;4(2):8–9.

20. Wilmot CB, Hall KM. The respiratory system. In: Whiteneck G, et al, eds. *Aging with Spinal Cord Injury*. New York: Demos Publications, Inc; 1993:93–104.

21. Bach JR. New approaches in the rehabilitation of the traumatic high level quadriplegia. *Am J Phys Med Rehabil*. 1991;70:13–19.

22. Colachis SC: Autonomic hyperreflexia with spinal cord injury. *J Am Paraplegia Soc*. 1992;15:171–186.

23. Green D, Lee MY, Ito V, et al. Fixed versus adjusted dose heparin in the prophylaxis of thromboembolism in spinal cord injury. *JAMA*. 1988;260:1255–1258.

24. Green D, Rossi EC, Yao JST, Flinn WR, Spies SM. Deep vein thrombosis in spinal cord injury: Effect of prophylaxis with cath compression, aspirin and dipyridamole. *Paraplegia*. 1982;20:227–234.

25. Merli GJ, Herbison GJ, Ditunno JF, et al. Deep vein thrombosis: Prophylaxis in acute spinal cord injured patients. *Arch Phys Med Rehabil*. 1988;69:661–664.

26. Todd JW, Frisbie JH, Rossier AB, et al. Deep vein thrombosis in acute spinal cord injury: A comparison of 125I fibrinogen leg scanning, impedance plethysmography and venography. *Paraplegia*. 1976;14:50–57.

27. Ragnarsson KT: The cardiovascular system. In: Whiteneck G, et al, eds. *Aging with Spinal Cord Injury*. New York: Demos Publications, Inc; 1993:73–92.

28. NIH Consensus Development Conference. Prevention of venous thrombosis and pulmonary embolism. *JAMA*. 1986;256:744–749.

29. Naso F. Pulmonary embolism in acute spinal cord injury. *Arch Phys Med Rehabil*. 1974;55:275–278.

30. Rossi EC, Green D, Rosen JS, Spies SM, Jao JST. Sequential changes in factor VIII and platelets preceding deep vein thrombosis in patients with spinal cord injury. *Br J Haematol.* 1980;45:143–151.

31. Green D, Lee MY, Lim AC, et al. Prevention of thromboembolism after spinal cord injury using low-molecular-weight heparin. *Ann Intern Med.* 1990;113:571–574.

32. Hirsh J. Oral anticoagulant drugs. *N Engl J Med.* 1991;324:1865–1875.

33. Naftchi NE, Viau AT, Sell GH, Lowman EW. Mineral metabolism in spinal cord injury. *Arch Phys Med Rehabil.* 1980;61:139–142.

34. Naftchi NE, Viau AT, Sell GH, Lowman EW. Pituitary testicular axis dysfunction in spinal cord injury. *Arch Phys Med Rehabil.* 1980;61:402–405.

35. Claus-Walker J, Halstead LS. Metabolic and endocrine changes in spinal cord injury, III: Less quanta of sensory input plus bedrest and illness. *Arch Phys Med Rehabil.* 1982;63:628–631.

36. Twist JT, Culpepper-Morgan JA, Ragnarsson KT, Petrillo CR, Creek MJ. Neuroendocrine changes during functional electrical stimulation. *Am J Phys Med Rehabil.* 1992;71:156–163.

37. Duckworth WC, Solomon SS, Jallepalli P, Heckemeyer C, Finnern J, Powers A. Glucose intolerance due to insulin resistance in patients with SCI. *Diabetes.* 1980;29:906–910.

38. Duckworth WC, Jallepalli P, Solomon SS. Glucose tolerance in spinal cord injury. *Arch Phys Med Rehabil.* 1983;64:107–110.

39. Nuhlicek DR, Spurr GB, Barboriak JJ, et al. Body composition of patients with spinal cord injury. *Eur J Clin Nutr.* 1988;42:765–773.

40. Mullinger LA, Spurr GB, Elghatit AZ, et al. Daily energy expenditure and basal metabolic rate of spinal cord injury patients. *Arch Phys Med Rehabil.* 1985;66:420–426.

41. Heldenberg D, Rubinstein A, Levtov O, Werbin B, Tamir I: Serum lipids and lipoprotein concentrations in young quadriplegic patients. *Atherosclerosis.* 1981;39:163–167.

42. Brenis G, Dearwater S, Shapera R, LaPorta RE, Collins E. High density lipoprotein cholesterol concentrations in physically active and sedentary spinal cord injured patients. *Arch Phys Med Rehabil.* 1986;67:445–450.

43. Bauman WA, Spungen AM, Zhong YG, Rothstein JL, Petry C, Gordon SK. Depressed serum high density lipoprotein cholesterol levels in veterans with spinal cord injury. *Paraplegia.* 1992;30:697–703.

44. Cardus D, Ribas-Cardus F, MacTaggart WG. Lipid profiles in spinal cord injury. *Paraplegia.* 1992;30:775–782.

45. Cardus D, Ribas-Cardus F, McTaggart WG. Coronary risk in spinal cord injury: Assessment following a multivaried approach. *Arch Phys Med Rehabil.* 1992;73:930–933.

46. Segal JH, Brunnemann SR. Clinical pharmacokinetics in patients with spinal cord injuries. *Clin Pharmacokinet.* 1989;17:109–129.

47. Segal JH, Gray DR, Gordon SK, Eltorai IM, Khonsari F, Patel J. Gentamicin disposition kinetics in humans with spinal cord injury. *Paraplegia.* 1985;23:47–55.

6

Pressure Ulcers

Gary M. Yarkony and Allen W. Heinemann

INTRODUCTION

Pressure ulcers continue to be a frequent complication of SCI. Charcot's postulation of a neurogenic trophic factor in pressure ulcer development is thought to have been responsible for the belief that their development in spinal cord–injured individuals was inevitable.[1] Brown-Séquard in 1853 published studies of spinal cord–injured guinea pigs and described the prevention and cure of pressure ulcers by elimination of compression and cleansing the skin.[1] Pressure ulcers were still a common problem as modern SCI care developed in Europe and the United States at the time of World War II. Munro[2] held the general view that bedsores were a natural accompaniment of spinal cord injuries, that "everybody talks about . . . but no one does anything about them." As late as 1955 Guttmann[3] commented on the belief that pressure ulcer development in persons with spinal cord injury was "natural and inevitable," and urged improvement in the education of medical and nursing students. Young and Burns,[4] in their initial review of Model Systems data, concluded that pressure ulcers are no longer inevitable, although their occurrence still remains a major problem. They described factors related to pressure ulcer development, including a higher incidence in delayed admissions to the Model Systems. Other relationships noted were an increased incidence in young persons, males, nonwhites, and persons with complete lesions.[4,5]

Pressure ulcers were initially called decubitus ulcers, from the Latin term *decubitus,* "lying down." Other terms used to describe them have been bedsores, ischemic ulcers, and pressure sores. An ulcer is a defect that results from the sloughing of necrotic tissue.[2] Consequently, *pressure ulcer* appears to be the most appropriate term.[1] There are numerous factors that are involved in the development of pressure ulcers, but pressure is the key factor.[6] Other factors include skin maceration due to moisture, poor nutrition, complete lesions, acute illness, and cigarette smoking.[7] For persons with an SCI, shear in combination with pressure is a major etiologic factor.[8–10]

The psychosocial adjustment of persons with SCI has a major impact on pressure ulcer development. Persons who do not follow through on self-care requirements due to depression, lack of motivation, or alcohol and substance abuse are at greatest risk of developing pressure ulcers.[11] In turn, pressure ulcers may have a negative impact on the psychosocial adjustment of the person after the injury.[12]

Traditionally, pressure ulcers are assigned a grade based on the depth of the pressure ulcer. The classification used to collect data for the Model Systems is described in Exhibit 6–1.[13]

MODEL SYSTEMS ANALYSIS OF PRESSURE ULCER DATA

The data analyses reported in this chapter address eight major questions:

1. What is the incidence of pressure ulcers during System hospitalization for persons admitted to Model Systems within 24 hours of injury?
2. What are the location and severity of pressure ulcers that occur during System hospitalization for persons admitted to Model Systems within 24 hours of injury?
3. What are the risk factors associated with development of pressure ulcers during System hospitalization for persons admitted to Model Systems within 24 hours of injury?

Exhibit 6–1 Classification of Pressure Ulcers for Model Systems Data Collection

Grade	Ulcer Depth
0	None
1	Limited to the superficial epidermal and dermal layers; includes redness that does not blanch to the touch and redness that requires intervention
2	Involves the epidermal and dermal layers and extends into the adipose tissue
3	Extends through superficial structures and adipose tissue down into and including muscle
4	Involves destruction of all soft tissue structures and communication with bone or joint structures

4. How do the occurrence and severity of pressure ulcers that develop during System hospitalization affect functional status at discharge from System care?
5. What are the prevalence and severity of pressure ulcers 1 and 2 years after System discharge?
6. What are the location and severity of pressure ulcers that develop 1 and 2 years after discharge from System care?
7. What are the risk factors associated with having pressure ulcers during the first 4 years after System discharge?
8. Have the rate and severity of pressure ulcers developing during System hospitalization among persons admitted to Model Systems within 24 hours of injury decreased over time?

It is important to analyze separately patients admitted promptly to a System hospital and patients admitted with some delay. This distinction is important for two reasons. First, the quality of nursing care has a direct impact on skin integrity; System facilities have greater experience in caring for patients with traumatic SCI and thus are better able to minimize skin problems. DeVivo et al.[14] demonstrated that patients admitted within the first day of injury to a Model System facility have a significantly lower rate of pressure ulcer development by rehabilitation discharge. Second, patients who develop ulcers early after SCI may be at risk for developing new ulcers at healed sites. This effect magnifies the consequences of poor care received early after SCI.

Patients with records in the Model System Database were admitted an average of 24.9 days postinjury (median = 11.0 days) with a range from 0 to 365 days. For the purposes of the analyses reported here, a cutoff of 1 day was selected to define prompt admission to the Model System; 38.3% met this criterion of prompt admission. Patients who were promptly admitted had a significantly lower rate of ulcers at admission (1.6%) than did patients admitted with some delay (28.9%; χ^2 [df = 1, N = 14,704] = 1,731.9, P < 0.00001), and a lower rate of severe ulcers, i.e., grades 3 and 4 (0.1% vs. 5.1%, χ^2 [df = 4, N = 14,260] = 1,455.6, P < 0.00001). Prompt admissions also had a lower rate of ulcers from injury to System discharge (33.1% vs. 41.8%, χ^2 [df = 1, N = 14,682] = 110.2, P < 0.00001). A clear benefit of prompt admission to a Model System is reflected in the drastically lower rate of pressure ulcers not only at System admission but continuing through to discharge.

Pressure Ulcer Incidence during Model Systems Care

For patients admitted within 1 day since 1973, the overall proportion who developed at least one pressure ulcer during System care (excluding ulcers at admission) was 31.7%. The number of pressure ulcers per patient during System care ranged from 0 to 11 with a median of 1.0 for patients who developed ulcers. One ulcer was reported for 62.5%, two ulcers for 21.3%, and three ulcers for 10.3%. The severity of the most serious ulcer, for patients with one or more ulcers, was grade 1 for 46.0% of the sample, grade 2 for 38.3%, grade 3 for 11.9%, and grade 4 for 3.8%.

Location and Severity of Pressure Ulcers during System Care

Figure 6–1 shows the most common sites of ulcers that developed during System care for patients admitted within 1 day of injury since 1973. Of all 2935 ulcers, the sacrum was the site of 37.4%; other common sites were heels (15.9%) and ischium (9.2%). Figure 6–2 shows the distribution of severe ulcers (grades 3 and 4). These occurred most often at the same sites: sacrum (50.9%), heels (12.5%), and ischium (6.3%).

Risk Factors Associated with Pressure Ulcers during Model Systems Care

Logistic regression was used to predict risk of developing pressure ulcers during System stays for prompt admissions since 1973. Indicator variables were level and completeness of injury; age; etiology (coded as motor vehicle crash, acts of violence, sports, falls, and other); education (coded as less than eighth grade, ninth to eleventh grades, high school graduate, or greater than high school); race (coded as white or African-American); preinjury employment; and gender. The relatively small number of patients from other races led us to exclude them from this analysis. Forward stepwise variable selection was used, with removal testing based on the probability of the Wald statistic. The selected variables correctly classified 89.9% of patients who did not develop ulcers and 23.5% of those who did (model χ^2 [df = 5] = 332.0, $P < 0.00001$). Men had an increased risk of pressure ulcers (odds = 1.73, $P < 0.0001$), as did patients with complete spinal lesions (odds = 1.26, $P < 0.0001$). Decreased risk of pressure ulcers was associated with paraplegia (odds = 0.53, $P < 0.0001$) and being white (odds = 0.81, $P < 0.01$).

The importance of prompt admission to pressure ulcer development at admission or during System care was evaluated by adding this variable to the logistic regression analysis described above, but for all cases. The same indicator variables were used. The selected variables correctly classified 85.8% of patients who did not develop ulcers and 30.3% of those who did (model χ^2 [df = 13] = 884.0, $P < 0.00001$). Prompt admission was associated with decreased risk of

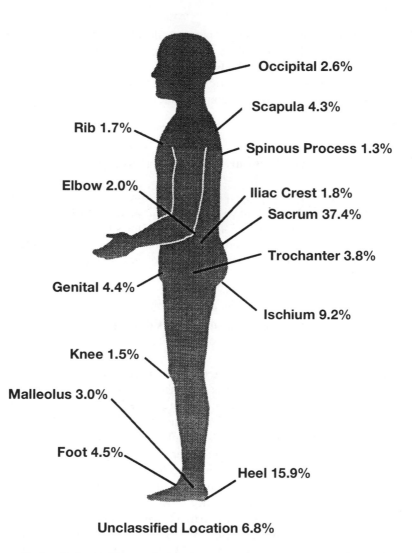

Occipital 2.6%

Scapula 4.3%

Rib 1.7%

Spinous Process 1.3%

Elbow 2.0%

Iliac Crest 1.8%

Sacrum 37.4%

Trochanter 3.8%

Genital 4.4%

Ischium 9.2%

Knee 1.5%

Malleolus 3.0%

Foot 4.5%

Heel 15.9%

Unclassified Location 6.8%

Note: Only patients admitted within 24 hours are included in this analysis.

Figure 6–1 Distribution of Pressure Ulcers That Developed during System Care

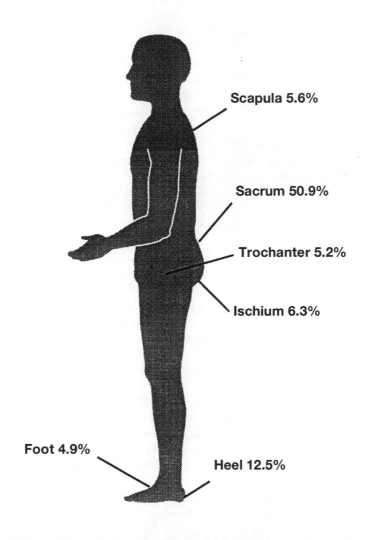

Note: Only patients admitted within 24 hours are included in this analysis.

Figure 6–2 Most Common Locations of Severe Ulcers (Grades 3 and 4) That Developed during System Care

pressure ulcers (odds = 0.72, $P < 0.00001$). As before, men had an increased risk of pressure ulcers (odds = 1.55, $P < 0.00001$), as did patients with complete lesions (odds = 1.23, $P < 0.00001$) and patients with less than an eighth-grade education (odds = 1.34, $P < 0.00001$), education between 9 and 11 years (odds = 1.29, $P < 0.001$), and high school education (odds = 1.16, $P < 0.05$) in contrast to the risk faced by persons with more than a high school education. Decreased risk of pressure ulcers was also associated with paraplegia (odds = 0.53, $P < 0.0001$); being white (odds = 0.90, $P < 0.05$); and injury resulting from falls (odds = 0.78, $P < 0.05$), sports (odds = 0.81, $P < 0.05$), and motor vehicle crashes (odds = 0.83, $P < 0.05$), in contrast to persons with other etiologies.

Functional Consequences of Pressure Ulcers

Analysis of covariance was used to evaluate the relationship between functional status at discharge from System rehabilitation and severity of pressure ulcers that developed during System admission for patients injured beginning in 1988, when Functional Independence Measure (FIM) scores were reported. Admission functional status and age were used as covariates, since earlier work has demonstrated the importance of these variables.[15]

The functional status measure used was the FIM. It was developed by the American Congress of Rehabilitation Medicine and the American Academy of Physical Medicine and Rehabilitation Task Force to Develop a National Uniform Data System for Medical Rehabilitation[16] to rate severity of patient disability and the outcomes of medical rehabilitation. The scaling characteristics of the FIM were described by Linacre et al.[17] and Heinemann et al.[18] Two measures derived from Rasch analysis of FIM items were used. The first measure assesses motor function and is based on the first 13 items that relate to self-care, sphincter management, mobility (transfers), and locomotion. The second measure assesses cognitive function and is based on the last five items that relate to communication and social cognition. Both measures demonstrate a sufficient range of item difficulty and good internal consistency.[17] The separate motor and cognitive measures function on an interval level with good clinical precision (i.e., reliability) and acceptable fit characteristics (i.e., validity). Each measure was scaled to range from 0 to 100.

Motor function at discharge from rehabilitation was related to severity of pressure ulcers when controlling statistically for motor function at admission and age at onset. Figure 6–3 shows that patients with more severe ulcer grades were discharged with lower levels of motor function. For example, patients with no pressure ulcers by System discharge had an average FIM motor measure of 57.7 (range 0 to 100), while patients with grade 2 ulcers had an average of 47.4. A

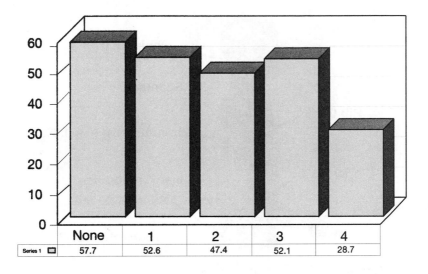

Series 1 ☐	None	1	2	3	4
	57.7	52.6	47.4	52.1	28.7

Figure 6–3 FIM Discharge Motor Measure across Score Severities

general downward trend in discharge motor function was observed with increasingly severe pressure ulcers (F[4,971] = 7.3, P < 0.001). This analysis also revealed that patients with lower admission motor function (F[1971] = 677.1, P < 0.001, r = 0.61) and those who were older (F[1971] = 22.3, P < 0.001, r = −0.14) were discharged with lower levels of motor function. These results suggest that pressure ulcers in combination with greater disability at admission and greater age are likely to reduce functional independence at discharge.

Pressure Ulcer Prevalence after Model Systems Discharge

Overall, the prevalence of pressure ulcers on visual inspection at the time of the first annual evaluation was 7.9% for patients admitted beginning in 1986. The number of pressure ulcers per patient at year 1 follow-up ranged from 0 to 10, with a mean of 1.6 for patients with ulcers. For patients with ulcers, one ulcer was reported for 64.3%, two ulcers for 24.9%, and three ulcers for 6.6%. At year 2 follow-up, the prevalence of pressure ulcers was 8.9%. The number of pressure ulcers per patient at System admission ranged from 0 to 20, with a mean of 1.6 ulcers per patient with ulcers. One ulcer was reported for 64.8%, two ulcers for 24.2%, and three ulcers for 4.7%.

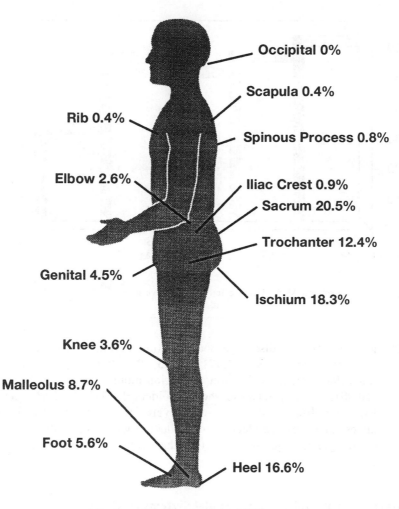

Occipital 0%

Scapula 0.4%

Rib 0.4%

Spinous Process 0.8%

Elbow 2.6%

Iliac Crest 0.9%

Sacrum 20.5%

Trochanter 12.4%

Genital 4.5%

Ischium 18.3%

Knee 3.6%

Malleolus 8.7%

Foot 5.6%

Heel 16.6%

Unclassified Location 4.7%

Note: All patients examined at year 1 are included
in this analysis.

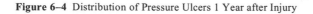

Figure 6–4 Distribution of Pressure Ulcers 1 Year after Injury

Location and Severity of Pressure Ulcers 1 and 2 Years after Discharge

Similar to what was found during System care, Figure 6–4 shows that the most common sites of ulcers at year 1 were the sacrum (20.5% of all ulcers at year 1), ischium (18.3%), heels (16.6%), and trochanters (12.4%). Figure 6–5 shows that the sites with the most severe ulcers were the sacrum (25.0% of grade 3 and grade 4 ulcers were at this site), trochanters (23.4%), ischium (22.7%), and heels (13.3%). The severity of the most serious ulcer, for patients with one or more ulcers, was grade 1 for 32.9% of the sample, grade 2 for 41.2%, grade 3 for 17.5%, and grade 4 for 8.3%.

Figure 6–6 shows at year 2 that the most common sites of ulcers were the ischium (24.3% of all ulcers at year 2), sacrum (20.3%), trochanters (12.5%), and heels (10.9%). Figure 6–7 shows that the sites with the most severe ulcers were the ischium (30.9% of grade 3 and grade 4 ulcers were at this site), trochanters (26.5%), and sacrum (17.6%). The severities of the most serious ulcers, for patients with one or more ulcers, were grade 1 for 29.5% of the sample, grade 2 for 40.1%, grade 3 for 18.5%, and grade 4 for 12.0%.

Risk Factors Associated with Development of Pressure Ulcers after Model Systems Discharge

Cox regression was used to evaluate the risk of pressure ulcer development from year 1 to year 4. The year after injury at which the first pressure ulcer developed was predicted, considering the year at which cases were lost to follow-up. Variables evaluated as risk factors were the occurrence of pressure ulcers during System stay, etiology of spinal cord injury, level and completeness of lesion; motor and cognitive function at discharge, age, race, education and employment status at time of injury, and gender. The entire set of variables did not predict pressure ulcer development (χ^2 [df = 16] = 20.7, P not significant), nor did any individual variable contribute to prediction of pressure ulcer risk.

Change in Pressure Ulcer Development across Time

The rate of pressure ulcer development during System care has remained constant across the 20-year history of Model Systems data collection for patients admitted within 24 hours. The rate across the entire 20 years is 31.9%, with a range from 30.0% in 1989–1992 to 34.7% in 1976–1979. Significant change in

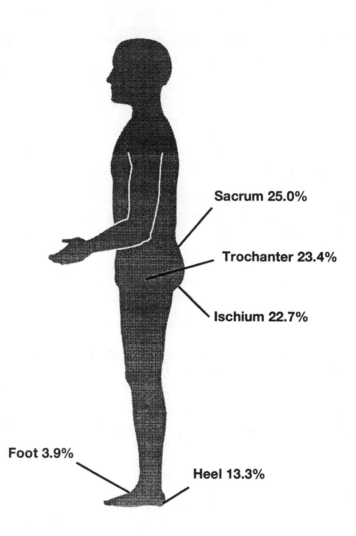

Sacrum 25.0%

Trochanter 23.4%

Ischium 22.7%

Foot 3.9%

Heel 13.3%

Note: All patients examined at year 1 are included in this analysis.

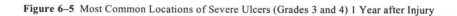

Figure 6–5 Most Common Locations of Severe Ulcers (Grades 3 and 4) 1 Year after Injury

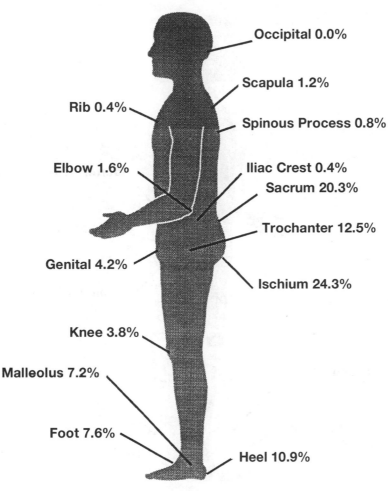

Occipital 0.0%

Scapula 1.2%

Rib 0.4%

Spinous Process 0.8%

Elbow 1.6%

Iliac Crest 0.4%

Sacrum 20.3%

Trochanter 12.5%

Genital 4.2%

Ischium 24.3%

Knee 3.8%

Malleolus 7.2%

Foot 7.6%

Heel 10.9%

Unclassified Location 4.8%

Note: All patients examined at year 2 are included in this analysis.

Figure 6–6 Distribution of Pressure Ulcers 2 Years after Injury

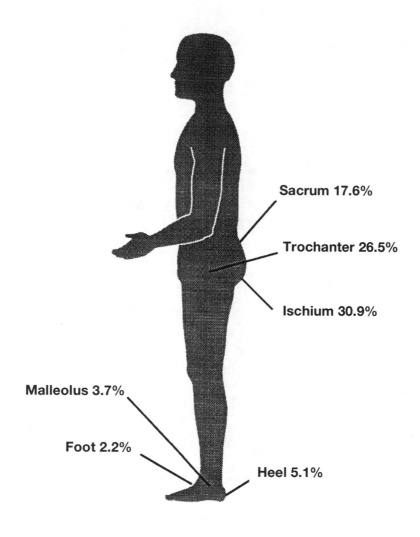

Note: All patients examined at year 2 are included in this analysis.

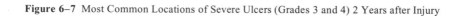

Figure 6–7 Most Common Locations of Severe Ulcers (Grades 3 and 4) 2 Years after Injury

the rate of severe ulcers (grades 3 and 4) did occur (χ^2 with Mantel-Haenszel test for linear association [$df = 1$, N = 5311] = 11.13, $P < 0.001$). While the rate of severe ulcers across 20 years was 4.4%, it was as high as 5.9% in 1986–1988 and as low as 3.0% in 1989–1992.

MEDICAL MANAGEMENT OF PRESSURE ULCERS

Model Systems data indicate the most common sites of pressure ulcer development and risk factors: the bony prominences in the sacrum, heels, and ischium. Persons who are older and those with complete lesions are also at greater risk, as well as persons with tetraplegia and African-Americans. While these risk factors are important to note, they are not modifiable. Medical management focuses on preventing the development of the conditions that lead to skin breakdown: prolonged pressure, shear, skin maceration, inadequate nutrition, and other risk factors.

The first step in the management of a pressure ulcer in persons with SCI is to remove the pressure. For persons with paraplegia this may involve their lying prone on a prone cart or turning from side to side to minimize pressure on their backs. For patients with tetraplegia who cannot tolerate lying prone, this often becomes more difficult, and occasionally special equipment is needed. Adequate nutrition is essential. Malnutrition can occur in hospitalized patients as well as in patients at home or in a nursing home.[19,20]

Debridement of the ulcer is essential to speed healing and determine the depth. Witkowski and Parish[21] have reviewed the numerous techniques to debride ulcers. These include surgical, mechanical, osmotic, chemical, enzymatic, and autolytic techniques, and the use of maggots. Necrotic tissue interferes with wound contraction and epithelialization and is a source of infection. It is our experience that surgical debridement is the quickest and most effective method. Debridement can often be done at the bedside or in the clinic. Wet to dry dressings will remove residual necrotic tissue or can be used to remove small amounts of necrotic tissue in wounds that do not require a scalpel. Once the wound is clean, wet to dry dressing should not be used because it will remove healthy epithelium.[22]

Wounds heal most efficiently in a moist environment. Occlusive dressings are one of the many ways to keep a wound moist. There is no evidence to suggest the use of one particular occlusive dressing out of the many available. Occlusive dressings decrease the need for frequent dressing changes and reduce the risk for infection.[23–26] Occlusive dressings should not be applied to grossly infected wounds. Use of occlusive dressings is not without difficulties.[27] Early removal of an occlusive dressing can cause epithelial damage and bleeding. Occasionally, granulating wounds that are covered with an occlusive dressing do not epithelialize; it should be removed and a different, nonadherent dressing applied. The dressing should not be placed over wounds that are surrounded by a dermatitis. There may be a minimal cost benefit to the use of occlusive dressings,[28] and occlusive dressings may not be more effective than gauze in lesions exposing muscles.[29]

Villian is credited with the saying, "you can put anything on the pressure ulcer except the patient"; however, this is not completely true.[30] One must be very careful about what is placed on a pressure ulcer. Povidone-iodine is a commonly used topical antiseptic. It can be absorbed systemically and can cause increased serum iodine levels,[31–34] which in turn can cause metabolic acidosis, hypernatremia, hyperosmolarity, renal failure, and hyper- and hypothyroidism. In addition, it is toxic to the wound and may stop the growth of fibroblasts. Hydrogen peroxide, sodium hypochlorite, and acetic acid also should not be used on ulcers, as they have similar toxicity. However, topical antibiotics such as bacitracin, silver sulfadiazine, and combinations of neomycin, bacitracin, and polymyxin B may enhance epidermal growth.[27,34,35] This enhancement of epidermal growth may not necessarily be explained by the antimicrobial activity, but it might occur as a result of the vehicle of the antibiotic or some other factors.[36] The clinical uses of topical antibiotics are not well established. It is our clinical experience that they are beneficial in superficial lesions involving the epidermis or dermis and when used in conjunction with a nonadherent gauze. They also are of value in areas where occlusive dressings cannot be applied, such as close to the rectum.

Growth factors are being studied to treat pressure sores and other skin lesions. Growth factors are proteins that are naturally occurring and are secreted from platelets and macrophages. They may direct the migration of cells into wounds and regulate repair processes.[37,38] Several growth factors have been described. Platelet-derived growth factor has been studied most extensively.[39–41] It is chemotactic for smooth muscle cells, neutrophils, and mononuclear cells. It encourages the synthesis of a matrix for wound healing and affects the differentiation of fibroblasts. It is available from recombinant DNA and as an autologous extract from the person's own blood.[42–44] The clinical utility of this growth factor has not as yet been determined, although it may play an important role in the future.

Pressure ulcers are often viewed incorrectly as a local problem occurring about the sacrum, ischium, or trochanters. There are numerous systemic complications of pressure ulcers that can be fatal. Pressure ulcers can lead to local infections such as cellulitis or local abscesses that extend to the bone and cause osteomyelitis.[45,46] Lewis and associates[47] demonstrated that a positive plain X-ray or a white cell count of 15,000/mm^3 or an erythrocyte sedimentation rate of 120 mm/h is good presumptive evidence of osteomyelitis. Biopsy is still the only way to determine a definitive diagnosis.[48–50] Nuclear medicine scans are often positive because of local pressure ulcer changes and generally are not helpful in diagnosis. Soft tissue abscess and pelvic abscesses can occur secondary to pressure ulcers. Sometimes they are not recognized until the abscess drains into the ulcer, although computed tomography can identify these abscesses.[45,46]

Bacteremia is a potentially fatal complication of pressure ulcers. Mortality rates tend to be quite high.[51] In patients with sepsis, pressure ulcers require debridement of the ulcers in addition to antibiotic treatment.[52]

A rare but potentially fatal complication of pressure ulcers is Marjolin's ulcer, a malignant degeneration of a pressure ulcer.[53] It generally occurs as a late complication of pressure ulcers that exist for more than 20 years. It is important to inform affected persons of these complications as part of their educational programs.

SURGICAL REPAIR OF PRESSURE ULCERS

When medical management fails, surgical repair is necessary. Large lesions are often surgically repaired, as the scar resulting from normal healing is prone to pressure ulcers. The ulcer must be excised, as well as the underlying bursae and the bony prominence. The most commonly used surgical procedure is a myocutaneous flap. A potential problem with myocutaneous flaps[54,55] is muscle atrophy. The need for surgical closure of pressure ulcers increases during follow-up years. For those patients with an annual evaluation performed after October 1, 1986, 3.3% of patients examined needed surgical closure during the first 5 years after discharge. From years 6 to 10, 6.5% of patients required surgical closure; and in years 11 through 18, 5.75% required surgical closure. Because variations in the number of patients reporting for follow-up, these data must be interpreted with caution.

PREVENTION

The best treatment for pressure ulcers is prevention. Of course, this is not possible for pressure ulcers that develop prior to the patient's arrival at the acute care hospital.[56] Prompt admission to a specialized spinal injury unit decreases the risk of pressure ulcers. During the acute care phase, proper bed positioning and frequent turning are essential. Generally this is done on an every-2-hour schedule.[57] Skin should be checked between turns and the frequency of turns increased if hyperemia persists for more than 30 minutes. This procedure changes when a person begins rehabilitation. If possible, the patient should be taught to lie prone, because this position decreases the risk of pressure sores.[58] Generally the turning schedule is from side to back to side at regular intervals. These intervals are slowly increased, but only if skin is checked carefully. Protective devices are available that totally prevent the heel from touching the bed.[59] As a person is mobilized and begins sitting, it is essential that this be done in a careful and consistent manner. Sitting is limited initially to 0.5 to 1 hour and increased only if the hyperemia resolves in 30 minutes.

Many individuals can increase their sitting periods quickly, but for others it progresses slowly. These tolerances can change. For example, a person who is hospitalized, becomes ill, suffers from malnutrition, or has had trauma to the ulcerated area will likely develop decreased tolerance. After a pressure ulcer heals, it is important to rebuild the patient's sitting tolerance slowly.

Wheelchair cushions help decrease pressure when sitting, and they increase comfort. However, they do not decrease pressure below capillary pressure and are not a cure. Numerous beds are available to prevent and treat pressure ulcers. Care should be given in selecting a bed that is similar to one that will be used at home. It is not realistic to discharge someone home from a specialized bed and expect him or her to have the same tolerance on a regular mattress.

Technology alone will not eliminate pressure ulcers. Cooperation of the patient and the caregiver and their ability to assess problems as they occur and to react to prevent further skin damage are critical. They should be taught to avoid simple technologies such as doughnut-shaped rings that decrease blood flow and increase ulcer risk.[60] Research at Model System members is evaluating prevention methods. One method, electrical stimulation, is being studied in Ann Arbor, Michigan. It may have two main effects: increased local blood flow and changes in the contour of the muscles of the buttocks.[60,61] Further work is needed to determine the benefits of this technology.

Model System investigators have studied prevention and treatment of pressure ulcers.[62] Early studies on occlusive dressings were conducted at a Model System facility.[63] Garber and associates at the Model System in Texas have studied wheelchair cushions, beds, and other pressure-relief methods and their relationship to body build.[64,65] Also in Texas, Rodriguez et al.[66] are studying collagen metabolite excretion as a predictor of skin and bone-related complications. Nursing manuals and patient education guidebooks have been published and disseminated to help prevent and treat pressure ulcers.[56,67] These efforts are needed in order to reduce further the incidence of a preventable complication.

REFERENCES

1. Gibbon JH, Freeman LW. The primary closure of decubitus ulcers. *Ann Surg.* 1940;124:1148–1164.

2. Munro D: Care of the back following spinal cord injuries: A consideration of bed sores. *N Engl J Med.* 1940;223:391–398.

3. Guttmann L. The problem of treatment of pressure sores in spinal cord paraplegics. *Brit J Plast Surg.* 1955;8:196–211.

4. Young JS, Burns PE. Pressure sores in the spinal cord injured. *Model Systems Dig.* 1981;3:9–18.

5. Young JS, Burns PE. Pressure sores in the spinal cord injured: Part II. *Model Systems Dig.* 1981;3:19–26.

6. Kosiak M. Etiology of decubitus ulcers. *Arch Phys Med Rehabil.* 1961;42:19–29.

7. Lamid S, El Ghatit AZ. Smoking, spasticity and pressure in spinal cord injured patients. *Am J Phys Med.* 1983;62:300–306.

8. Rochin P, Beaudet MP, McGinchley-Berroth R, et al. Risk assessment for pressure ulcers: An adaptation of the national pressure ulcer advisory panel: Risk factors to spinal cord injured patients. *J Am Paraplegia Soc.* 1993;16:169–177.

9. Reichel SM. Shearing force as a factor in decubitus ulcer in paraplegics. *JAMA.* 1958;166:762–763.

10. Bennett L, Kavner D, Lee BY, Trainer FA. Shear vs pressure as causative factors in skin blood flow occlusion. *Arch Phys Med Rehabil.* 1979;60:309–314.

11. Anderson TP, Andberg MM. Psychosocial factors associated with pressure sores. *Arch Phys Med Rehabil.* 1979;60:341–346.

12. Gordon WA, Harasymiw S, Bellile S, Lehman L, Sherman B. The relationship between pressure sores and psychosocial adjustment in persons with spinal cord injury. *Rehabil Psychol.* 1982;27:185–191.

13. Enis JE, Sarmiento A. The pathophysiology and management of pressure sores. *Orthop Rev.* 1973;2:25–34.

14. DeVivo MJ, Kartus PL, Stover SL, Fine PR. Benefits of early admission to an organized spinal cord injury care system. *Paraplegia.* 1990;28:545–555.

15. Heinemann AW, Linacre JW, Wright BD, Hamilton BB, Granger C. Prediction of rehabilitation outcomes with disability measures. *Arch Phys Med Rehabil.* 1994;75:133–143.

16. Hamilton BB, Granger CV, Sherwin FS, Zielezny M, Tashman JS. A uniform national data system for medical rehabilitation. In: Fuhrer MJ, ed. *Rehabilitation Outcomes: Analysis and Measurement.* Baltimore: Paul H. Brookes Publishing Co; 1987.

17. Linacre JW, Heinemann AW, Wright BD, Granger C, Hamilton BB. The structure and stability of the functional independence measure. *Arch Phys Med Rehabil.* 1994;75:127–132.

18. Heinemann AW, Linacre JW, Wright BD, Hamilton BB, Granger C. Relationships between impairment and disability as measured by the functional independence measure. *Arch Phys Med Rehabil.* 1993;74:566–573.

19. Bristian BR, Blackburn GL, Vitale J, Cochran D, Naylor J. Prevalance of malnutrition in general medical patients. *JAMA.* 1976;235:1567–1570.

20. Bruslow RA, Hallfrish J, Goldberg AP. Malnutrition in tube fed nursing home patients with pressure sores. *J Parenter and Enteral Nutr.* 1991;15:663–668.

21. Witkowski JA, Parish LC. Debridement of cutaneous ulcers: Medical and surgical aspects. *Clin Dermatol.* 1992;9:585–591.

22. Alvarez OM, Mertz PM, Eaglstein WH. Effect of occlusive dressings on collagen synthesis and re-epithelialization in superficial wounds. *J Surg Res.* 1983;35:142–148.

23. Varghese ML, Balin AK, Carter M, Caldwell D. Local environment of chronic wounds under synthetic dressings. *Arch Dermatol.* 1986;122:52–57.

24. Katz S, McGinley K, Leyden JT. Semipermeable occlusive dressing. *Arch Dermatol.* 1986;40:58–62.

25. Mertz PM, Marshall D, Eaglstein WH. Occlusive wound dressings to prevent bacterial invasion and wound infection. *J Am Acad Dermatol.* 1985;12:662–668.

26. Hutchinson JT, McGuckin M. Occlusive dressings: A microbiologic and clinical review. *Am J Infect Control.* 1990;18:257–268.

27. Falanga V. Occlusive wound dressings: Why when which? *Arch Dermatol.* 1988;124: 872–877.

28. Xakellis GC, Chrischilles EA. Hydrocolloid vs. saline-gauze dressings in treating pressure ulcers: A cost-effectiveness analysis. *Arch Phys Med Rehabil.* 1992;73:463–469.

29. Seburn MD. Pressure ulcer management in home health care:Efficacy and cost effectiveness of moisture vapor permeable dressing. *Arch Phys Med Rehabil.* 1986;67:726–729.

30. Constantian MB. *Pressure Ulcers: Principles and Techniques of Management.* Boston: Little, Brown & Co; 1987.

31. Dela Cruz F, Brown DH, Leikin JB, Franklin C, Hrehorczuli DO. Iodine absorption after topical administration. *West J Med.* 1987;146:43–45.

32. Shetty KR, Duthie EH Jr. Thyrotoxicosis induced by topical iodine application. *Arch Intern Med.* 1990;150:2400–2401.

33. Aronott GR, Friedman SJ, Doedeus DJ, Lavelle KJ. Increased serum iodide concentration from iodine absorption through wounds treated topically with povidone-iodine. *Am J Med Sci.* 1980;279:173–176.

34. Lineaweaver W, Howard R, Soucy D, et al. Topical antimicrobial toxicity. *Arch Surg.* 1985;120:267–270.

35. Baxter CR, Rodeheaver GT. Interventions: Hemostasis, cleansing, topical antibiotics, debridement and closure. In: Eaglstein WH, ed. *New Directions in Wound Healing.* Princeton, NJ: ER Squibb & Sons; 1990:71–82.

36. Geronemus RG, Mertz PM, Eaglstein WH. Wound healing: The effects of topical antimicrobial agents. *Arch Dermatol.* 1979;115:1311–1314.

37. Rudolph R, Shannon ML. The normal healing process. In: Eaglstein WH, ed. *New Directions in Wound Healing.* Princeton, NJ: : ER Squibb & Sons; 1990.

38. Hotta SS, Holohan TV. *Procuren: A Platelet-Derived Wound Healing Formula.* Health Technology Rev #2. Agency for Health Care Policy and Research, Department of Health and Human Services; August 1992. AHCOR Pub No. 92-0065.

39. Pierce GF, Vande Berg T, Rudolph R, Torpley T, Mustoe TA. Platelet-derived growth factor and transforming growth factor beta selectively modulate glycosaminoglycans, collagen and myofibroblasts in excisional wounds. *Am J Pathol.* 1991;138:629–646.

40. Antoniades HN, Scher CD, Stiles CD. Purification of human platelet-derived growth factor. *Proc Natl Acad Sci USA.* 1979;76:1809–1813.

41. Robson MC, Phillips LG, Thomason A, Robson LE, Pierce GF. Platelet-derived growth factor BB for the treatment of chronic pressure ulcers. *Lancet.* 1992;339:23–25.

42. Knighton DR, Ciresi K, Fiegel VD, et al. Classification and treatment of chronic nonhealing wounds: Successful treatment with autologous platelet-derived wound healing factors (PDWHF). *Ann Surg.* 1986;204:322–330.

43. Knighton DR, Ciresi K, Fiegel VD, et al. Stimulation of repair in chronic, nonhealing, cutaneous ulcers using platelet-derived wound healing formula. *Surg Gynecol Obstet.* 1990;170: 56–60.

44. Atri SC, Misra J, Bisht D, Misra K. Use of homologous platelet factors in achieving total healing of recalcitrant skin ulcers. *Surgery.* 1990;108:508–512.

45. Firooznia H, Rafii M, Golimbu C, Lom S, Sokolow J, Kung JS. Computerized tomography of pressure sores, pelvic abscess, and osteomyelitis in patients with spinal cord injury. *Arch Phys Med Rehabil.* 1982;63:545–548.

46. Firooznia H, Rafii M, Golimbu C, Sokolow J. Computerized tomography in diagnosis of pelvic abscess in spinal-cord-injured patients. *Comput Radiol.* 1983;7:335–341.

47. Lewis VL Jr, Bailey MH, Pulawski G, Kied G, Bashicum MD, Hendrix R. The diagnosis of osteomyelitis in patients with pressure sores. *Plast Reconstr Surg.* 1988;81:229–232.

48. Sugarman B. Pressure sores and underlying bone infection. *Arch Intern Med.* 1987;147: 553–555.

49. Thornhill-Joynes M, Gonzales F, Stewart CA, et al. Osteomyelitis associated with pressure ulcers. *Arch Phys Med Rehabil.* 1986;67:314–318.

50. Sugarman B. Osteomyelitis in spinal cord injury. *Arch Phys Med Rehabil.* 1984;65:132–134.

51. Bryan CS, Dew CE, Reynolds KL. Bacteremia associated with decubitus ulcers. *Arch Intern Med.* 1983;143:2093–2095.

52. Galpin JE, Chow AW, Bayer AS, Guze LB. Sepsis associated with decubitus ulcers. *Am J Med.* 1976;61:346–350.

53. Berkwits L, Yarkony GM, Lewis V. Marjolin's ulcer complicating a pressure ulcer: Case report and literature review. *Arch Phys Med Rehabil.* 1986;67:831–833.

54. Nola GT, Vistnes LM. Differential response of skin and muscle in the experimental production of pressure sores. *Plast Reconstr Surg.* 1980;66:728–733.

55. Daniel RK, Faibusoff B. Muscle coverage of pressure points: The role of myocutaneous flaps. *Ann Plast Surg.* 1982;8:446–452.

56. Mawson AR, Biundo PR Jr, Neville P, Linares HA, Winchester Y, Lopez A. Risk factors for early occurring pressure ulcers following spinal cord injury. *Am J Phys Med Rehabil.* 1988;67: 123–127.

57. Matthews PJ, Carlson CE. *Spinal Cord Injury: A Guide to Rehabilitation Nursing.* Gaithersburg, Md: Aspen Publishers, Inc; 1987.

58. Lindan O, Greenway RM, Piozza JM. Pressure distribution on the surface of the human body, I. Evaluation in lying and sitting positions using a "bed of springs and nails." *Arch Phys Med Rehabil.* 1965;46:378–385.

59. Pinzur MS, Schumacher D, Reddy N, Osterman H, Havey R, Patuardin A. Preventing heel ulcers: A comparison of prophylactic body-support systems. *Arch Phys Med Rehabil.* 1991;72:508–510.

60. Allman RM. Pressure ulcers among the elderly. *N Engl J Med.* 1989;320:850–853.

61. Levine SP, Kett RL, Gross MD, Wilson BA, Cederna PS, Juni JE. Blood flow in the gluteus maximus of seated individuals during electrical muscle stimulation. *Arch Phys Med Rehabil.* 1990;71:682–686.

62. Levine SP, Kett RL, Cederna PS, Brooks SV. Electrical muscle stimulation for pressure sore prevention: Tissue shape variation. *Arch Phys Med Rehabil.* 1990;71:210–215.

63. Yarkony GM, Kramer E, King R, Lukanc C, Carle TV. Pressure sore management: Efficacy of a moisture reactive occlusive dressing. *Arch Phys Med Rehabil.* 1984;65:597–600.

64. Garber SL, Krouskop TA. Body build and its relationship to pressure distribution in the seated wheelchair patient. *Arch Phys Med Rehabil.* 1982;63:17–20.

65. Garber SL, Campion LJ, Krouskop TA. Trochanteric pressure in spinal cord injury. *Arch Phys Med Rehabil.* 1982;63:549–552.

66. Rodriguez GP, Claus-Walker J, Kent MC, Garza HM. Collagen metabolite excretion as predictor of bone and skin related complications in spinal cord injury. *Arch Phys Med Rehabil.* 1989;74:442–444.

67. Rehabilitation Institute of Chicago, Division of Nursing. *Rehabilitation Nursing Procedures Manual.* Gaithersburg, Md: Aspen Publishers, Inc; 1990:179–203.

7

Management of Gastrointestinal, Genitourinary, and Sexual Function

Diana D. Cardenas, Lisa Farrell-Roberts,
Marca L. Sipski, and Deborah Rubner

GASTROINTESTINAL MANAGEMENT

Introduction

Acute and chronic gastrointestinal (GI) problems are less common and less dramatic after spinal cord injury than the profound sensory and motor deficits frequently experienced. There has been a limited number of investigations into the GI system and changes in the GI tract after SCI. This is likely due to the subtlety of such impairments. Acute ileus is common immediately after SCI, while chronic constipation is a frequent problem in the postacute stages. The following section focuses on early GI complications, late GI complications, the Functional Independence Measure (FIM), and GI management outcomes after SCI.

Early Complications

Gastrointestinal Hemorrhage

Gastrointestinal hemorrhage is a problem experienced by varying numbers of SCI survivors. Data compiled by the NSCISC indicate the incidence of GI hemorrhage during the initial hospitalization after SCI to be very low. In individuals who were treated within the system from day 1 of their injury, 50 (3.2%) of 1566 suffered GI hermorrhage during initial hospitalization. These data did not include infomation on the time from injury that the GI hemorrhage occurred; thus, cases may include early (less than 1 month) as well as late (more than 1 month) hemorrhage. Of these injuries, both complete and incomplete, 1.2% had paraplegia and 2.0% had tetraplegia. These findings are consistent with past investigations, which have indicated an increased incidence of GI hemorrhage with increased level of injury as well as the completeness of the SCI.[1]

Soderstrom and Ducker[1] identified 9 patients out of 408 (2.2%) with SCI who developed peptic ulcerations: six gastric and three duodenal lesions. Albert et al.[2] identified GI hemorrhage in 6.2% (n = 950) of SCI patients over a 10-year period. This retrospective study postulated that the low occurrence was secondary to global use of ulcer prophylactics and heightened awareness of ulcer prevention at the treatment center. Other acute GI complications, although infrequent, reported to be experienced in the first month post-SCI include ileus, gastric dilatation, superior mesenteric artery syndrome, and pancreatitis.[3] Another factor that has been considered in the occurrence of GI hemorrhage after SCI is the use of steroids.[4] Soderstrom and Ducker,[1] however, did not find this to be a contributing factor in the occurrence of GI hemorrhage in patients with cervical cord lesions. All patients under their protocol did, however, receive standard antacid therapy.

Late Complications

Gastrointestinal problems that occur more than 1 month post-SCI are considered late complications. Data regarding late complications per se have not been collected by the NSCISC; thus the following information is a review of the literature. Paralytic ileus is common immediately after SCI and typically resolves over several days. In very rare cases paralytic ileus has a late onset after SCI. Watson[5] reported two case studies of paralytic ileus at 5 weeks and 6 weeks post-SCI. Both cases were difficult to treat, and the cause was considered to be sympathetic overactivity accompanied by severe vasomotor disturbances. The precipitating factor in triggering the autonomic imbalance was not determined.

A second complication that is increased after SCI is gallstone disease. The most frequent cause of emergency abdominal surgery in people with SCI is cholecystitis or cholelithiasis.[6] Apstein and Dalecki-Chipperfield[7] reported the results of an autopsy study that indicated that gallstones were three times as likely to occur in individuals with SCI than in the control group. They postulated that the causes may be abnormal gallbladder motility, abnormal enterohepatic circulation, and altered intestinal motility leading to abnormal biliary secretion.

Esophageal problems post-SCI appear to be more frequent than commonly recognized. Stinneford et al.[8] investigated the frequency and severity of esophagitis and esophageal dysfunction in males at least 1 year postinjury. Spinal cord injury levels ranged from C5 to T10. In comparison with a control group, persons with SCI reported a higher number of GI complaints. The most common complaints were of heartburn, dysphagia, esophageal chest pain, and abdominal pain. Forty-five percent of SCI subjects showed evidence of mild esophagitis, and 91% showed histologic evidence of esophagitis. The exact mechanism for the increase in this symptomatology post-SCI is unclear; however, the occurrence indicates a greater need for attention to diagnosis and treatment of esophagitis post-SCI.

The most frequent late GI complication reported and investigated after SCI is altered bowel elimination.[9-13] Difficulties contributing to problems with elimination may be due to a variety of mechanisms, including altered colonic compliance, impaired transit time, chronic constipation, incontinence, and poor dietary management.

An investigation by Stone et al.[13] identified through interviews of 127 SCI persons that 27% had significant chronic gastrointestinal problems. Gastrointestinal problems reported were localized abdominal pain (14%), difficulty with bowel evacuation (20%), hemorrhoids (74%), abdominal distention (43%), and autonomic dysreflexia arising from the GI tract (43%). In this investigation, the presence of GI symptoms was related to increased time since injury and completeness of injury.

Gastrointestinal hemorrhage after SCI may provide an increased challenge in diagnosis. Multiple signs may be present, but may also mimic other acute medical crises. Neumayer et al.[6] reported the findings of 22 patients with SCI reviewed for correct diagnosis associated with acute abdomen. Presenting signs and symptoms were abdominal pain, bloating, shoulder pain, autonomic dysreflexia, abdominal tenderness, abdominal distention, and rigidity/spasticity.

Gastric dilatation has been evidenced in persons with SCI in both acute and chronic phases. Initially, gastric dilatation may or may not be accompanied by ileus.[3] Extreme cases in which fatality results may be caused by vagally mediated respiratory arrest, aspiration pneumonia, or gastric rupture. Although the exact mechanism is unclear, there is believed to be an imbalance between sympathetic and parasympathetic innervation to the bowel.

Superior mesenteric artery (SMA) syndrome is a condition in which the duodenum is compressed by the SMA. Symptoms include emesis of green material, distention, and abdominal discomfort. Accurate diagnosis is made by completion of a GI series showing an abrupt cessation of barium in the third part of the duodenum. Persons with SCI that appear more susceptible to SMA syndrome are those in body casts, those with severe weight loss, and those with spinal deformity. Treatment is typically effective with the use of a lumbrosacral corset that pushes the abdomen upward, remaining in a position with the head elevated after meals, and replacement of weight lost. Surgical intervention is rarely necessary.[3]

Functional Independence Measure

The Functional Independence Measure (FIM) was developed by multi-disciplinary researchers across the nation to provide a consistent measurement system for patient-related activities and functions. The FIM was incorporated into the National Database in 1988. According to the FIM for sphincter control, bowel management includes complete intentional control for bowel movements and use of equipment or agents necessary for bowel control. At discharge from the Model Systems, 20.4% (n = 1758) of individuals with complete or incomplete injury demonstrated complete independence with bowel management and 30.4%, modified independence. Total assistance with bowel management was required by 24.4% (Figure 7–1). These data represent only those patients discharged from 1988 through 1992. As expected, the higher-level injuries required total assistance. Seventy-eight percent of individuals with complete tetraplegia required total assistance. Of individuals with complete paraplegia, the majority (53.3%) managed their bowel care with modified independence, while 11.8% required total assistance. It is anticipated that the number of individuals with paraplegia requiring total assistance with bowel management will decrease at the 1-year follow-up, but since FIM scores are not available at follow-up, this cannot be verified.

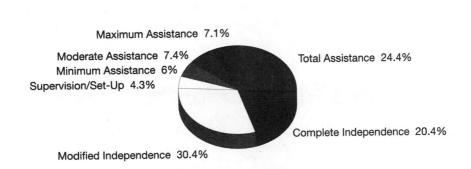

Maximum Assistance 7.1%

Moderate Assistance 7.4%
Minimum Assistance 6%
Supervision/Set-Up 4.3%

Total Assistance 24.4%

Complete Independence 20.4%

Modified Independence 30.4%

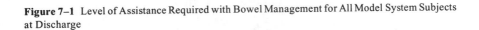

Figure 7–1 Level of Assistance Required with Bowel Management for All Model System Subjects at Discharge

Data from 1988 to 1992 indicate that a greater level of independence, as shown by a higher FIM score, correlates with greater neurologic preservation. Those with higher-level tetraplegia require more assistance with bowel management than those with tetraplegia at a lower level or those with paraplegia. More specifically, in looking at the percentage of individuals with complete or incomplete tetraplegia who require total assistance with bowel management, 42.3% had C1 to C4 injuries (Table 7–1). There were slightly more individuals with complete injuries requiring total assistance than those with incomplete injuries.

The FIM score for mobility in relation to toileting functionally defines the individual's ability to get on and off the toilet. At discharge, 27.3% of 1852 individuals with SCI demonstrated complete independence and 23.0% demonstrated modified independence in transfers to and from a toilet. Total assistance was required by 19.9% (Figure 7–2). These data represent only those individuals discharged from 1988 through 1992.

Another significant variable assessed was the individual's place of residence. Traditionally, individuals with heavy care needs that cannot be provided at home live in alternative sites such as group homes and skilled nursing facilities. At the time of discharge from a Model System, the majority (92.9%) of all individuals were discharged to a private residence (Table 7–2). Among persons requiring total assistance, 87.7% were discharged to a private residence and 8.9% went to a nursing home. Specifically, looking at persons discharged to a private residence, 28.2% required total or maximal assistance with bowel elimination and 54.5% evidenced either modified or complete independence. In contrast, of the persons discharged to a nursing home, 65.7% required total or maximal assistance while 21.5% demonstrated either modified or complete independence. The data indicate two trends: (1) the majority of individuals, regardless of assistance required with bowel management, are discharged to a private residence; (2) persons discharged to a nursing home require more assistance with bowel management.

Table 7–1 Percentage Distribution of Persons with Tetraplegia Who Require Total Assistance with Bowel Management by Level of Injury

Level of Injury	Neurologic Impairment (n = 345)		
	Incomplete	Complete	Total
C1–C4	19.1	23.2	42.3
C5	10.7	14.5	25.2
C6	9.0	10.7	19.7
C7	2.3	7.3	9.6
C8	2.6	0.6	3.2

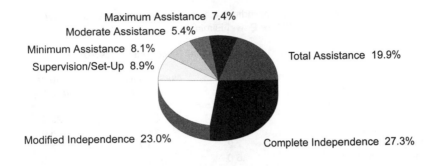

Maximum Assistance 7.4%
Moderate Assistance 5.4%
Minimum Assistance 8.1%
Supervision/Set-Up 8.9%

Total Assistance 19.9%

Modified Independence 23.0%

Complete Independence 27.3%

Figure 7–2 Level of Assistance Required for Toileting Mobility in All Model System Subjects

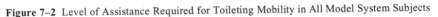

Management Outcomes

The acute management of GI problems after SCI has had little investigation. Again, this is most likely due to the low frequency of occurrence of such problems. It is, however, important to be aware of the signs and symptoms of GI problems in the SCI population and of effective treatment options. As with the general population, the population of persons with SCI also experiences an increased incidence of GI problems with aging.

Ileus after acute SCI usually lasts 2 to 5 days. In some individuals this time may be prolonged. Miller and Fenal[14] reported a single case involving acute tetraplegia with prolonged ileus that responded to metoclopramide. Other treatments during the acute stage that have been found to be effective for ileus include nasogastric decompression, injections of neostigmine methylsulfate and transabdominal neurostimulation.[3,15]

Gastrointestinal hemorrhage, as discussed previously, provides a challenge for accurate diagnosis. However, once an accurate diagnosis has been made, the treatment of GI hemorrhage is the same for all persons, including the SCI individual. Histamine H_2 blockade with drugs, such as cimetidine, is frequently prescribed. Research supports the use of nutritional support as prophylaxis against stress bleeding after SCI. Kuric et al.[16] found a significant reduction in bleeding stress ulcers when total parental nutrition was started if the patient was not tolerating an oral diet by day 5 after SCI. There is no literature indicating the incidence of esophageal ulceration per se after SCI.

Bowel elimination is achieved on a long-term basis through the implementation of a routine bowel program early in the acute phase to develop routine evacuation. Although such a bowel program is individualized, the basic program for an individual with an upper motor neuron lesion consists of insertion of a bisacodyl suppository after a meal at the same time daily or every other day,

Table 7–2   Place of Residence for Individuals at Discharge and the Associated
Percentage for FIM for Bowel Elimination

Functional Independence Level of Assistance	Place of Residence at Discharge		
	Private Residence (n = 1723)	Nursing Home (n = 70)	Other (n = 60)
Total Assistance	21.6	54.3	23.4
Maximal Assistance	6.6	11.4	5.0
Moderate Assistance	7.2	5.7	5.0
Minimal Assistance	6.0	2.9	8.3
Supervision Set-up	4.1	4.3	3.3
Modified Independence	30.5	8.6	41.7
Complete Independence	24.0	12.9	13.3

followed 20 minutes later by digital stimulation. If elimination is not successful, the same program is repeated the following day. However, some individuals do well with digital stimulation without the use of a suppository. Persons with lower motor neuron lesions evacuate by increasing intra-abdominal pressure through the Valsalva maneuver or, if unsuccessful, by manual removal. Suppositories are used if there is no success with manual removal, but they have a risk of creating incontinence with a flaccid sphincter.

The consistency of stool is controlled by food and fluid intake, the use of supplemental fibers such as psyllium hydrophilic mucilloid (Metamucil), stool softeners (docusate sodium, docusate calcium), and stimulant laxatives (senna). A problematic area for persons with SCI is the amount of time required for bowel elimination, which is reported to range from 5 minutes to 2 hours.[17]

Gastrointestinal problems post-SCI provide a challenge for both patients and practitioners. Impairments of the GI tract post-SCI typically are subtle. Clinical research is needed to investigate problematic areas further and determine effective treatment approaches, particularly in regard to management of bowel elimination.

BLADDER MANAGEMENT

Introduction

One of the most potentially deleterious effects of SCI is the loss of normal genitourinary function. Although renal failure is no longer the leading cause of death after SCI, urinary tract infection continues to pose a threat to the health and welfare of persons with SCI. The NSCISC has collected data regarding urinary tract infection, methods of bladder management, urologic complications and procedures, and functional outcomes that are discussed briefly in the following portions of this chapter. The sample is from individuals discharged from the Model Systems from 1986 through 1992 unless otherwise stated.

Urinary Tract Infection

The most frequent secondary medical complication reported by the Model Systems during acute care or rehabilitation is urinary tract infection (UTI), defined by the NSCISC as a colony count of (1) 1 to 100,000 colonies; or (2) over 100,000 colonies. Since the definition does not include symptoms, this might be referred to as bacteriuria. Data on UTI collected from 1986 through 1992 indicate the presence of UTI or bacteriuria in 80.4% (n = 4107) of individuals overall. This ranged from a low of 73.8% in persons with incomplete paraplegia to 87.4% in those with complete tetraplegia. The percentage of persons developing secondary medical complications during each postinjury year also indicated that UTI or bacteriuria remains the most common complication after discharge, ranging from 56.6% (n = 946) in the first postinjury year to 80.4% (n = 49) in year 16. However, because of the bias introduced by losses to follow-up, the occurrence of UTI or bacteriuria may be slightly overestimated.

Treatment of UTI is aimed at eradicating the infection and preventing complications. Thus, symptomatic UTI should be treated with the appropriate antibiotics for 7 to 14 days. It is not clear whether longer courses of treatment are beneficial except in cases complicated by abscess formation or prostatitis. There is no controversy regarding the need for treatment of symptomatic UTI; however, symptoms may differ from those expected. A person with SCI may not experience dysuria or urgency but may complain of increased spasticity or general malaise. Other signs and symptoms of UTI that may or may not be present include pyuria, discomfort or pain over the kidney or bladder, onset of urinary incontinence, fever, and autonomic dysreflexia. Treatment of asymptomatic bacteriuria has been somewhat controversial.[18-20] The difficulty lies in localizing asymptomatic infection to the upper or lower urinary tract.[21-23] Pyuria has been advocated by some to determine which asymptomatic bacteriuric individuals to treat, but pyuria is a poor indicator of tissue invasion in this group.[24] The general consensus is that asymptomatic bacteriuria need not be treated routinely with antibiotics in otherwise healthy persons with SCI; however, the presence of urease-producing organisms that are associated with stone formation may warrant antibiotic treatment.[25] There is little evidence to support the use of prophylactic antibiotics at the present time.

Methods of Bladder Management

The decline in reported cases of renal failure has been attributed in large part to the use of intermittent catheterization, which by the mid-1970s replaced the indwelling catheter as the major mode of bladder management. Better medical care, the continued development of antibiotics, and improvements in catheter materials may also be contributing factors. Data from the Model Systems indicate that 30.1% of persons were discharged on intermittent catheterization from 1973 through 1985.[26] Data since 1986 indicate that 51.5% (n = 3426) of all individuals are discharged on intermittent catheterization and only about 12.5% are discharged with an indwelling urethral catheter.

Indwelling catheterization continues to be used in the acute stage after SCI and in some, especially women, becomes the chronic method of management. Of the surgical approaches, external sphincterotomy, with or without bladder neck resection, was performed in 0.4% of all persons by discharge.

The four general categories of neurologic impairment, (1) paraplegia, incomplete; (2) paraplegia, complete; (3) tetraplegia, incomplete; and (4) tetraplegia, complete, are related to method of bladder management in Table 7–3. Intermittent catheterization was the most common method used at discharge from the Model Systems for all four categories. For those with incomplete paraplegia or incomplete tetraplegia, the next most common method was normal micturition, found in about one-third at discharge. For those with complete paraplegia or complete tetraplegia, the second most common method at discharge was the

Table 7–3 Method of Bladder Management at Discharge by Neurologic Impairment

Method of Management	Neurologic Impairment				
	Paraplegia, Incomplete (n = 731)	Paraplegia, Complete (n = 885)	Tetraplegia, Incomplete (n = 1019)	Tetraplegia, Complete (n = 593)	Total (n = 3228)
None	3.0	0.4	2.8	0.3	2.0
Indwelling Catheter	4.5	10.8	13.4	25.3	13.0
Catheter Free with External Collector	4.4	7.4	11.5	12.1	9.0
Catheter Free without External Collector	3.4	0.6	1.1	—	1.0
Normal Micturition	33.2	—	31.5	—	17.0
Intermittent Catheter	50.6	78.2	36.2	51.5	54.0
Conduit	—	0.1	—	—	<1.0
Suprapubic Cystostomy	0.7	1.6	3.1	9.7	3.0
Other	0.1	0.3	0.3	0.5	<1.0

indwelling urethral catheter, which was also the third most common method for incomplete paraplegia or incomplete tetraplegia. The third most common method for complete paraplegia or complete tetraplegia was catheter free with an external collector.

Trends in Bladder Management

Examining the method of bladder management over time, using 15 years of follow-up data from the Model Systems, the most predominate trend for men was a decline in the use of intermittent catheterization from 36.4% at discharge to 6.8% at 15 years (Table 7–4). There was a concomitant increase in the use of condom drainage from 22.2% at discharge to 35.6% at 15 years. There also appears to be an increase in suprapubic cystostomies over the follow-up years, but this apparent trend does not represent a large increase in people getting suprapubic cystostomies but instead an increasing share of the follow-up population (8.5% at discharge; 30.8% at 15 years) of a center that does more than 80% of all suprapubic cystostomies.

The use of intermittent catheterization declined in women also, from 38.6% at discharge to 18.5% at 15 years (Table 7–5). There was a concurrent increase in the use of indwelling urethral catheterization from 33.2% at discharge to 52.3% at 15 years. The apparent increase in suprapubic cystostomies is artificial for the same reasons as stated above for the men.

Table 7–4 Method of Bladder Management for Males at Discharge and at 1-, 5-, 10-, 15-Year Follow-Up

Method of Management	*Time of Data Collection*				
	Discharge (n = 12,083)	Year 1 (n = 8820)	Year 5 (n = 4000)	Year 10 (n = 1322)	Year 15 (n = 236)
None	0.6	1.2	2.1	2.2	4.7
Indwelling Catheter	12.0	8.8	7.2	9.6	8.1
Catheter Free with External Collector	22.2	31.4	41.1	40.5	35.6
Catheter Free without External Collector	3.4	3.8	3.5	2.2	2.5
Normal Micturition	16.3	19.0	12.5	10.1	7.6
Intermittent Catheter	36.4	24.2	12.8	6.1	6.8
Conduit	0.0	0.1	0.5	1.4	2.5
Suprapubic Cystostomy	8.5	10.8	19.9	26.8	30.8
Other	0.6	0.8	0.6	1.1	1.3

Table 7–5 Method of Bladder Management for Females at Discharge and at 1-, 5-, 10-, and 15-Year Follow-Up

Method of Management	Time of Data Collection				
	Discharge (n = 2612)	Year 1 (n = 1844)	Year 5 (n = 866)	Year 10 (n = 263)	Year 15 (n = 65)
None	2.1	2.6	4.3	3.8	3.1
Indwelling Catheter	33.2	31.8	40.5	46.4	52.3
Catheter Free with External Collector	0.1	0.0	0.0	0.0	0.0
Catheter Free without External Collector	4.8	5.2	5.7	4.9	3.1
Normal Micturition	19.4	23.6	18.0	12.2	6.2
Intermittent Catheter	38.6	33.7	23.9	20.5	18.5
Conduit	0.0	0.1	1.0	1.5	3.1
Suprapubic Cystostomy	1.8	2.8	6.0	8.7	12.3
Other	0.0	0.2	0.6	1.9	1.5

Method of Management Related to Place of Residence and Gender

Table 7–6 shows the distribution of the method of bladder management for complete or incomplete SCI for men and women who were discharged to a private residence or a nursing home from 1986 to 1992. When discharged to a private residence, both men and women are most likely to be using intermittent catheterization for their method of bladder management. When discharged to a nursing home, men are still more likely to be using intermittent catheterization, but the incidence of other methods, such as an indwelling catheter or suprapubic cystostomy, is greatly increased. This is probably related to a greater degree of disability and the inability to perform independent intermittent catheterization, since 78% of men discharged to nursing homes had tetraplegia. In contrast, women discharged to a nursing home are more likely to be using an indwelling catheter than intermittent catheterization for their method of bladder management, but only 55% of women discharged to a nursing home had tetraplegia. Data from the NSCISC indicate that 62% of women with paraplegia who are discharged to a nursing home are managing their bladders using an indwelling catheter compared to 23% of men with paraplegia. The percentages of men and women with tetraplegia discharged to a nursing home using an indwelling catheter are approximately the same, 21% and 25%, respectively.

Differences among the Model Centers

The differences in choice of mode of bladder management at discharge among the Model Systems are most striking for two methods (i.e., suprapubic cystostomy

Table 7-6 Percentage Distribution for the Method of Bladder Management for Males and Females Discharged to a Private Residence or Nursing Home

Method of Management	Private Residence		Nursing Home	
	Male (n = 2382)	Female (n = 526)	Male (n = 99)	Female (n = 29)
None	1.3	3.4	1.0	6.9
Indwelling Catheter	7.8	20.5	21.2	41.4
Catheter Free with External Collector	10.7	—	16.2	—
Catheter Free without External Collector	1.2	1.9	—	—
Normal Micturition	18.4	18.3	11.1	13.8
Intermittent Catheter	57.0	53.8	38.4	31.0
Suprapubic Cystostomy	3.2	2.1	10.1	6.9
Other	0.3	—	2.0	—

and indwelling urethral catheterization). First, suprapubic cystostomy is seldom used as a method of management. Data since 1986 indicate that only 3.2% (n = 3426) of all individuals used this method at discharge; however, 63.1% of all cases came from a single Model System. On the other hand, 7 of 17 Systems did not report any cases of suprapubic cystostomy at initial discharge. Second, 63.3% (n = 427) of all cases with indwelling urethral catheterization were from three Systems, but all Systems used this method to some degree, which accounted for 12.5% of all cases. Use of intermittent catheterization was fairly evenly distributed across all Systems, ranging from 18% to 78%, and accounted for 51.1% of all cases. If subject mix is considered when interpreting these data, the three Systems that frequently used indwelling urethral catheterization had 32.9% (n = 593) of all persons with complete tetraplegia, who would be less likely to perform self-catheterization. Two of these three Systems used intermittent catheterization less than 20% of the time for persons with complete tetraplegia, while other Systems averaged 53% intermittent catheterization use at discharge for individuals with complete tetraplegia.

The use of a particular method also varied according to neurologic impairment, as one would expect (Table 7–3). However, differences were found among the different Systems for the same neurologic category. For example, in individuals with complete tetraplegia (n = 593), intermittent catheterization was used in 51.5% and indwelling urethral catheterization in 25.3%. In those Systems that seldom used either of these two methods in complete tetraplegia, one System used suprapubic cystostomy in 73.2% and two Systems used an external collector in 65.2% and 68.8% of all their persons with complete tetraplegia.

Indwelling urethral catheterization was used at discharge in 10.8% of all individuals with complete paraplegia (n = 885). Approximately half (51%) of these 96 were from one System. This System also used indwelling urethral catheterization in 59% of all its individuals with complete paraplegia (n = 90). All other Systems used intermittent catheterization in the majority (61.5% to 100%) of individuals with complete paraplegia.

Almost half (48.5%) of all cases of persons with incomplete paraplegia using indwelling urethral catheterization at discharge (n = 33) were from one System, which used indwelling urethral catheterization 27.1% of the time, as often as it did intermittent catheterization for this group. The remaining Systems used intermittent catheterization anywhere from 30.8% to 78.8% in persons with incomplete paraplegia.

These differences point out the lack of uniformly applied methods of bladder management. The majority of Systems, however, appear to limit the use of indwelling catheters. Institutional and professional presuppositions are therefore still important in advocating various methods of bladder management until further research provides guidance to the efficacy of the various methods.

Urologic Complications

Urologic complications can be divided anatomically into two categories: upper and lower tract complications. Those of the upper tract (i.e., vesicoureteral reflux, hydronephrosis, pyelocaliectasis, renal calculi, renal and perirenal infection, and renal insufficiency and failure) are considered more serious to long-term health and survival.

Upper Tract Complications

The data on upper tract complications collected in the NSCISC Database include results of glomerular filtration rate, renal scan results, excretory urogram/intravenous pyelogram (EU/IVP) or renal ultrasound, and calculi of the kidneys or ureters. No data have been collected in the NSCISC Database about the occurrence of renal failure, although a collaborative study was conducted on cause of death, including diseases of the urinary system (see Chapter 14). The information on glomerular filtration rate has been collected in less than 2% of patients at discharge from initial hospitalization or during all subsequent annual follow-up visits. Renal scan results have been obtained in only about 10% of all patients at initial discharge and in only 20% of all subjects during subsequent years of follow-up, primarily by two Model Systems.

The traditional imaging modality, EU/IVP, which provides an anatomic description of the renal calyces, renal pelvis, and the ureters, was performed in

60.1% (n = 3401) of individuals by discharge from initial hospitalization since 1986 and in 9.8% (n = 4790) of individuals during follow-ups. The EU/IVP remains the best imaging study capable of demonstrating small lesions such as papillary necrosis, ureteral strictures, uroepithelial tumors, and ureteral stones.[27] The EU/IVP data collected by the NSCISC were divided broadly into four categories: (1) normal calyces or mild pyelocaliectases with mild caliceal blunting, (2) definitely abnormal caliceal blunting, (3) unable to grade, and (4) absent or nonfunctioning kidney. Using these criteria, EU/IVP was abnormal (category 2) in only 0.3% (n = 1752) at initial discharge and in 2.5% (n = 467) at follow-up visits.

Although the EU/IVP provides a better definition of cortical scarring than does renal ultrasonography,[28] the invasive nature of the EU/IVP is a drawback to its use as a screening device. Renal ultrasonography, using the same definition for normal and abnormal as for EU/IVP, was abnormal in 0.3% (n = 286) of individuals who had the procedure during the initial stay and in 0.8% (n = 378) at annual follow-up visits.

Calculi

Calculi in the kidney were found in 1.0% (n = 3394) of persons at initial discharge and in 1.8% (n = 4561) of all follow-up visits. Calculi in the ureter were found in 0.1% (n = 3395) of patients at initial discharge and in about 0.2% (n = 4563) of all follow-up visits. Calculi of the kidneys or ureters were seen more frequently in individuals using an indwelling urethral catheter than in those using other methods of bladder management.[29]

Based on data from the NSCISC, a low frequency of upper tract complications has been found. Currently renal calculi are considered the most serious complication of the upper tracts.[30] Untreated calculi can lead to abscess formation, septicemia, and even death.[30] Although calculi of the kidneys or ureters have been found less frequently in individuals using an external collector or intermittent catheterization than with an indwelling urethral catheter, causation cannot be assumed, since some individuals may have had an indwelling catheter placed because of known calculi. The lack of completed studies of the upper tract may be due in part to an expected low yield of findings by physicians, cost, refusal by patients, or lack of consensus as to which test is best. Lloyd et al.[31] reported that in comparing radionucleotide renal scans with EU/IVP, no severe EU/IVP findings were undetected by renal scans in 200 patients. However, the EU/IVP appears to be utilized more frequently than scans.

A case-controlled study at one Model system determined that those who developed renal calculi were more likely to have complete cervical lesions ($P < 0.025$), vesicoureteral reflux ($P < 0.01$), and a history of bladder calculi ($P < 0.05$).[32] In this same study, patients with renal calculi were somewhat more likely to use an indwelling urethral catheter, although this finding was not statistically significant. A low frequency of upper urinary tract problems has been found by others in long-term follow-up studies in individuals managed with intermittent catheterization.[33-35] However, three recent reviews have reported upper tract changes in 17% to 30% of patients over 5 to 10 years from injury. [36-38]

Data from the NSCISC on stone removal indicate that 74.1% (23/31) of the stones in either the kidney or the ureter, present during initial stay, were not removed by discharge, but only 3.0% (2/66) of the stones found in the bladder were not removed by discharge. Thus, location is one of the factors determining stone removal. A small number of stones present in either location or in an unknown location, 11.7% (12/103), passed spontaneously. The remaining 66 stones of the 103 known stones were removed by a variety of methods. Stone removal was performed by cystolitholapaxy in 78.0% (46/59) of the bladder calculi. The second most common method for bladder stone removal was lithotripsy, 11.9% (7/59). Lithotripsy was the primary method used for the removal of kidney or ureteral stones, 66.7% (4/6).

During follow-up years, the incidence of renal and bladder stones increased from 3.0% (62/2054) at year 1, to 4.0% (52/1274) at year 2, and 4.6% (35/748) at year 3; however, this may not represent an increase in stones but a greater follow-up rate among persons with stones in the kidney or ureter which usually were not removed. At year 1, 58.1% of all stones were located in the bladder, as compared with 64.1% for initial stay. Since the majority of stones in the bladder were removed by discharge, this suggests new or recurrent cases of bladder stones.

Lower Urinary Tract Complications

Lower urinary tract complications, other than bladder calculi (see above), examined by the NSCISC are orchitis/epididymitis and urethral fistula/false passage. Since 1986, during the initial hospitalization phase 2.2% (n = 2804) of males sustained episodes of orchitis/epididymitis, while data from first-year follow-up (from discharge to first anniversary) indicate that 1.9% (n = 1720) of males had an episode of orchitis/epididymitis. During initial hospitalization only 0.4% (14/3442) of individuals developed a urethral fistula or false passage, while data from the first-year follow-up indicate that 0.2% (5/2109) developed a urethral fistula. At 2- and 3-year follow-up visits, 0.2% and 0.1% of patients (n = 1303 and 769, respectively) developed this problem, thus indicating that urethral fistula/false passage is probably a rare complication in persons cared for within the Model Systems.

Follow-Up

Periodic evaluation of the urinary system is important to preserve renal function and to reduce morbidity/mortality. The evaluation may include attention to catheterization or voiding schedules and techniques, frequency of urinary tract infections, care of any urinary appliance, use of recommended drugs, and studies of the upper urinary tract and the bladder, including urodynamics when indicated.[39] Such evaluations may necessitate changing the system of drainage during the individual's lifetime. Changes may include addition of appropriate drugs or more intensive changes such as surgical interventions. No data have been collected in the NSCISC Database on pharmacologic agents used for bladder management.

Surgical interventions have been examined by the NSCISC, including external sphincterotomy and bladder neck resection. Table 7–7 shows the percentage of sphincterotomy and bladder neck resection by follow-up year.

Another related complication studied at follow-up is autonomic dysreflexia. Using only those persons with the same method of bladder management at discharge as at the first-year follow-up, 9.3% (n = 1537) reported autonomic dysreflexia at first-year follow-up. In those persons using catheter techniques for bladder management, episodes of autonomic dysreflexia were reported at first-year follow-up in the Model Systems by individuals using suprapubic tubes or indwelling urethral catheters almost twice as often as those on intermittent catheterization (Table 7–8).

Functional Independence Measure

The FIM for sphincter control: bladder management includes complete intentional control of the urinary bladder and use of equipment or agents

---

Table 7–7 Number and Percentage of Total Individuals: Frequency of Having an External Sphincterotomy and/or a Bladder Neck Resection by Year Postinjury

	Year Postinjury*									
Procedure	1	2	3	4	5	6	7	8	9	10
External Sphincterotomy										
No.	22	52	42	45	25	15	12	10	10	10
%	0.7	1.9	1.6	1.9	1.3	0.9	0.8	0.8	1.0	1.1
Bladder Neck Resection										
No.	5	11	4	8	4	5	7	5	6	5
%	0.2	0.4	0.2	0.3	0.2	0.3	0.5	0.4	0.6	0.5

*Data from NSCISC Annual Reports 9 and 10 for Model Spinal Cord Injury Care Systems, June 1992, Table 34B.

Table 7–8 Percentage of Individuals Using the Same Method of Bladder Management at Discharge As at First-Year Follow-Up Who Reported Episodes of Autonomic Dysreflexia during the First-Year Postinitial Discharge

Method of Management (Same at Discharge and First-Year Follow-Up)	% Reporting Autonomic Dysreflexia: First-Year Follow-Up (n = 143)
None	3.0
Indwelling Catheter	18.6
Catheter Free: External Collector	12.6
Catheter Free: No External Collector	0.0
Normal Micturition	0.9
Intermittent Catheterization	10.0
Conduit	0.0
Suprapubic Cystostomy	19.2
Other	0.0

necessary for bladder control. Future research is needed to help those with the greatest degree of neurologic impairment to increase their independence in this area.

Although there was no gender difference in the percentage of individuals by the four major neurologic categories who achieved total independence in bladder management by discharge, men were more likely to require no helper (modified independence or independence) in all four categories. Total assistance was needed by only 4% of men with complete paraplegia, yet 13% of women with complete paraplegia required total assistance. The reason for this gender difference is not known.

Since there are different methods of bladder management, an analysis of method by FIM score was made (Table 7–9). Of all individuals on intermittent catheterization (n = 1059), 58.7% required no helper (modified or complete independence) and only 18.4% required total assistance. Of all individuals using an indwelling urethral catheter (n = 180), only 19.4% required no helper and 51.1% required total assistance. The use of an external collector was about the same whether the individual needed total or maximal assistance or had modified or complete independence. Of those individuals requiring total assistance (n = 374), 52.1% were on intermittent catheterization and 24.5% were on indwelling urethral catheterization; thus, despite the need for total assistance, intermittent catheterization was the more common method of management.

SEXUAL FUNCTION

Sexual function relies on similar nervous pathways to the bladder and bowel and is altered after SCI. Because of the large number of variables necessary to

Table 7-9 Method of Bladder Management and Associated Percentage of Functional Independence Measure

Functional Independence Level of Assistance	Method of Bladder Management								
	None (n = 44)	Indwelling Catheter (n = 180)	Catheter Free: External Collector (n = 20)	Catheter Free: No External Collector (n = 20)	Normal Micturition (n = 359)	Intermittent Catheter (n = 1059)	Conduit (n = 1)	Suprapubic Cystostomy (n = 67)	Other (n = 5)
Total Assistance	2.3	51.1	35.9	0.0	1.9	18.4	0.0	53.7	40.0
Maximal Assistance	0.0	10.6	4.3	0.0	0.8	5.9	0.0	14.9	0.0
Moderate Assistance	2.3	7.2	3.4	0.0	1.1	7.1	0.0	1.5	0.0
Minimal Assistance	0.0	5.0	1.7	10.0	1.4	4.4	0.0	4.5	20.0
Supervision Set-up	2.3	6.7	7.7	15.0	3.5	5.5	0.0	0.0	0.0
Modified Independence	9.1	11.1	39.3	25.0	7.2	46.7	100.0	25.4	40.0
Complete Independence	84.1	8.3	7.7	50.0	84.1	12.0	0.0	0.0	0.0

obtain significant information about the topic, only select data have been collected in the Model Systems Database. Information that has been collected includes the occurrence of orchitis/epididymitis (see Urologic Complications) and the insertion of a penile prosthesis. Data indicate that very few men have insertion of a penile prosthesis after SCI, with only 14 of 2780 follow-up forms since 1986 indicating a prosthesis inserted within 2 years of injury. Of these, four prostheses were of the silicone rod type and nine were of the inflatable type.

Similar to the Model Systems data, most other information available regarding sexual function after SCI pertains to males. This is primarily due to the high ratio of males with SCI to females with SCI; however, it may also be due to the external nature of men's genitalia or previous societal bias that women's sexual function is limited to procreation. The remainder of this chapter provides a review of current knowledge available about sexual function and SCI.

The effect of SCI on erection and ejaculation is known primarily through self-report data. Bors and Comarr[40] classified men based on the type of neurologic damage in the sacral reflex arc. They noted that 93% of men with an upper motor neuron (UMN) complete SCI had reflex erections, while none could have psychogenic erections and 4% achieved ejaculations. With incomplete UMN SCI, 80% had reflex erections, 19% had some type of combination reflex and psychogenic erections, and 32% had ejaculations. Among individuals with a lower motor neuron (LMN) complete SCI, none achieved reflex erections, 26% achieved psychogenic erections, and 18% achieved ejaculation. Finally, with LMN incomplete SCI, 90% achieved combined reflex and psychogenic erections and 70% were able to ejaculate.

The parallel event to erection in women is known to be lubrication, whereas uterine and vaginal contractions are thought to be the parallel to ejaculation.[41] It has been postulated that after SCI women should undergo changes in sexual response similar to those of men.[42–44] However, only one report questioned women with SCI of identified neurologic status about their ability to lubricate.[45] The study concluded that further laboratory analyses using plethysmography are necessary to understand the physiologic effects of SCI on female sexual response.[45]

In addition to the physiologic effects of SCI on sexual response, the sexuality of males and females is greatly affected. After SCI, sexual desire has been noted to decrease in both sexes.[45,46] Similarly, frequency of activity and satisfaction were noted to decrease in both sexes.[45–48] Types of sexual activities engaged in have been found to be unchanged after SCI.[45,46]

Sexual Function in Males

Treatment of sexual dysfunction in the SCI population has focused on restoration of erectile function. Although penile prostheses were the primary available means of treating erectile dysfunction 10 years ago, today there are multiple methods one can utilize to manage impotence. In one of these methods, known as intracavernous injections, men are taught to inject vasoactive medications into the corpora of the penis. Erections occur after approximately 5 minutes and generally last for 1 to 1.5 hours. Intracavernous injection of vasoactive drugs into the corpus cavernosa of the penis was compared with the use of the penile prosthesis to determine the type and frequency of adverse occurrences.[49] Complications occurred in 22 of 72 men using intracavernous injections.[49] In contrast, of 19 men who used the penile prosthesis, mechanical failures occurred 15 times, infection occurred 9 times, and late erosion occurred 3 times. Because of these complications, the men required the use of a total of 30 prostheses, and only 14 men reported satisfactorily functioning implants at their last office visit.[49]

Even less invasive, vacuum constriction devices have been used therapeutically since 1986.[50] A vacuum tube is placed over the penis and suction is used to create an erection. Afterward, a constricting band is placed at the base of the penis and should be kept in place no longer than 30 minutes. Complications have been noted to include skin irritation, edema, sweating,[51] and penile erythema[52]; however, the technique is generally considered safe and is well tolerated. Most recently, the surface application of nitroglycerin has been shown to be useful in treating impotence in spinal cord–injured men.[53]

SCI results in diminished concentration and motility of sperm,[54] in addition to causing ejaculatory dysfunction. Because of this, assistive techniques aimed at producing ejaculation have been developed to allow men with SCI to father children. Electroejaculation, one technique used to harvest sperm from men with SCI, is performed by transrectal electrical stimulation of myelinated sympathetic efferent fibers of the hypogastric plexus.[55] The procedure is performed in a hospital or clinic setting, because anoscopy must be performed before and after the electroejaculation[56] to evaluate for any mucosal damage that could have been produced by the stimulation. The procedure causes emission to occur. Once produced, the semen is milked from the urethra, in addition to the bladder being catheterized for any ejaculate that may have traveled retrograde. Electroejaculation has been coupled with artificial insemination[56] and with in vitro fertilization and embryo transfer[57] to produce pregnancies. Although relatively safe, electroejaculation is also known to cause autonomic dysreflexia.

Alternatively, electrovibration has been recommended to stimulate ejaculation.[56] Varying types of vibratory stimulation of the penis generally will result in ejaculation within 4 minutes.[55] Electrovibration has the advantage of being able to be performed in the home; however, the ability to produce an ejaculate is less consistent than with electroejaculation. Moreover, men can also experience autonomic dysreflexia with electrovibration. It should be noted that, despite the widespread clinical availability of electrovibration and electroejaculation, few pregnancies have been reported with these techniques.

Female Fertility

Early studies reported 3 to 6 months of amenorrhea post-SCI, along with an absence of dysmenorrhea.[58,59] More recent reports reveal that approximately 60% of women exhibit amenorrhea for 5 months and that dysmenorrhea is as common as prior to injury.[47,60] Hyperprolactinemia with or without galactorrhea has been noted to occur in association with amenorrhea post-SCI,[61] and autonomic dysreflexia has also been noted to occur in association with the menstrual cycle.[62]

Pregnancy

Previous reports have noted that risks associated with pregnancy in the SCI female include decubitus ulcers, UTIs, and anemia.[44] Difficulty with transfers as the pregnancy progresses has also been reported.[63] Premature and small-for-date infants were felt to occur at increased rates as compared with rates for the general population.[63,64] Labor has been noted to be difficult to appreciate with SCI above T10; however, concomitant sympathetic symptoms such as back pain, difficulty breathing, or strong spasms have been noted to occur often and allow the women to sense that labor is approaching.[65] Labor has also been reported to be shorter with stronger contractions,[66] and Caesarean delivery has been noted to be more common, occurring in 38 of 96 reported pregnancies.[63,65,67,68] Finally, autonomic dysreflexia has been noted to occur commonly during labor in women with SCI above the level of T6. It has also been associated with induction of labor and has been shown to result in death secondary to misdiagnosis and confusion with preeclampsia.[69] In a recent review of 13 pregnancies in 11 spinal cord–injured women decubitus ulcers, UTIs, and difficulty in transferring were noted as complications during pregnancy[70]; however, anemia was not. Preterm delivery was not noted, as has been reported in the past, and both the mean duration of labor and the incidence of Caesarean delivery were noted to be similar to those in the able-bodied population.

REFERENCES

1. Soderstrom G, Ducker T. Increased susceptibility of patients with cervical cord lesions to peptic gastrointestinal complications. *J Trauma.* 1990;25:1030–1038.

2. Albert T, Levine M, Balderston R, Cotler J. Gastrointestinal complications in spinal cord injury. *Spine.* 1991;16(suppl):S522–S525.

3. Gore R, Mintzer R, Calenoff L. Gastrointestinal complications of spinal cord injury. *Spine.* 1981;6:538–544.

4. Bracken M, Bracken B, Shepard M, et al. A randomized controlled trial of methylprednisolone or naloxone in the treatment of acute spinal cord injury. *JAMA.* 1990;322:1406–1411.

5. Watson N. Late ileus in paraplegia. *Paraplegia.* 1981;19:13–16.

6. Neumayer L, Bull L, Mohr J, et al. The acutely affected abdomen in paraplegic spinal cord injury patients. *Ann Surg.* 1990;212:561.

7. Apstein M, Dalecki-Chipperfield K. Spinal cord injury as a risk factor for gallstone disease. *Gastroenterology.* 1987;92:966.

8. Stinneford J, Deshwarzian A, Nemchasky A, Doria M, Durkin M. Esophagitis and esophageal motor abnormalities in patients with chronic spinal cord injury. *Paraplegia.* 1993;31: 384–392.

9. Binnie R, Creasey G, Edmond P, Smith A. The action of cisapride on the chronic constipation of paraplegia. *Paraplegia.* 1988;26:151–158.

10. Binnie R, Smith A, Creasey G, Edmond P. Constipation associated with chronic spinal cord injury: The effect of pelvic parasympathetic stimulation by the Brindley stimulator. *Paraplegia.* 1991;29:463–469.

11. Menardo G, Bausano G, Corazziari E, et al. Large-bowel transit in paraplegic patients. *Dis Colon Rectum.* 1987;30:924–928.

12. Nino-Murcia M, Friedland G. Functional abnormalities of the gastrointestinal tract in patients with spinal cord injuries: Evaluation with imaging procedures. *AJR.* 1992;158:279–281.

13. Stone J, Nino-Muracia M, Wolfe V, Perkash I. Chronic gastrointestinal problems in spinal cord injury patients: A prospective analysis. *Am J Gastroenterol.* 1990;85:1114–1119.

14. Miller F, Fenal T. Prolonged ileus with acute spinal cord injury responding to metoclopramide. *Paraplegia.* 1981;19:43–45.

15. Guttman L. Disturbances of intestinal function. In: *Spinal Cord Injuries: Comprehensive Management and Research.* 2nd ed. New York: Blackwell Scientific Publications; 1976.

16. Kuric J, Lucas C, Ledgerwood A, Kiraly A, Salciccioli G, Sugawa C. Nutritional support: A prophylaxis against stress bleeding after spinal cord injury. *Paraplegia.* 1989;27:140–145.

17. Weingarden S. The gastrointestinal system and spinal cord injury. *Phys Med Rehabil Clin North Am.* 1992;3:765–781.

18. Maynard FM, Diokno AC. Urinary infection and complication during clean intermittent catheterization following spinal cord injury. *J Urol.* 1984;132:943–946.

19. Mohler JL, Cowen DL, Flanigan RC. Suppression and treatment of urinary tract infection in patients with intermittently catheterized neurogenic bladder. *J Urol.* 1987;138:336–340.

20. Stickler DJ, Chawla JC. An appraisal of antibiotic policies for urinary tract infections in patients with spinal cord injuries undergoing long-term intermittent catheterization. *Paraplegia.* 1988;26:215–225.

21. Kuhlemeier KV, Lloyd LK, Stover SL. Failure of antibody-coated bacteria and bladder washout tests to localize infection in spinal cord injury patients. *J Urol.* 1983;130:729–732.

22. Merritt JL, Keys TF. Limitations of the antibody-coated bacteria test in patients with neurogenic bladders. *JAMA.* 1982;247:1723–1725.

23. Hooton TM, O'Shaugnessy EJ, Clowers D, Mack L, Cardenas DD, Stamm WE. Localization of urinary tract infection in patients with spinal cord injury. *J Infect Dis.* 1984;150:85–91.

24. Gribble MJ, Puterman JL, McCallum NM. Pyuria: Its relationship to bacteriuria in spinal cord injured patients on intermittent catheterization. *Arch Phys Med Rehabil.* 1989;70:376–379.

25. National Institute on Disability and Rehabilitation Research Consensus Statement, January 27–29, 1992. The prevention and management of urinary tract infections among people with spinal cord injuries. *J Am Paraplegia* Soc. 1992;15:194–207.

26. Stover SL, Fine PR, eds. *Spinal Cord Injury: The Facts and Figures.* Birmingham, Ala: University of Alabama; 1986.

27. Linsenmeyer TA. The potential contribution of urodynamics and imaging studies in urinary tract infections in spinal cord injured patients. NIDRR Consensus Validation Conference; January 1992.

28. Palubisnskas AJ. Imaging of the urinary tract. In: Tanagho EA, McAninch JW, eds. *General Urology.* 12th ed. Norwalk, Conn. Appleton & Lange; 1988:57–109.

29. Maynard FM, Karunas R. Bladder management and urologic complications after spinal cord injury. *Arch Phys Med Rehabil.* 1992;73:954.

30. Stover SL, Lloyd LK, Waites KB, Jackson AB. Urinary tract infections in spinal cord injury. *Arch Phys Med Rehabil.* 1989;70:47–54.

31. Lloyd LK, Dulovsky EV, Bueschen AJ, et al. Comprehensive renal scintillation procedures in spinal cord injury patients. *J Urol.* 1981;126:10–13.

32. DeVivo MJ, Fine PR. Predicting renal calculus occurrence in spinal cord injury patients. *Arch Phys Med Rehabil.* 1986;67:722–725.

33. Maynard FM, Glass J. Management of the neuropathic bladder by clean intermittent catheterization: 5 year outcomes. *Paraplegia.* 1987;25:106–110.

34. McGuire E, Savastino JA. Long-term follow-up of spinal cord injured patients managed by intermittent catheterization. *J Urol.* 1983;123:775–776.

35. Timoney AG, Shaw PJR. Urological outcome in female patients with spinal cord injury: The effectiveness of intermittent catheterization. *Paraplegia.* 1990;28:556–563.

36. Dewire DM, Owens RS, Anderson GA, Gottlieb MS, Lepor H. A comparison of the urological complications associated with long-term management of quadriplegics with and without chronic indwelling urinary catheters. *J Urol.* 1992;147:1069–1072.

37. Gerridzen RG, Thijssen AM, Dehoux E. Risk factors for upper tract deterioration in chronic spinal cord injury patients. *J Urol.* 1992;147:416–418.

38. Killorin W, Gray M, Bennett JK, Green BG. The value of urodynamics and bladder management in predicting upper urinary tract complications in male spinal cord injury patients. *Paraplegia.* 1992;30:437–441.

39. Cardenas DD. Neurogenic bladder. *Phys Med Rehabil Clin North Am.* 1992;3:751–763.

40. Bors E, Comarr AE. Neurological disturbances of sexual function with special reference to 529 patients with spinal cord injury. *Urol Surv.* 1960;110:191.

41. Griffith ER, Trieschmann RB. Sexual functioning in women with spinal cord injury. *Arch Phys Med Rehabil.* 1975;56;18–21.

42. Comarr AE, Vigue M. Sexual counseling among male and female patients with spinal cord injury and/or cauda equina injury. *Am J Phys Med.* 1978;57:215–227.

43. Berard EJJ. The sexuality of spinal cord injured women: Physiology and pathophysiology: A review. *Paraplegia.* 1989;27:99–112.

44. Sipski ML, Alexander CJ. Sexual function and dysfunction after spinal cord injury. *Phys Med Rehabil Clin North Am.* 1992;3:811–828.

45. Sipski ML, Alexander CJ. Sexual activities, response and satisfaction in females pre- and post-spinal cord injury. *Arch Phys Med Rehabil.* 1993;74:1025–1029.

46. Alexander CJ, Sipski ML, Findley TW. Sexual activities, desire and satisfaction in males pre- and post-spinal cord injury. *Arch Sex Behav*. 1993;22:215–226.

47. Charlifue SW, Gerhard KA, Menter RR, Whiteneck GG, Scott Manley M. Sexual issues of women with spinal cord injuries. *Paraplegia*. 1992;30:192–199.

48. Berkman AH, Weissman R, Frielich MH. Sexual adjustment of spinal cord injured veterans living in the community. *Arch Phys Med Rehabil*. 1978;59:29–33.

49. Dietzen CJ, Lloyd LK. Complications of intracavernous injections and penile prosthesis in spinal cord injured men. *Arch Phys Med Rehabil*. 1992;73:652–655.

50. Nadig PW, Ware JC, Blumoff R. Noninvasive device to produce and maintain an erection-like state. *Urology*. 1986;27:126–131.

51. Lloyd EE, Toth LL, Perkash I. Vacuum tumescence: An option for spinal cord injured males with erectile dysfunction. *SCI Nursing*. 1989;6:25–28.

52. Zasler ND, Katz PG. Synergist erection system in the management of impotence secondary to spinal cord injury. *Arch Phys Med Rehabil*. 1989;70:712–716.

53. Sonksen J, Biering-Sorensen F. Transcutaneous nitroglycerin in the treatment of erectile dysfunction in spinal cord injured. *Paraplegia*. 1992;30:554–557.

54. Linsenmeyer TA, Perkash I. Infertility in men with spinal cord injury. *Arch Phys Med Rehabil*. 1991;72:747–754.

55. Yarkony GM. Enhancement of sexual function and fertility in spinal cord injured males. *Am J Phys Med Rehabil*. 1990;69:81–87.

56. Bennett CJ, Ayers JWT, Randolph JF, et al. Electroejaculation in paraplegic males followed by pregnancies. *Fertil Steril*. 1987;48:1070–1072.

57. Ayers JWT, Moinipanah R, Bennett CJ, Randolph JF, Peterson EP. Successful combination therapy with electroejaculation and in vitro fertilization-embryo transfer in the treatment of a paraplegic male with severe oligosthenospermia. *Fertil Steril*. 1988;49:1089–1090.

58. Comarr AE. Observations of menstruation and pregnancy among female spinal cord injury patients. *Paraplegia*. 1966;3:263–272.

59. Durkan JP. Menstruation after high spinal cord transection. *Am J Obstet Gynecol*. 1968;100:521–524.

60. Axel SJ. Spinal cord injured women's concerns: Menstruation and pregnancy. *Rehabil Nursing*. 1982;7(5):10–15.

61. Jackson AB, Varner ER. Hyperprolactinemia in females following spinal cord injury. *J Am Paraplegia Soc*. 1992;15:94.

62. Allen JB, Stover SL, Jackson AB, et al. Autonomic dysreflexia and the menstrual cycle in a woman with spinal cord injury. *Neurorehabilitation* 1991;1(4):58–62.

63. Verduyn WH. Spinal cord injured women, pregnancy and delivery. *Paraplegia*. 1986;24:231–240.

64. Goller H, Paeslack V. Pregnancy damage and birth complications in the children of paraplegic women. *Paraplegia*. 1972;10:213–217.

65. Wanner MB, Rageth CJ, Zach GA. Pregnancy and autonomic hyperplexia in patients with spinal cord lesions. *Paraplegia*. 1987;25:482–490.

66. Young BK, Katz M, Klein SA. Pregnancy after spinal cord injury: Altered maternal and fetal responses to labor. *Obstet Gynecol*. 1983;61:59–63.

67. Cross LL, Meythaler JM, Tuel SM, et al. Pregnancy after traumatic paraplegia and quadriplegia. *J Am Paraplegia Soc*. 1991;14:72.

68. Turk R, Turk M, Assejev V. The female paraplegic and mother-child relations. *Paraplegia.* 1983;21:186–191.

69. McGregor JA, Meeuwsen J. Autonomic hyperreflexia: A mortal danger for spinal cord damaged women in labor. *Am J Obstet Gynecol.* 1985;151:330–333.

70. Baker ER, Cardenas DD, Benedetti TJ. Risks associated with pregnancy in spinal cord injured women. *Obstet Gynecol.* 1992;80:425–428.

8

Management of the Neuromusculoskeletal Systems

Frederick M. Maynard, Rosalie S. Karunas, Rodney H. Adkins,
J. Scott Richards, and William P. Waring III

INTRODUCTION

Management of the neuromusculoskeletal systems is directed at preserving and enhancing voluntary muscle strength, maintaining muscle and joint flexibility, and preventing secondary conditions that interfere with limb function, such as spasticity, contracture, pain, post-traumatic syringomyelia, osteoporosis with limb fracture, and heterotopic ossification. In this chapter, the frequencies among persons in the National SCI Database affected by these medical and rehabilitative problems of the neuromusculoskeletal systems are presented, and factors associated with their occurrence are analyzed. For data collection purposes, specific definitions of these entities were developed that identify the more severe forms of these conditions. Results are discussed in relationship to available literature about methods for prevention and optimal management of these problems.

TREATED SPASTICITY

Spasticity is a neurophysiologic condition characterized by hyperactive deep tendon reflexes and increased muscle tone. It is an expected manifestation of the pathophysiology of injury to the spinal cord above the conus medullaris. The mere presence of spasticity should not be viewed as a complication of SCI, since it can have some beneficial effects on the health and function of persons with spinal paralysis. Nevertheless, spasticity often becomes problematic. Involuntary movements and severely increased resistance to passive movement of joints from muscle hypertonus may interfere with or prevent performance of functional activities. Spasms may also be painful.

145

The following definition is used to code the occurrence of spasticity in persons entered into the National SCI Database: "spasticity that is severe enough to have warranted a trial of medication or surgical treatment" at admission, at discharge, and at annual follow-up. All references to spasticity in this chapter are to the "treated" spasticity of this definition unless otherwise noted. Figure 8–1 shows that 32.2% of persons in the National SCI Database developed spasticity before discharge from initial hospitalization and 42.7% reported spasticity occurring between initial discharge and first anniversary of injury. The proportion with spasticity in subsequent years after injury gradually declines, remaining under 35% after 10 years of follow-up. Declining frequency of spasticity during long-term follow-up may result from gradual neurochemical alterations in the chronically injured spinal cord, from improving functional adaptation of individuals with chronic SCI, or from growing reluctance to take medications because of their perceived ineffectiveness.

Table 8–1 compares rates of spasticity during the first year of follow-up among persons grouped by demographic and neurologic characteristics. Gender, but not race, is significantly related to spasticity rates. A significant difference among age groups, with persons older than 60 and under 16 reporting spasticity less often than those aged 16 to 60, suggests that indications for treatment are related to expectations for independent performance of functional activities. Expectations may be lower in older and younger ages. Persons with tetraplegia are more likely to have spasticity than those with paraplegia. This result may be explained

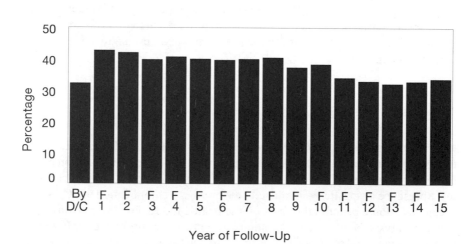

Figure 8–1 Percentages of Persons Developing Spasticity (Treated) by Time of Discharge from Initial Hospitalization and during Follow-Up Years

Table 8-1 Demographic and Neurologic Characteristics of Persons with SCI with Treated Spasticity during the First Year of Follow-Up

Characteristic	% with Treated Spasticity
Male	43.5
Female	38.9‡
White	42.5
Nonwhite	43.2
Age	
0–15 Years	26.1
16–30 Years	42.9
31–45 Years	44.9
46–60 Years	45.6
>60 Years	37.1†
Tetraplegia at Discharge	53.5
Paraplegia at Discharge	31.9†
Frankel Grade at Discharge	
A	46.4
B	56.6
C	46.6
D	30.6†

†$P < 0.01$.
‡$P < 0.05$.

Note: P values for age and Frankel grade at discharge are the results of χ^2 tests among all groups in these categories.

partially by differential rates of spasticity development in lesions above and below the conus medullaris, since lower motor neuron damage is the usual consequence of injury to the conus medullaris or to the cauda equina.

In a study of the epidemiology of spasticity in persons with SCI at one Model System,[1] a significantly lower incidence of clinical signs of spasticity (increased reflexes, increased tone, and/or involuntary spasms), regardless of treatment, was found in persons with paraplegia below T7, compared with those with levels of T7 and above. This study also reported a lower rate of spasticity in persons in the National SCI Database with paraplegia below T7 levels, compared with those with levels of T7 and above. A significant relationship between discharge Frankel grade of neurologic impairment and incidence of spasticity during initial hospitalization was also found among persons with tetraplegia and paraplegia of T7 and above. Persons with Frankel grades B and C were more likely to have spasticity. A similar analysis (Table 8–2) of current Model SCI Systems' persons with tetraplegia at discharge reveals a significant relationship between discharge Frankel grade and spasticity during first year of follow-up. Again, the highest incidences of spasticity occur in persons who are classified as Frankel grades B (67.9%) and C (64.6%).

Table 8–2 Percentage of Persons with Tetraplegia Who Have Treated Spasticity during First Year of Follow-Up, by Frankel Grade

Characteristic	% with Treated Spasticity
Frankel Grade at Discharge	
A	59.5
B	67.9
C	64.6
D	37.8[†]

[†]$P < 0.01$.

One of the inherent limitations in the Model SCI Systems data on spasticity is the absence of uniform clinical indications for treatment, since data are based on individualized clinical decisions of persons with SCI and their physicians. Customary indications include the following: (1) spasticity preventing or interfering with performance of activities of daily living, including transfers, bed mobility, stable seating posture, and driving; (2) spasticity-related pain that prevents or interferes with these activities; and (3) spasticity interfering with sleep. While it has been proposed that aspects of early management of SCI (such as operative or nonoperative handling of spinal fractures) and presence of bowel, bladder, and skin complications may influence the development of problematic spasticity,[2,3] no empirical evidence has been presented in support. Any study of relationships among occurrence of spasticity and complications and types of treatment should account for the differential spasticity rates relating to level and severity of SCI and to demographic characteristics.

When spasticity remains problematic in spite of treatment with medications or local nerve blocks, destructive or ablative surgical procedures such as rhizotomy and myelotomy may be performed. The frequency of "surgical ablation or destruction of spinal cord or nerve root tissue to reduce spasticity or spasms" is very low among persons in the National SCI Database.

Only three persons (less than 0.1%) have undergone such a procedure during initial hospitalization, with a total of 162 surgical ablations occurring in 124 persons from time of injury through 15 years of follow-up. Two thirds of these subjects had ablations performed at one Model System, which suggests limited availability of the procedures and/or a lack of consensus about their effectiveness. The annual rate of occurrence of these procedures among all persons with recorded follow-up data between years 2 and 15 postinjury varies between 0% and 1.6% (Table 8–3).

While there is no trend toward higher rates after many years with SCI, a trend did appear in an analysis of proportions of persons who had surgery. This analysis

Table 8–3 Rate of Occurrence of Surgery for Spasticity at Discharge from Initial Hospitalization and during Follow-Up Years

Time	Rate of Occurrence (%)	No. of Occurrences	Total Persons at Time Point
At Discharge	0.1	3	4357
During Follow-Up			
Year 1	0.4	14	3456
Year 2	0.9	28	2960
Year 3	1.0	27	2753
Year 4	0.8	19	2473
Year 5	0.7	15	2080
Year 6	0.6	11	1697
Year 7	0.9	14	1494
Year 8	0.4	5	1288
Year 9	0.5	5	1079
Year 10	0.7	7	955
Year 11	0.4	3	798
Year 12	—	0	648
Year 13	0.6	3	490
Year 14	1.6	6	365
Year 15	0.7	2	294

was performed using only those persons in the National SCI Database who had complete data during initial hospitalization and during successive follow-up years and using only the person's *first* surgery, if he or she underwent repeated procedures. Therefore, the persons included in any year must also have had data collected through all previous years. For example, persons included with year 2 data are a subset of persons with year 1 data. Five follow-up years were studied in this way, because surgery for spasticity has been collected in the National SCI Database only since 1986.

A year-by-year examination of these groups shows few persons with surgery in each group. This small number remains relatively stable, but because the numbers of persons for whom complete data are available decline yearly, the proportion that has had at least one destructive surgical procedure for spasticity rises steadily until follow-up year 5, when it reaches 4.4% of persons with complete data (Table 8–4.) Although this finding may be biased by differential rates of consistent follow-up related to severity of injury, it suggests that a substantial number and an increasing proportion of persons with SCI do not achieve satisfactory control of spasticity with medications and/or peripheral nerve procedures, and it also suggests a real need to develop other effective measures.

Table 8–4 Proportions with Surgery for Spasticity in Persons with SCI

Time	Proportion with Surgery	No. with Surgery	Total Persons with Complete Data*
Through:			
Discharge	0.1	3	4319
Year 1	0.5	15	2924
Year 2	1.4	26	1850
Year 3	2.4	29	1225
Year 4	2.7	20	739
Year 5	4.4	17	388

*Note: Includes only those persons for whom complete data are available through discharge from initial hospitalization and each of the first 5 years of follow-up.

Table 8–5 compares percentages of subjects, grouped by demographic and neurologic characteristics, with at least one destructive surgery for spasticity at any time during initial hospitalization or follow-up. Procedures were significantly less frequent among persons over age 45 at injury and in nonwhites. Procedures were more common among persons with tetraplegia than those with paraplegia and significantly so among those with motor complete (Frankel grade A or B) injuries, compared with those with motor incomplete (Frankel grade C or D) injuries.

In recent years other invasive methods for treating severe spasticity have been developed. Dorsal column stimulators have been implanted into the spinal cord distal to an injured level. Results have shown limited effectiveness.[4] Another approach has been implantation of intrathecal infusion pumps that deliver very small doses of antispasticity medications, such as baclofen, directly to the spinal cord. Early results of these procedures show dramatic reduction in spasticity,[5] although data pertaining to their long-term use are not yet available.

SURGICAL TREATMENT FOR POST-TRAUMATIC SYRINGOMYELIA

Cystic cavities commonly form in the glial scar that develops in the spinal cord following traumatic injury. Occasionally these cysts enlarge and they may be associated with loss of sensation and strength above and below the level of injury. Surgical drainage of these cystic cavities and placement of permanent shunts can sometimes reverse neurologic losses. These procedures are considered success-

Table 8–5 Demographic and Neurologic Characteristics of Persons with SCI and with Surgery for Spasticity

Characteristics	% with Surgery for Spasticity*
Men	1.5
Women	1.0
White	1.7
Nonwhite	0.9[†]
≤45 Years	1.6
>45 Years	0.7[‡]
Tetraplegia at Discharge	1.6
Paraplegia at Discharge	1.2
Frankel Grade at Discharge	
Motor Complete (A or B)	2.1
Motor Incomplete (C or D)	0.5[†]
All Patients	1.4

[†]$P < 0.01$.

[‡]$P < 0.05$.

Note: Surgery for spasticity performed at any time during initial hospitalization or during 15 years of follow-up.

ful when they prevent further enlargement of the cysts and arrest progressive neurologic loss.[6,7]

In the National SCI Database since 1986, any occurrence of "surgical treatment of syringomyelia," defined as "drainage of a spinal cord cyst to promote decompression of the cavity," has been recorded at admission to initial hospitalization, at discharge, and at annual follow-up. Only six such procedures have occurred before discharge ($<0.1\%$), and 115 procedures are reported during all annual follow-up visits, an overall incidence of 0.5%. The rate of occurrence of this procedure during individual follow-up years varies between 0% and 1.1%, and there is no apparent trend toward a rising rate with time postinjury (Table 8–6). However, an analysis of proportions with surgery for syringomyelia was conducted, using only those persons in the National SCI Database with complete data during initial hospitalization and during successive follow-up years, as described earlier. Again, the proportion of persons who have had surgery for syringomyelia since the onset of SCI rises steadily, reaching 3.4% by follow-up year 5 (Table 8–7).

In order to gain insight into potential risk factors for occurrence of progressive post-traumatic syringomyelia requiring surgical treatment, Table 8–8 displays data for persons who have had surgery for syringomyelia during initial hospitalization or any follow-up year, contrasting various demographic and neurologic characteristics. Analysis of relative risks shows significantly lower risks for women, for nonwhites, for persons injured by gunshots, for those with

Table 8–6 Rate of Occurrence of Surgery for Syringomyelia at Discharge from Initial Hospitalization and during Follow-Up

Time	Rate of Occurrence (%)	No. of Occurrences	Total Persons at Time Point
At Discharge	0.1	6	4355
During Follow-Up			
Year 1	0.3	11	3458
Year 2	0.3	8	2959
Year 3	0.4	12	2754
Year 4	0.6	14	2473
Year 5	0.6	13	2081
Year 6	0.5	9	1697
Year 7	0.7	10	1493
Year 8	—	0	1289
Year 9	0.7	8	1079
Year 10	0.6	6	955
Year 11	0.9	7	798
Year 12	1.1	7	649
Year 13	0.8	4	490
Year 14	0.8	3	365
Year 15	0.7	2	294
Year 16	0.7	1	151

incomplete paraplegia, and for those classified as Frankel grade D, regardless of level.

A review of the literature concerning post-traumatic syringomyelia confirms that only a small proportion of persons with SCI develop progressive cystic enlargement with symptoms, as estimates of incidence vary from 1% to 3% in various clinical series.[8] In one study of 370 persons followed over 10 years, the

Table 8–7 Proportions with Surgery for Syringomyelia in Persons with SCI

Time	Proportion with Surgery	No. with Surgery	Total Persons with Complete Data*
Through:			
Discharge	0.1	6	4316
Year 1	0.4	13	2925
Year 2	0.8	14	1850
Year 3	1.2	15	1224
Year 4	2.0	15	738
Year 5	3.4	13	387

*Note: Includes only those persons for whom complete data are available through discharge from initial hospitalization and each of the first 5 years of follow-up.

Table 8–8 Demographic and Neurologic Characteristics of Persons with SCI Who Have Surgery for Syringomyelia at Any Time during Initial Hospitalization or during 16 Years of Follow-Up

Characteristics	% with Surgery for Syringomyelia	Relative Risk	95% Confidence Intervals
Male	1.3		
Female	0.7	1.96	1.02, 3.76
White	1.5		
Nonwhite	0.5	2.95	1.68, 5.17
Etiology			
All Other	1.3		
Gunshot Wounds	0.5	2.64	1.23, 5.67
16–60 Years of Age	1.3		
< 16 or > 60 Years of Age	0.5	2.62	0.97, 7.09
Neurologic Category at Discharge			
Tetraplegia or Complete Paraplegia	1.4		
Incomplete Paraplegia	0.5	2.96	1.44, 6.07
Frankel Grade at Discharge			
A or B or C	1.5		
D	0.6	2.57	1.47, 4.50

incidence was 1.6%.[9] Recent advances in neurologic imaging of the spinal cord, particularly magnetic resonance imaging (MRI), have enabled clinicians to document readily the presence of focal cystic changes in the spinal cord. One recent MRI study on a random sample of persons with chronic paraplegia found that 64% had cystic changes.[10] In another MRI study, 67% of persons with SCI admitted for rehabilitation (mean of 2.2 years postinjury) were found to have cysts.[11] Therefore, while prevalence of cystic progression with symptoms may well be higher than has previously been reported, the causal relationship between cystic changes and clinical symptoms is not clear at this time.

The gradually rising proportions of persons who had surgery in the data displayed in Table 8–7 indeed suggest that individuals with SCI are at considerably greater risk of developing this condition over their lifetime than has been previously recognized, even though number of years postinjury may not be an independent risk factor. It has recently been suggested that tethering of the cord at the site of spinal trauma may be associated with progressive syringomyelia.[12] In view of changing methods of surgical management of spinal trauma, further investigation of risk factors for this condition is clearly needed.

Unfortunately, the benefit of surgical treatment for syringomyelia cannot be assessed from current Model SCI Systems data. Knowledge is not sufficient to define indications clearly for surgery when early symptoms develop. A collaborative Model SCI Systems study is currently under way in order to gain more detailed information about short-term and long-term results of surgical interventions and about the natural history of cystic myelopathy, from early symptoms to definite motor and sensory loss.

SURGICAL TREATMENT FOR NEUROGENIC PAIN

A number of classification schemes for SCI pain have been proposed. The one most widely adopted is that of Donovan et al.,[13] but lack of a standardized and agreed-upon classification scheme limits the comparability of reports in the literature.[14] All such classifications of SCI pain, however, include mention of what can be termed neurogenic pain, generally agreed to be the most problematic type of pain postinjury. A variety of other terms have been used for neurogenic pain, including central pain, phantom pain, deafferentation pain, dysesthetic pain, central dysesthesia syndrome, and spinal cord pain. All of these terms generally refer to the same phenomenon—burning, tingling, or aching diffuse pain below the level of injury.

The only data collected in the National SCI Database relative to pain refer to surgical procedures for pain relief. The definition for this variable is "partial or complete surgical ablation or destruction of spinal cord or nerve root tissue to reduce pain." This can include myelotomy, cordotomy, surgical or percutaneous posterior rhizotomy, and the dorsal root entry zone procedures, but peripheral nerve blocks or other procedures performed on the peripheral nerves are not coded in this variable. Information is recorded at admission, at discharge, and at annual follow-up. Examination of data for all of these time points revealed that only 39 persons in the database have ever had surgery for pain, less than 0.5% of the more than 8500 subjects for whom information on this variable was obtained at least one time.

The rarity of this procedure, at least as it is carried out in the Model SCI Systems, is striking, given the attention such procedures have been given in the SCI literature. Given this very small series, definitive investigations of factors associated with the probability of surgical procedures for pain relief cannot be carried out. Sex and etiology do not appear to be related to the occurrence of surgery for pain relief. The proportion with surgery is slightly lower for nonwhites than for whites and tends to rise with age, declining after age 60. Surgery was somewhat more likely to occur in persons with complete injuries (either paraplegia or tetraplegia) than in those with some degree of preserved function.

Seventy-two percent of persons who underwent these procedures were classified as having complete injuries, contrasted to approximately 50% of complete injuries in the general SCI population. It is also noteworthy that procedures for

62% of these persons occurred in only 1 of the 13 centers. This probably reflects both the diversity of opinion within the Model SCI Systems about the efficacy of surgery for pain and variability across centers in expertise available to execute such procedures.

Table 8–9 shows the proportions of persons who had surgery for pain relief, counting only those who had complete data during initial hospitalization and during successive follow-up years, as has been described earlier. A year-by-year examination of these groups indicates only a few persons with surgery in each group and a rising proportion with increasing time since injury. As has been stated earlier, such an increase could result from differential rates of consistent follow-up related to severity of SCI, with a loss to follow-up of persons without complications and therefore a lower likelihood of surgery for pain relief. The data suggest that there may be some hesitancy to resort immediately to surgical procedures for pain relief until all of the more conservative procedures have been pursued.

The reported prevalence of pain following SCI varies widely in the literature, partly due to the variety of research methods used to investigate this topic. In his review of the literature, Mariano[15] found that the estimated prevalence of disabling pain ranged from 18% to 63% in the SCI population. In an earlier Model SCI Systems project, Nepomuceno et al.[16] surveyed 200 persons with SCI. They reported an 80% prevalence of pain or discomfort, with 43% describing their pain as mild, moderate, or severe. Twenty-three percent (high thoracic or cervical) to 37% (low thoracic or lumbosacral) of those surveyed stated that they would be willing to trade loss of sexual and/or bowel and bladder functions, as well as the hypothetical possibility for cure, in order to obtain pain relief.

While most investigators have suggested a relatively low prevalence of severe and disabling neurogenic pain in the SCI population, this problem has been cited

---

Table 8–9 Proportions with Surgery for Pain Relief in Persons with SCI

Time	Proportion with Surgery	No. with Surgery	Total Persons with Complete Data*
Through:			
Discharge	0.0	2	4318
Year 1	0.1	4	2925
Year 2	0.3	6	1850
Year 3	0.6	7	1224
Year 4	0.9	7	738
Year 5	1.0	4	387

*Note: Includes only those persons for whom complete data are available through discharge from initial hospitalization and each of the first 5 years of follow-up.

as the single most important factor responsible for lowered ratings of quality of life, when it occurs.[17] A variety of medications has been used for treating neurogenic pain,[18,19] with virtually no consensus on effectiveness. Similarly, although a number of surgical procedures have been utilized, reports of their efficacy vary[19] and long-term benefits remain questionable. Increased prevalence of SCI pain has been associated with injuries caused by gunshot wounds, but in two separate Model SCI Systems investigations, surgical removal of the bullet has had no demonstrable impact on subsequent pain perception.[20,21]

MUSCULOSKELETAL PAIN

Musculoskeletal pain is known to be a common problem among people with SCI[13]; however, no data on musculoskeletal pain problems have been collected in the National SCI Database. Although it has been estimated that up to 70% of persons with SCI have chronic pain,[16,22] studies have not separated pain problems into musculoskeletal and neurogenic. As expected with spinal trauma, some type of pain is present in almost all newly injured persons with SCI.

In addition to acute pain expected at the site of spinal trauma and surgery, shoulder pain also commonly occurs among people with cervical injuries and tetraplegia. Shoulder pain among persons with new SCI is of special interest because of their dependence on use of upper limbs when learning to perform basic activities of daily living, such as wheelchair propulsion, transfers, eating, and dressing. Weakness of shoulder muscles can cause imbalance of the force coupling of the rotator cuff, deltoid, biceps, and trapezius muscles that keeps the humeral head depressed and in the glenoid fossa of the shoulder joint.

Fleming and Dawson reported in 1958 that 14 of 18 (78%) persons with tetraplegia admitted for initial rehabilitation had shoulder or neck pain.[23] A later study also identified a high prevalence (75%) of shoulder pain during initial hospitalization for SCI but found that the improvement or disappearance of shoulder pain was common by discharge from rehabilitation.[24] Besides traditional approaches for preventing shoulder pain following acute SCI, such as range of motion exercises, Scott and Donovan have described a special positioning technique believed to be more effective for preventing this pain, although it has not gained wide acceptance in the United States.[25]

Reports of upper-limb, musculoskeletal pain problems due to chronic overuse and age-related degenerative processes in tendons and joints have risen as life spans for people with SCI have increased. Unlike the shoulder-pain problems common among people with recent tetraplegia, upper-limb pain among those with paraplegia has been the focus of recent reports dealing with secondary musculoskeletal pain problems associated with long-term survival. One of the first reports of this problem came in 1979 from people with SCI in England who experienced a 50% prevalence of chronic shoulder pain.[26] In 1987, Gellman et al. reported a prevalence of 68% for any complaint of upper-limb pain and 34.5% specifically for shoulder pain among a follow-up clinic population with chronic paraplegia in California.[27]

Bayley et al. noted a 33% prevalence of shoulder pain during transfers among a group of 94 persons with chronic paraplegia.[28] Further testing revealed that 16% had aseptic necrosis of the humeral head and 74% had a chronic impingement syndrome with subacromial bursitis. Those with a clinical syndrome of chronic impingement were given arthrograms, and rotator cuff tears were found in 65% of the cases. Osteoarthritis of the shoulder joint seems to be an infrequent finding.[29,30]

Other common sites of pain in the upper limb for people with chronic paraplegia are the hand and wrist. One degenerative process that leads to wrist pain is osteoarthritis at the base of the thumb or at the first metacarpal head.[31] Another common cause of hand and wrist pain is median neuropathy at the wrist, or the carpal tunnel syndrome. Several studies have reported a prevalence of 60% for carpal tunnel syndrome based on electromyographic evidence, although only 30% to 40% have clinical symptoms.[32,33]

Pain problems at the elbow appear to be less frequent than at the shoulder and hand/wrist. Lateral epicondylitis or tennis elbow resulting from strain of wrist muscles is probably the most common diagnosis for elbow pain. Pain may also accompany contracture of the elbow flexor muscles, particularly among persons with recent tetraplegia. The incidence of degenerative spinal processes such as osteoarthritis, herniated discs, or failure of previous fusions is not known, but these can also be serious long-term musculoskeletal complications.

No studies have described musculoskeletal pain in lower limbs of persons with chronic SCI. Further work is needed to investigate effective treatments for early musculoskeletal-pain problems of the limbs and to study risk factors, treatment methods, and prevention strategies for chronic musculoskeletal pain in people with SCI.

CONTRACTURES AFFECTING FUNCTIONAL LIMITATIONS

Contractures of muscles and joints are a well-known complication of immobilization, paralysis, and increased muscle tone, although they can usually be prevented by active and passive movements. For persons entered into the National SCI Database, contracture is defined as a "reduction in joint range of motion severe enough to have warranted or recommended specific stretching exercises," which usually also involves "treatment with physical agents (e.g., cold, heat, etc.), splinting or surgery" and which precludes "functional ability consistent with level of injury." Development of contractures is recorded at admission, discharge, and annual follow-up.

Note that persons recorded as having developed contractures include only those who lose a sufficient degree of joint range of motion to have potential functional consequence, as evidenced by their receiving specific treatment, an incidence of 4.5% by the time of discharge from initial hospitalization. Figure 8–2 shows that the incidence of contracture rises somewhat after discharge, remaining relatively constant after several follow-up years.

The rate of occurrence of contracture by discharge among persons admitted to Model SCI Systems on the day of injury was 3.7% and among those admitted between 2 and 60 days after injury was 5.4%. This difference is significant ($P < 0.01$) and supports the hypothesis that early treatment in Model SCI Systems can reduce the rate of this preventable complication, which leads to increased costs of hospitalization and may continue to affect negatively a person's functional ability even after the contracture is treated.

Lower rates of contracture among persons receiving early treatment in Model SCI Systems compared with those referred later have also been reported by Yarkony et al.[34] In that study, the range of motion of all major limb joints was measured and compared with normal values. At discharge, early-referral persons had normal range of motion in 78% of joint motions, compared with 68% for late-referral persons ($P < 0.05$). The study also found that in late-referral persons, 17% of joint motions were significantly reduced, and in early-referral persons, 13% of joint motions were significantly reduced, with "significant" reduction specifically defined in measured degrees of movement for each joint. The average number of joints with contracture per person was 7.5. The results of this

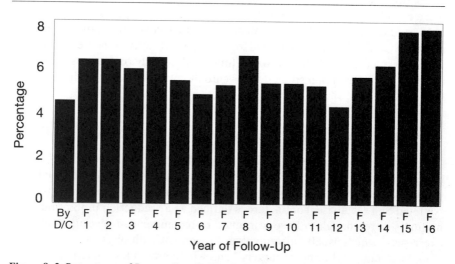

Figure 8–2 Percentages of Persons Developing Contractures by Time of Discharge from Initial Hospitalization and during Follow-Up Years

study suggest that the data from the National SCI Database do indeed represent only cases with severe contractures.

Because the National SCI Database definition for contracture is based on clinical judgment rather than routine measurement of joint range of motion, considerable variation among reported rates at individual centers exists, and this limitation probably further contributes to the relatively low proportion (4.5%) of persons with contracture by time of discharge, as noted in Figure 8–2.

Table 8–10 shows differences in occurrence of contractures during initial hospitalization and first-year follow-up for persons grouped by gender, race, age, level of SCI, Frankel grade of SCI severity, presence of spasticity, and heterotopic ossification, as defined in the next section. A smaller proportion of nonwhites have contractures by discharge, but during first-year follow-up, their proportion

Table 8–10 Demographic and Neurologic Characteristics of Persons with SCI with Contractures by Time of Discharge from Initial Hospitalization and during the First Year of Follow-Up

	% with Contractures	
Characteristic	By Discharge	During Follow-Up Year 1
Male	4.5	6.0
Female	4.4	7.7
White	4.8	5.7
Nonwhite	3.5	7.2
Age (y)*		
0–15	3.5	5.2
16–30	4.3	4.8
31–45	4.1	6.9
46–60	5.5	11.4
>60	5.5	9.6[†]
Tetraplegia at Discharge	6.4	7.7
Paraplegia at Discharge	2.5[†]	4.9[†]
Frankel Grade at Discharge		
A, B, or C	5.0	6.4
D	3.4[‡]	6.1
With Spasticity	7.9	
Without Spasticity	2.8[†]	
With Heterotopic Ossification	17.4	
Without Heterotopic Ossification	3.7[†]	

[†]$P < 0.01$.
[‡]$P < 0.05$.

*Note: P value for age category is result of χ^2 test comparing ages $\leq$ 45 and > 45.

is higher than that of whites. Women also have a higher rate of contracture than men at first-year follow-up. Fewer younger persons have contractures by discharge, and examination of follow-up data reveals that older persons have higher rates of contracture than younger ones during the first several follow-up years.

The proportion of persons who have had contractures by the time of their discharge from initial hospitalization and the proportion of persons with contractures during the first year of follow-up are significantly higher among those with tetraplegia at discharge than among those with paraplegia. This proportion remains higher for persons with tetraplegia throughout the first 9 follow-up years, reflecting the greater number of limbs with weakness in persons with tetraplegia (four), compared with those with paraplegia (two).

Table 8–10 shows a greater rise in rate of contracture from discharge to first-year follow-up among those with paraplegia. A significantly smaller proportion of persons classified as having Frankel grade D have contractures by discharge, compared with those classified as having Frankel grades A, B, and C, but this significance is no longer present at first-year follow-up. Contracture by discharge was also found to be significantly more likely among persons who had spasticity and among those who had developed heterotopic ossification during initial hospitalization.

In the study by Yarkony et al.[34] of early- and late-referral persons cited previously, higher rates of joint contracture were also found among persons with tetraplegia than among those with paraplegia, and there were no significant differences based on Frankel grades. Surprisingly, the presence of coexisting limb fractures was not found to be a predisposing factor for contracture development.

Although the results of analysis of contracture rates among persons in the National SCI Database during follow-up years must be interpreted cautiously because of inherent limitations in these data, the finding of higher rates among nonwhites is disturbing. Perhaps it relates to less successful education and/or less frequent performing of routine range of motion/stretching exercises after discharge. It could also be related to availability of less adequate outpatient and in-home services among this population. Certainly, further study of factors related to higher rates of contracture during follow-up years and better documentation of the impact of contracture on the development of other medical complications (e.g., pressure sores) and on functional skills are needed.

HETEROTOPIC OSSIFICATION

Heterotopic ossification (HO) has been reported to occur in 16% to 53% of persons with new SCI.[35] It affects joints distal to the level of SCI, most commonly the hips and knees. When HO is extensive, it can restrict joint range of motion and limit functional abilities. It can also predispose a person with SCI to pressure sores.

Persons in the National SCI Database are coded as to whether they have developed HO "documented by X-ray or bone scan with flexion of the hip and/ or knee restricted to less than 90 degrees" at admission, discharge from initial hospitalization, and at annual follow-up. This syllabus definition was chosen because it is based on objective criteria, which should increase the reliability of case ascertainment when routine radiographic studies are not conducted and should provide useful information about the incidence of HO that is likely to have an impact on health and/or function.

Figure 8–3 shows the rates of occurrence of HO among persons in the National SCI Database. While 4.9% of subjects develop HO by discharge, rates decline among persons seen in follow-up years, perhaps as a result of reporting only cases with functional limitation and documented by X-ray or bone scan. These findings are compatible with previous reports that about 3% of persons with SCI have severe limitations in joint motion caused by HO.[36] The actual incidence of HO that is less extensive and does not restrict hip and knee motion or that is present in other locations is undoubtedly higher.

Table 8–11 shows proportions of persons with HO grouped by various demographic and neurologic characteristics. Significantly higher proportions were reported among men than among women, among persons aged 45 and under, among those admitted more than 1 day after injury, and among those with complete injuries.

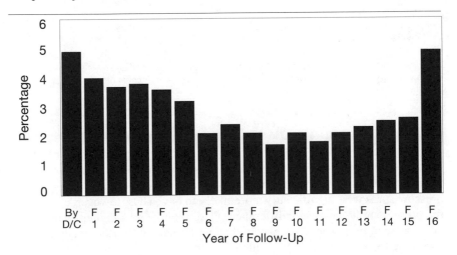

Figure 8–3 Percentages of Persons with SCI Developing Heterotopic Ossificiation by Time of Discharge from Initial Hospitalization and during Follow-Up Years

Table 8–11 Demographic and Neurologic Characteristics of Persons with SCI Who Have Heterotopic Ossification by Time of Discharge from Initial Hospitalization

Characteristic	% with Heterotopic Ossification
Male	5.2
Female	3.4[‡]
White	4.7
Nonwhite	5.2
Age (y)*	
0–15	4.9
16–30	5.6
31–45	5.7
46–60	2.1
>60	1.2[†]
Tetraplegia at Discharge	5.5
Paraplegia at Discharge	4.3
Day 1 Admission	3.6
Days 2–60 Admission	6.3[†]
Frankel Grade at Discharge*	
A	7.6
B	6.2
C	4.0[†]
D	1.2[†]
With Spasticity	6.7
Without Spasticity	4.0[†]
With Contractures	19.2
Without Contractures	4.2[†]

[†]$P < 0.01$.
[‡]$P < 0.05$.

*Note: P value in age category is result of χ^2 test comparing ages ≤ 45 and > 45; P value in Frankel grade category is result of χ^2 test comparing Frankel grade A with Frankel grades B, C, and D.

These findings generally confirm results of a study of risk factors for HO that used a case definition of clinical signs and X-ray evidence of HO in any part of the body.[37] It found that persons with complete lesions, with spasticity, and with pressure sores were significantly more likely to have HO. However, contrary to the present study, no gender differences were found, and a higher incidence of HO was seen in persons over age 30 than under age 30. Further study of these demographic differences is warranted.

In a double-blind, placebo-controlled study of persons with SCI, disodium etidronate was shown to be effective in the prevention of HO.[38] It is possible that the lower incidence of HO among persons admitted to a Model SCI System on the day of injury compared with those admitted later is due to greater prophylactic use of disodium etidronate or due to earlier recognition with prompt treatment. The number of persons provided with prophylactic treatment is not known in this database. It may also be explained by the higher rate of pressure sores among late-referral persons and a higher proportion of complete injuries among the late-referral group.

Current research clearly supports the usefulness of prophylactic disodium etidronate in persons with motor complete SCI. Anti-inflammatory medications may also be of some benefit, but this has not yet been proven in persons with SCI. Early initiation of frequent stretching exercises to maintain joint range of motion and muscle flexibility at sites of HO is also recommended in order to avoid the disabling consequences of reduced motion at the hips and knees.

OSTEOPOROSIS

Osteoporosis is pathologic bone loss. It has been defined as a condition in which there is lack of bone tissue, and the tissue that remains is fully calcified.[39] More recent definitions include: "a lower bone mass than might be expected from age and sex norms and that produces an increased risk of fractures"[40] and "an absolute decrease in the amount of bone, leading to fractures after minimal trauma."[41] Fracture threshold, defined as the bone mineral density below which the risk of fracture increases in the absence of major trauma, has been established as 1.0 g/cm^2 at the hip and vertebrae.[42] While the primary focus of the clinical study of osteoporosis has been the elderly, particularly women,[41] osteoporosis has also been noted as a common sequela of SCI.[43–55]

Persons in the National SCI Database are coded at admission, discharge, and annual follow-up as having had "fracture resulting from osteoporosis." Only "pathologic fractures resulting from osteoporosis in a long bone in the lower extremity (i.e., femur, tibia, fibula)" are coded, with instructions to "document only those fractures secondary to osteoporosis." Examination of the current Model SCI Systems data reveals somewhat variable, but certainly low, reported rates within each of 16 follow-up years (Figure 8–4).

Examination of proportions of persons with fractures due to osteoporosis among only those with complete data during initial hospitalization and successive follow-up years again reveals small but steadily rising proportions (Table 8–12). These figures undoubtedly underestimate actual values, because fractures secondary to any trauma, fractures of other than lower-extremity sites, or fractures occurring where medical documentation did not specifically address osteoporosis as a contributing factor were not reported. In a collaborative study among Model SCI Systems designed to examine issues related to aging in SCI,

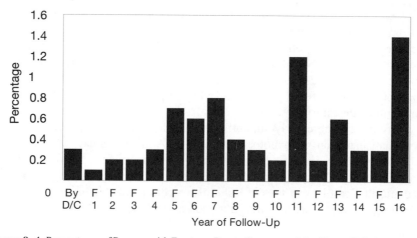

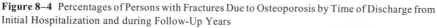

Figure 8–4 Percentages of Persons with Fractures Due to Osteoporosis by Time of Discharge from Initial Hospitalization and during Follow-Up Years

the response of participants indicated a much higher incidence of fractures. Among those who had been injured 5 years, 14% reported that they had experienced fractures; among those injured 10 years, 28%; and for those 15 years postinjury, 39% (this study is described in Chapter 13).

In another study of fracture incidence in a chronic SCI population, Ragnarsson and Sell[48] argued that their estimated incidence was probably low (4%) because fractures were not always treated in the SCI center from which their data were gathered. This explanation may well contribute to the discrepancy between the rate in the National SCI Database and other reports.

Table 8–12 Proportions with Fracture Due to Osteoporosis in Persons with SCI

Time	Proportion with Fracture	No. with Fracture	Total Persons with Complete Data*
Through:			
Discharge	0.3	12	4120
Year 1	0.4	10	2652
Year 2	0.6	9	1629
Year 3	0.5	5	1032
Year 4	0.9	5	572
Year 5	2.4	6	254

Note: Includes only those persons for whom complete data are available through discharge from initial hospitalization and each of the first 5 years of follow-up.

While estimates of fracture incidence may be low within the Model SCI Systems, the distribution of characteristics for those who have had fractures at any time during initial hospitalization or 15 follow-up years seems logical. The data show a higher rate for complete versus incomplete injuries, 1.3% versus 0.8%, respectively, for paraplegia, and 1.3% versus 0.9%, for tetraplegia. Similarly, findings related to Frankel grade are as expected: persons classified as having Frankel grades A and B had higher rates (1.3% and 1.7%, respectively) than those classified as having Frankel grades C and D (0.9% and 0.5%, respectively). Women had higher rates (1.7%) of fractures resulting from osteoporosis than did men (0.9%).

Analogous to the gender data, age at onset is logically distributed for ages 16 to 30, 31 to 45, and 46 to 60, with reported fracture rates of 0.8%, 1.2%, and 2.0%, respectively. However, the rate for persons under age 16 at injury was the highest, 2.5%. This is consistent with the concept that injury not only causes a decline in existing bone, but retards bone development in younger persons with SCI. Surprisingly, persons aged 61 to 75 at injury had the lowest fracture rate, 0.8%. While this appears to be inconsistent, it is probably due to shorter life expectancy, and thus a shorter duration of follow-up, for these individuals.

The findings regarding etiology, race, and injury completeness appear to be confounded. Among etiologies of SCI, violence was associated with the lowest follow-up fracture rate, 0.8%, compared with 1.1% for motor vehicle accidents and falls, and 1.2% for sports. Yet gunshot wounds (accounting for 88% of the patients comprising the violence category) result in a higher incidence of complete injuries,[56] which have a higher fracture rate. Spinal cord injuries due to gunshot wounds, however, tend to occur to a greater extent among nonwhites[57]; and nonwhites show a fracture rate that is less than half that of whites, 0.6% versus 1.3%. From this perspective, the data suggest that nonwhites have either higher premorbid bone density or greater resistance to bone loss following SCI.

Early studies attempting to quantify osteoporotic bone loss associated with SCI have been mainly biochemical, based on the imbalance between anabolic and catabolic functions, or occasionally histomorphometric.[44–47,49,50] While periods of negative calcium, phosphorus, and nitrogen balance have been documented, the majority of these studies have been less than definitive. The basic reason for these ambiguous results is that neither research design nor statistical methodology has accounted for such factors as gender, age, completeness of spinal cord lesion, level of injury, and time after injury.

While earlier studies have not always been well designed, they also lacked the technology to measure bone loss adequately. Therefore, regional differences in bone loss (e.g., hip versus spine), profiles of loss over time, or definitive steady state of bone status in this population could not be assessed adequately. Dual photon absorptiometry (DPA) represented a major advance in the noninvasive measurement of total bone mineral content or total bone mass and bone mineral density in selected regions of the body.[58] Since the advent of DPA, a number of studies have used the technique to examine bone character and loss and change in SCI individuals.[51–54]

Garland et al.[53] reported the first comprehensive study of osteoporosis in the SCI population that employed DPA and that also controlled for gender, extent of injury, and injury acuity. Results confirmed that bone loss in the lower extremities following complete lesions of the spinal cord is relatively rapid. In the first 3 months after injury, the bone is depleted by approximately 22%. An additional 5% is lost between the third and fourth months postinjury, and at 14 months postinjury approximately 32% of the bone has been lost. However, perhaps the most striking finding is that bone depletion at 16 months postinjury is essentially equal to that found 10 years postinjury, approximately 37%. While these percentages of loss appeared to be about equal, 25% of the subjects had a bone mineral density below the established fracture threshold at the distal femur 16 months postinjury, compared with 40% of the subjects 10 years postinjury. At the proximal tibia, the comparable percentages were 50% and 90%, respectively. Nevertheless, none of the 16-month or the 10-year participants had experienced any fractures in the lower extremities postinjury.

In an attempt to examine the issue of fractures associated with osteoporosis in persons with SCI, Garland et al.[55] more recently investigated bone density using dual-energy X-ray absorptiometry. The knees of two comparable groups of individuals with SCI were examined. The bone about the knee was chosen because it is the most common fracture site in persons with chronic SCI. Members of one group presented with fractures at the time of enrollment. Members of the other group had never had a fracture. In addition, comparisons of an analogous able-bodied control group were incorporated. The mean bone density of the knees of the fracture group was found to be significantly lower ($P < 0.04$) than that of the nonfracture group. However, the means for both groups were well below the fracture threshold of 1.0 g/cm^2. Compared with the able-bodied controls, the fracture group's mean bone mineral density was 49% of "normal."

While further clarification of the nature of osteoporosis and associated fractures in persons with SCI has been provided by the recent studies discussed above, the pathophysiology is still not fully understood, nor is the magnitude of the problem of osteoporosis among this population. Early estimates of the overall incidence of pathologic fractures are 1.4% to 6.0%.[43,48] In 1982, Young et al.[59] reported fracture incidence rates of 3.6% among hospitalized patients and 1.1% among nonhospitalized persons with SCI followed in Model SCI Systems from 1975 to 1981. Data in the current National SCI Database indicate a low incidence, but one that may be rising steadily with time. However, the collaborative investigation described by Menter and Hudson in Chapter 13 indicates a high rate that increases dramatically with time. While rapid bone loss is noted very early following SCI, it is not clear whether the loss continues or is altered further by other physiologic changes associated with aging. As the SCI population grows older, the problem of osteoporosis, which is specifically related to aging, may become very serious, a hypothesis supported by the findings of Menter and Hudson described in Chapter 13.

REFERENCES

1. Maynard FM, Karunas RS, Waring WP. Epidemiology of spasticity after spinal cord injury. *Arch Phys Med Rehabil.* 1990;71: 566–569.

2. Merritt J. Management of spasticity in spinal cord injury. *Mayo Clin Proc.* 1981;56:614–622.

3. Katz RT. Management of spasticity. *Am J Phys Med Rehabil.* 1988;67:108–116.

4. Dimitrijevic MM, Dimitrijevic MR, Illis LS, et al. Spinal cord stimulation for control of spasticity in patients with chronic spinal cord injury, I: Clinical observations. *Cent Nerv Syst Trauma.* 1986;3:129–144.

5. Loubser PG, Narayan RK, Sandin KJ, Donovan WH, Russell KD. Continuous infusion of intrathecal baclofen: Long-term effects on spasticity in spinal cord injury. *Paraplegia.* 1991;29: 48–64.

6. Edgar RE. Surgical management of spinal cord cysts. *Paraplegia.* 1976;14:21–27.

7. La Haye PA, Botzdorf U. Post-traumatic syringomyelia. *West J Med.* 1988;148:657–663.

8. Barnett HJM, Jousse AT. Post-traumatic syringomyelia (cystic myelopathy). In: Vinken PJ, Bruyn EM, eds. *Handbook of Clinical Neurology.* Amsterdam: North Holland; 1976;26(pt 2): 113–157.

9. Vernon JD, Silver JR, Ohry A. Post-traumatic syringomyelia. *Paraplegia.* 1982;20: 339–364.

10. Hussey RW, Ha C, Vijay M, Lipper M, Kubota R. Prospective study of the occurrence of post-traumatic cystic degeneration of the spinal cord utilizing magnetic resonance imaging. In: *Abstracts Digest.* Chicago: American Spinal Injury Association; 1990:86.

11. Backe HA, Betz RR, Mesgarzadeh M, Clancy M, Steel HH. Post-traumatic spinal cord syrinx: An evaluation by MRI. In: *Abstracts Digest.* Chicago: American Spinal Injury Association, 1990:85.

12. Caplan LR, Norohna AB, Amico LL. Syringomyelia and arachnoiditis. *J Neurol Neurosurg Psychiatry.* 1990;53:106–113.

13. Donovan WH, Dimitrijevic MR, Dahm L, Dimitrijevic MM. Neurophysiological approaches to chronic pain following spinal cord injury. *Paraplegia.* 1982;20:135–146.

14. Richards JS. Chronic pain and spinal cord injury. *Clin J Pain.* 1992;8:119–122. Review and Comment.

15. Mariano AJ. Chronic pain and spinal cord injury. *Clin J Pain.* 1992;8:87–92.

16. Nepomuceno C, Fine PR, Richards JS, et al. Pain in patients with spinal cord injury. *Arch Phys Med Rehabil.* 1979;60:605–608.

17. Lundqvist C, Siosteen A, Blomstrand C, Lind B, Sullivan M. Spinal cord injuries: Clinical, functional, and emotional status. *Spine.* 1991;16:78–83.

18. Davidoff G, Guarracini M, Roth E, Sliwa J, Yarkony G. Trazodone hydrochloride in the treatment of dysesthetic pain in a traumatic myelopathy: A randomized, double-blind, placebo-controlled study. *Pain.* 1987;29:151–161.

19. Balazy TE. Clinical management of chronic pain in spinal cord injury. *Clin J Pain.* 1992;8:102–110.

20. Waters RL. Gunshot wounds to the spine: The effects of bullet fragments in the spinal canal. *J Am Paraplegia Soc.* 1984;7:30–33.

21. Richards JS, Meredith RL, Nepomuceno C, Fine PR, Bennett G. Psychosocial aspects of chronic pain in spinal cord injury. *Pain.* 1980;8:355–366.

22. Burke DC. Pain in paraplegia. *Paraplegia.* 1973;10:297–313.

23. Fleming W, Dawson AR. Shoulder pain in quadriplegic patient: A theory as to its cause. *South Med J.* 1958;51:1460–1463.

24. Waring WP, Maynard FM. Shoulder pain in traumatic quadriplegia. *Paraplegia.* 1991;29:1.

25. Scott J, Donovan W. The prevention of shoulder pain and contracture in the acute tetraplegic patient. *Paraplegia.* 1981;19:313–319.

26. Nichols PJR, Norman PA, Ennis JR. Wheelchair users' shoulder? *Scand J Rehabil Med.* 1979;11:29–32.

27. Gellman H, Sie I, Waters RL. Late complications of the weight-bearing upper extremity in the paraplegic patient. *Clin Orthop.* 1987;233:132–135.

28. Bayley JC, Cochran TP, Sledge CB. The weight-bearing shoulder. *J Bone Joint Surg.* 1987;69A(5):676–678.

29. Wing PC, Tredwell SJ. The weight-bearing shoulder. *Paraplegia.* 1983; 21: 107–113.

30. Wylie EJ, Chakera TM. Degenerative joint abnormalities in patients with paraplegia of duration of greater than 20 years. *Paraplegia.* 1988;26:101–106.

31. Blankstein A, Shmueli R, Weingarten I, Engel J, Ohry A. Hand problems due to prolonged use of crutches and wheelchairs. *Orthop Rev.* 1985;14(12):29–34.

32. Aljure J, Eltorai I, Bradley WE, Lin JE, Johnson B. Carpal tunnel syndrome in paraplegic patients. *Paraplegia.* 1985;23:182–186.

33. Davidoff G, Werner R, Waring W. Compressive mononeuropathies of the upper extremity in chronic paraplegia. *Paraplegia.* 1991;29:17–24.

34. Yarkony GM, Bass LM, Keenan V, Meyer PR. Contractures complicating spinal cord injury incidence and comparison between spinal cord centre and general hospital acute care. *Paraplegia.* 1985;23:265–271.

35. Finerman GA, Stover SL. Heterotopic ossification following hip replacement or spinal cord injury: Two clinical studies with EHDP. *Metab Bone Dis Relat Res.* 1981;3:337–342.

36. Wharton GW, Morgan TH. Ankylosis in the paralyzed patient. *J Bone Joint Surg.* 1970;52A:105–112.

37. Lal S, Hamilton BB, Heinemann AW, Betts HB. Risk factors for heterotopic ossification in spinal cord injury. *Arch Phys Med Rehabil.* 1989;70:387–390.

38. Stover SL, Hahn HR, Miller JM. Disodium etidronate in the prevention of heterotopic ossification following spinal cord injury: Preliminary report. *Paraplegia.* 1976;14:146–156.

39. Albright F, Burnett CH, Cope O, Parson W. Acute atrophy of bone (osteoporosis) simulating hyperparathyroidism. *J Clin Endocrinol Metab.* 1941;1:711–716.

40. Woolf A, Dixon AS. *Osteoporosis: A Clinical Guide.* Philadelphia: JB Lippincott Co; 1988.

41. Riggs L, Melton LJ. Involutional osteoporosis. *N Engl J Med.* 1986;314:1676–1686.

42. Riggs BL, Wahner HW, Seeman E, et al. Changes in bone mineral density of proximal femur and spine with aging: Differences between the postmenopausal and senile osteoporosis syndromes. *J Clin Invest.* 1982;70:716.

43. Comarr AE, Hutchinson RH, Bors E. Extremity fractures of patients with spinal cord injuries. *Am J Surg.* 1962;104:732–739.

44. Chantraine A. Clinical investigations of bone metabolism in spinal cord lesions. *Paraplegia.* 1971;8:253–259.

45. Claus-Walker J, Carter RE, Campos RJ, Spencer WA. Hypercalcemia in early traumatic paraplegia. *J Chronic Dis.* 1975;28:81–90.

46. Bergmann P, Heilporn A, Schoutens A, Paternot J, Tricot A. Longitudinal study of calcium and bone metabolism in paraplegic patients. *Paraplegia.* 1977;15:147–159.

47. Chantraine A. Actual concept of osteoporosis in paraplegia. *Paraplegia.* 1978;16:51–58.

48. Ragnarsson KT, Sell GH. Lower extremity fractures after spinal cord injury: A retrospective study. *Arch Phys Med Rehabil.* 1981;62:418–423.

49. Stewart AF, Adler M, Byers CM, Segre GV, Broadus AE. Calcium homeostasis in immobilization: An example of resorptive hypercalciuria. *N Engl J Med.* 1982;306:1136–1140.

50. Chantraine A, Nusgens B, Lapiere CM. Bone remodeling during the development of osteoporosis in paraplegia. *Calcif Tissue Int.* 1986;38:323–327.

51. Garland DE, Rosen CD, Stewart CA, Adkins RH, Hung G. Bone mineral distribution five years or more after spinal cord injury. *J Nucl Med.* 1989;30:857.

52. Leeds EM, Ganz W, Serafini A, Klose KJ, Green BA. Bone mineral density after FES cycle ergometry training. In: *Abstracts Digest.* Chicago: American Spinal Injury Association; 1989:11.

53. Garland DE, Stewart CA, Adkins RH, et al. Osteoporosis after spinal cord injury. *J Orthop Res.* 1992;10:371–378.

54. Kunkel CF, Scremin AME, Eisenberg B, Garcia JF, Roberts S, Martinez S. Effect of "standing" on spasticity, contracture, and osteoporosis in paralyzed males. *Arch Phys Med Rehabil.* 1993;74:73–78.

55. Garland DE, Maric Z, Adkins RH, Stewart CA. Bone mineral density about the knee in spinal cord injured patients with pathological fractures. *Contemp Orthop.* 1993;26:375–379.

56. Waters RL, Adkins RH, Yakura J, Sie I. Profiles of spinal cord injury and recovery after gunshot injury. *Clin Orthop.* 1991;267:14-21.

57. Stover SL, Fine PR. *Spinal Cord Injury: The Facts and Figures.* Birmingham, Ala: The University of Alabama at Birmingham; 1986.

58. Sartoris DJ, Resnick D. Osteoporosis: Update on densitometric techniques. *J Musculoskel Med.* 1989;6:108–124.

59. Young JS, Burns PE, Bowen AM, McCutchen R. *Spinal Cord Injury Statistics: Experience of the Regional Model Spinal Cord Injury Systems.* Phoenix, Ariz: Good Samaritan Medical Center; 1982.

9

Functional Outcomes

John F. Ditunno, Jr., Michelle E. Cohen, Christopher Formal, and Gale G. Whiteneck

INTRODUCTION

The word *function* is used in this chapter in two clinical contexts. First, it applies to altered activity of neural structures as measured by muscle weakness and sensory loss, which are the major impairments in spinal cord injury (SCI). Second, function also applies to altered activities of daily living such as self-care and mobility, which represent the major disabilities in severe SCI. Changes in social role functions such as vocation, marital status, and avocational interests, which represent handicaps, are discussed in the following chapters of this book. The first publication from the Database[1] reported Frankel grades[2] at admission and discharge and frequency of neurologic levels at admission and discharge, and compared functional abilities in self-care and mobility based on Frankel grades. In 1986, Stover and Fine[3] reported data on changes in category of neurologic impairment, frequency of neurologic levels, Frankel grades at admission and discharge, and categories of neurologic impairment related to etiology and age at time of injury.

The Functional Independence Measure (FIM), the most widely accepted functional assessment measurement in use today, was introduced into the Database following reliability testing in 1988 because of the need to have a measure of disability. The most recent revision of the American Spinal Injury Association (ASIA) Standards[4] in 1992 incorporated the FIM as the disability measure to complement the revised impairment measures. Since its inception, the National SCI Database has collected data on neurologic level and extent of injury on system admission, discharge, and follow-up. In 1986 the ASIA Motor Score was incorporated. While changes have recently been made in the Database to incorporate the 1992 standards for neurologic and functional classification of SCI (adopted by ASIA and endorsed by the International Medical Society of

Paraplegia), the impairment data presented in this chapter represent earlier versions of the ASIA Standards.[5,6]

IMPAIRMENT OUTCOMES

Impairment of neurologic function is one of the most objective measures of SCI, and virtually every chapter in this book examines relationships among a variety of variables and the neurologic impairment category, Frankel grade, or neurologic level. Neurologic impairment (the classification of injuries into four categories of tetraplegic complete and incomplete and paraplegic complete and incomplete) represents one of the earliest and simplest methods of classification.[7] Frankel et al.[2] introduced the system of classifying impairment in 1969 (grade A for complete injury, grade B for preserved sensation only, grade C for preserved nonfunctional motor, grade D for preserved functional motor, and grade E for normal). Almost every study on neurologic outcome that compares changes from admission to discharge utilizes Frankel grades. In 1982, ASIA defined neurologic levels precisely. This system of classification was incorporated into the Model SCI Systems' Database, but emphasis was placed on determining a single neurologic level in which all neurologic function (motor and sensory) was intact. The ASIA motor index score was added to the Database in 1986 in an effort to refine further the precision of measuring neurologic impairment. In the assessment of persons with SCI, key muscles and sensory points are examined from which the neurologic impairment category, Frankel grade, neurologic level, and motor index score are derived. This chapter considers outcomes in order from category of neurologic impairment to motor index scores. This order also represents a progression of increased precision of measurement from a four-category nominal scale (categories of neurologic impairment) used primarily for epidemiologic description to a more precise 100-point ordinal scale (motor index scores) used to demonstrate change in neurologic status.

Category of Neurologic Impairment

In this Database of 14,791 persons with SCI, neurologic impairment is categorized by four groups, tetraplegia complete (23.8%), tetraplegia incomplete (29.8%), paraplegia complete (27.0%) and paraplegia incomplete (19.0%). Over the past 20 years, the percentage of persons with complete injuries has decreased from 59.5% in 1972–1976 to 47.9% in 1989–1992; for the same period, the percentage of persons with neurologically incomplete injuries has increased from 40.5% to 50.9%. Stover[8] has suggested that this may be due to improved treatment at the scene of injury and subsequent care in the center. When this change in types of injuries is examined by neurologic impairment categories (Table 9–1), it can be seen that tetraplegic incomplete (TI) and paraplegic complete (PC) injuries have not shown any consistent trend, but there has been a steady decrease in tetraplegic complete (TC) injuries (28.9% to 18.9%) and an increase in paraplegic incomplete (PI) injuries (15.7% to 21.7%). When the distributions of injuries among these groups are compared from admission to discharge there is little change in the percentage of injuries in each category and none at subsequent follow-up intervals for the total sample. It therefore appears that these categories lack sensitivity for determining improvement in outcome and are best used for determining epidemiologic patterns over time.

Frankel Classification of Degree of Completeness

The Frankel grade indicates the degree of motor and sensory preservation below the level of injury. Among all the 14,791 persons in the Database, the

Table 9–1 Category of Neurologic Impairment at Admission

Years	Type of Injury			
	PI	PC	TI	TC
1972–1976				
No.	284	555	450	523
%	15.7	30.6	24.8	28.9
1977–1980				
No.	696	1054	1090	968
%	18.3	27.7	28.6	25.4
1981–1984				
No.	734	965	1232	919
%	19.0	25.0	31.9	23.8
1985–1988				
No.	684	873	1076	743
%	20.1	25.7	31.6	21.9
1989–1992				
No.	395	528	532	345
%	21.7	29.0	29.2	18.9
Total				
No.	2793	3975	4380	3498
%	19.0	27.0	29.8	23.8

Note: Table excludes those patients in the Database not given a classification and those classified as normal or as having minimal deficit (145 patients).

distribution for Frankel grade on admission is as follows: grade A (complete) 50.5%; grade B (incomplete, preserved sensation only), 13.2%; grade C (incomplete, preserved motor nonfunctional), 12.9%; and grade D (incomplete, preserved motor functional), 21.6%. Comparison between individuals within the Database admitted within 24 hours of injury and those admitted later showed that those admitted within 24 hours had greater improvement than those admitted after 24 hours. This is especially important to note, since the distribution of Frankel grades on admission were the same for both sets of patients. Across all Frankel grades, 19.7% of persons admitted within 24 hours improved while only 15% of the total group improved.

Table 9–2 shows percentage of change in Frankel grades from the 5658 individuals admitted within 24 hours. For example, in the Frankel grade A category 88.8% remained grade A from admission to discharge, 5% changed to grade B, 2.9% to grade C, and 2.8% to grade D. The degree of improvement was greatest for those admitted with a Frankel grade C, where a majority (53.3%) improved from nonfunctional to functional status. Similarly, 43.9% of persons admitted with a Frankel grade B (sensory only) improved, with 27.6% improving to functional status. Only 10.7% of those admitted with Frankel grade A improved, and only 6.5% with Frankel grade D improved to Frankel grade E (normal motor and sensory function). It must be noted that slightly over 1% declined in function. For the 9133 patients admitted after 24 hours postinjury, of those classified as Frankel grade A, 94.4% remained grade A from admission to discharge. Of those in the Frankel grade B category, 70.2% remained unchanged at discharge. The majority of those classified as Frankel grade C (52.3%) remained grade C on discharge, and only 1.3% of those classified as Frankel grade D improved to Frankel grade E (95.1% remained unchanged). These data suggest that although the impairments are the same on admission, those admitted to the system within 24 hours of injury are less impaired at discharge than those admitted later.

Table 9–2 Percentage Change in Frankel Grades from Admission to Discharge: Admissions within 24 Hours of Injury, 1972–1992

Admission Grade	Discharge Grade					
	A	B	C	D	E	Unknown
A	**88.8**	5.0	2.9	2.8	0	0.6
B	4.9	**48.9**	15.6	27.6	0.7	2.3
C	1.9	0.8	**41.4**	53.3	1.3	1.3
D	0.5	0.5	0.8	**90.3**	6.5	1.4
E	33.3	33.3	0	0	**33.3**	0
Unknown	11.1	8.7	6.4	25.4	4.0	**44.4**

In 1991, a study[9] on drug intervention in acute SCI utilized an improvement of two Frankel grades as indicative of a beneficial outcome. An analysis of the data in the Model SCI Systems Database showed that an improvement of two Frankel grades occurred only in Frankel grade A (4%) and Frankel grade B (19%) injuries, whereas in Frankel grade C it was less than 1% and not possible in Frankel grade D injuries, illustrating a ceiling effect. Improvement determined by changes in Frankel grade is confined to improvement distal to the zone of injury and is not quantitative, nor does it demonstrate improvement within the zone of injury. Improvement within the zone of injury may be functionally significant in a complete injury.[10] Therefore other means of classification may be more useful in determining improvement for complete injuries.

Neurologic Level

Figure 9–1 indicates the distribution of neurologic level of injury in the Database. The most frequently reported neurologic level of injury at discharge is C5 (15.7%). The next most frequent levels are C4 (12.7%) and C6 (12.6%). For persons with paraplegia the most frequent level is T12 (7.6%), followed by L1 (4.7%) and T10 (4.0%). For 84% of persons with SCI, the neurologic level of injury is symmetrical (left equals right) on admission and remains so on discharge; 8% of persons are asymmetrical at admission and remain so at discharge. In 8% of persons with SCI, there is a shift from asymmetrical to symmetrical or vice versa. Examination of those admitted within 24 hours showed that 82% remained symmetrical, 10% were asymmetrical, with an 8% shift. A recent study[11] of 55 persons with complete tetraplegia indicated that 38% were asymmetrical at 1 month and 56% at 1 year, with a 40% shift. The reason for the great disparity between the Database and that study is that in the study by Waters et al.,[11] asymmetry is a reflection of motor index scores (discussed below), which as a 100-point scale will yield greater differences than the 26 individual neurologic levels.

Patterns of change of neurologic level within individuals are useful in predicting functional recovery soon after injury. The Database provides the frequencies of discharge level for each admission level. Overall, for those individuals admitted within 24 hours of injury, 76.2% remain at the same neurologic level from admission to discharge, 12.5% increase one neurologic level, 4.5% increase two levels, and 3.7% decrease one level. This information is most important for admission levels of C4, C5, and C6 (Table 9–3), as these are the most frequent admission levels and relatively small changes at these levels can have great functional implications. In addition, change in level is most important in cases with Frankel grades A and B, since a majority of patients

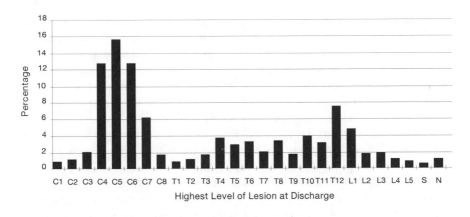

Figure 9–1 Percentage of Patients by Highest Neurologic Level of Lesion at Discharge

admitted with Frankel grades C and D develop functional strength in the lower limbs, making the level less important.

For persons admitted with motor complete C4 injuries (grades A and B) and discharged with motor complete injuries, the two most common discharge levels are C4 (78%) and C5 (18%). For C5, the most common discharge levels are C5 (79%) and C6 (16%); for C6, the most common discharge levels are C6 (84%) and C7 (11%). Thus, the majority of persons admitted with single neurologic

Table 9–3 Admission and Discharge Levels for C4 to C6 Frankel Grades A and B on Admission and at Discharge

	Discharge Level						
Admission Level	C3	C4	C5	C6	C7	C8	Total
C4							
No.	15	691	157	17	2	0	882
%	1.7	78.0	17.7	1.9	0.2	0.0	34.3
C5							
No.	2	33	817	165	12	1	1030
%	0.2	3.2	79.2	16.0	1.2	0.1	40.0
C6							
No.	1	5	20	560	71	4	661
%	0.2	0.8	3.0	84.5	10.7	0.6	25.7
Total							
No.	18	729	994	742	85	5	2573
%	0.7	28.3	38.6	28.8	3.3	0.2	100.0

levels of C4, C5, or C6 motor complete injuries do not change levels when classified by a single neurologic level, despite the commonly held belief that such patients will "gain a level." The single neurologic level in the Database most often reflects the most proximal sensory level, which is usually higher than the motor level. This was illustrated in a recent report[12] showing that of 19 individuals with a single C4 neurologic level, five were C4 motor level, seven were C5 motor level, six were C6 motor level, and one was C7 motor level. Since most investigators[13-15] utilize the motor level rather than the single neurologic or sensory level in predicting functional outcome, use of the single neurologic level may be misleading and represent a less optimistic prognosis.

Studies using classifications other than the single neurologic level suggest that many persons with tetraplegia may indeed improve. Ditunno et al.,[10] Mange et al.,[16,17] and Stauffer[18] all demonstrated a gain of a motor level in subsets of persons admitted with motor complete tetraplegia. However, Eschbach et al.[19] found that a minority of persons with Frankel grade A tetraplegia gain a sensory level.

In summary, it appears likely that only a minority of persons admitted and discharged with motor complete tetraplegia gain a neurologic level. However, this is probably due to lack of sensory recovery. Most persons in this group probably gain a motor level that is functionally important.[12] The database represented here provides only the single neurologic level. Individual motor and sensory level will be reported in the future.

Motor Index Scores

ASIA motor index scores were introduced to the Database as a measure of motor function in 1986, and 3444 cases have been reported that include admission and discharge scores. These data, when divided into individual neurologic levels and Frankel grades, are insufficient to examine motor recovery from admission to discharge. They do, however, allow comparison of larger groups, such as neurologic impairment categories and grouped Frankel grades and grouped neurologic levels. For the entire Database, total motor index scores increased from a mean of 39.8 on admission to 48.6 on discharge, or approximately 9 points per case. This included both complete and incomplete tetraplegic and paraplegic cases.

In an analysis of the increase in motor index scores for the neurologic impairment categories, the improvement from admission to discharge was least for paraplegic complete (mean = 3, median = 1), more for tetraplegic complete (mean = 6, median = 4), greater still for paraplegic incomplete (mean = 11, median = 13), and most for tetraplegic incomplete (mean = 18, median = 13). The largest increase among individuals with incomplete tetraplegia usually reflects both upper and lower extremity improvement at the zone of injury and distal to it. For this reason, it is difficult to estimate how much of this results in muscles achieving a functional grade. The paraplegic complete group, however, showed little improvement (this is probably diminished by the large number of persons with thoracic paraplegia who gain only a sensory level at best), suggesting little if any functional improvement, whereas an 8-point improvement in the legs of a person with incomplete paraplegia should have functional significance for ambulation. The 4-point improvement in complete tetraplegia is not helpful for prognostication unless the initial motor power of a muscle is known. For example, a symmetrical improvement of 2 points each in two 0/5 wrist extensors does not result in increased function. The same improvement, however, in one muscle from 0/5 to 4/5 or in two muscles from 2/5 to 4/5 would yield either unilateral or bilateral functional strength by adding an additional motor level.

A recent study[11] reported a 4.3-point motor score increase in subjects over the initial 4-month postinjury period, which is comparable to the Database. Motor index scores alone, however, do not reflect the number or level of functioning muscles. Although at present no studies have been done that characterize the range of motor index scores for a given neurologic level, Ditunno et al.[10,20] and Waters et al.[11] have determined the number of subjects within a given neurologic level who achieve a functional muscle grade of 3/5. Furthermore, these studies have shown that it may take up to 2 years for individual muscles to achieve a functional grade.

Table 9–4 shows the changes in ASIA motor index scores grouped by Frankel grade (A and B vs. C and D) and grouped neurologic level. There is a consistent

Table 9–4 Average Change in ASIA Motor Index Scores Grouped by Frankel Grades and Neurologic Level

	Level				
Frankel Grades	C1–C4	C5–C8	T1–T6	T7–T12	L1–L5
A and B					
Mean	7.4	9.0	3.8	3.2	7.1
Median	3	6	1	1	5
No.	322	687	400	595	138
C					
Mean	23.1	22.3	17.7	13.3	12.4
Median	17	18	15	10	9.5
No.	107	199	335	105	94
D					
Mean	17.7	16.1	13.3	10.0	9.7
Median	15	13	10	8	8
No.	167	279	105	75	148

trend for persons classified as Frankel grades C and D to show greater improvement in ASIA motor index scores than individuals with motor complete lesions (Frankel grades A and B). For the high tetraplegic grades A and B group, of which 95% are C4, the median improvement is 3 points as compared with 6 points for the low tetraplegic group. Improvement scores in grades C and D groups for persons with high and low tetraplegia are 17 and 15 and 18 and 13 points, respectively, and appear similar to those for the incomplete group as a whole. High thoracic and low thoracic levels yield only a 1-point improvement in the A and B group. The overall increase for persons with complete paraplegia is small, primarily because improvement for this group of individuals is in the sensory levels. Persons with lumbar-level A and B lesions on average improve 5 points, which is probably a functionally significant gain. There were only 11 persons with sacral-level lesions in the Database who had both admission and discharge motor index scores, and these yield too few data points on which to base conclusions. However, since the majority of these persons had motor index scores of 90 points or greater, a ceiling effect for change scores would be seen.

Motor index scores are used as a clinical end point in neuropharmacologic studies.[9,21,22] Virtually all multicenter studies in progress are utilizing the 1992 revised standards of classification and the same motor index score method to document changes in neurologic status. Recent studies[11,23,24] have been reported on motor index score changes during the course of recovery. Motor index scoring is the most quantitative measure of motor function in the Database. As stated above, motor scores have been and will be used in major studies involving intervention. Motor scores are ordinal, rather than interval, and care must be taken to avoid misuse in data interpretation and analysis. Furthermore, different levels of injury have different potential for improvement in motor scores. Therefore, outcome studies involving motor index scores must compare subjects with similar levels.

DISABILITY OUTCOMES

The major goal of rehabilitation is to reduce disability by increasing the independence with which individuals perform activities of daily living. While many measures of functional independence exist, the instrument selected for inclusion in the National SCI Database—the FIM—is currently the most widely used disability measure within rehabilitation. The FIM is an 18-item measure that assesses the degree of independence in areas of self-care, sphincter control, mobility, locomotion, communication, and social cognition.[25,26] Statistical analysis of the FIM has identified two independent measures within the FIM[27]: (1) a motor dimension, including self-care, sphincter control, mobility, and locomotion items, and (2) a cognitive dimension, including the communication and social cognition items. The FIM is an ordinal scale. Formulas for converting raw score totals to 100-point scales employing Rasch analysis have been developed for both the motor and cognitive dimensions.[28] The advantage of utilizing these transformed scores over the raw score totals is based on the ability of Rasch analysis to produce a measure with equal intervals so that assessment of change and parametric statistical analyses can be performed.

Table 9–5 presents the average discharge FIM scores and Rasch measures by level and extent of SCI. Table 9–5 quantifies the degree of independence that is achieved by various groups of individuals with SCI who have been rehabilitated

Table 9–5 Mean Discharge FIM Scores and Measures by Level and Extent of Spinal Cord Injury

Items/Level	Frankel Grades A, B, and C			Frankel Grade D		
	No.	Raw Score	Rasch Measure	No.	Raw Score	Rasch Measure
FIM Motor Items						
C1–C3	48	17.2	15.3	33	67.9	59.5
C4	161	23.8	25.4	93	70.1	62.7
C5	185	32.9	35.4	104	70.2	62.5
C6	145	41.8	41.7	82	70.9	63.2
C7	83	53.2	48.5	53	75.9	66.4
C8	21	65.1	56.3	18	78.4	69.6
Thoracic	716	72.1	60.9	123	80.9	70.1
Lumbar/Sacral	141	75.4	63.8	160	78.8	68.9
FIM Cognitive Items						
C1–C3	48	31.5	84.7	34	32.0	84.9
C4	161	32.1	83.8	98	33.1	87.1
C5	186	32.9	86.2	106	32.8	88.2
C6	151	32.8	86.1	84	33.3	89.3
C7	83	32.8	86.6	53	33.6	90.3
C8	22	34.1	93.8	19	34.3	95.4
Thoracic	728	33.4	89.9	124	33.9	93.4
Lumbar/Sacral	145	33.6	90.5	165	33.5	89.9
FIM Total						
C1–C3	46	48.8		33	100.0	
C4	158	55.9		92	103.7	
C5	184	65.7		103	103.0	
C6	145	74.5		82	104.3	
C7	80	85.5		52	109.4	
C8	21	99.2		18	112.7	
Thoracic	712	105.7		121	114.9	
Lumbar/Sacral	141	108.9		157	112.9	

within the Model Systems program. Tetraplegia is presented by each individual cervical level between C4 and C8 because of substantial FIM differences between these cervical levels. Paraplegia is divided into only two groups, thoracic and lumbar/sacral, because of the similarity in functional outcomes within the individual levels of these two groupings. Similarly, Frankel grades A, B, and C are combined into one category representing all individuals without functional motor preservation because their functional outcomes are similar. On the other hand, Frankel grade D, representing functional motor preservation below the level of injury, is separated because of dramatic differences in functional outcomes occurring within this group.

On discharge, for FIM motor items, clear differences exist at each neurologic level within the Frankel grades A, B, and C classification. Raw scores range from 17.2 at C1 to C3 to 75.4 at the lumbar/sacral level, while Rasch measures range from 15.3 at C1 to C3 to 63.8 at the lumbar/sacral level. In contrast, relatively small differences exist in FIM discharge motor scores by level within the Frankel grade D classification. In either raw score or Rasch measure terms, there is only about a 10-point variation by neurologic level among the Frankel grade D group, and their scores do not vary substantially from individuals with Frankel grade A, B, or C paraplegia.

In comparison to the motor items, the discharge FIM cognitive items show less difference by either level of injury or Frankel grade. All scores are high, indicating that most individuals with SCI have little continuing cognitive deficit. However, persons with high-level tetraplegia have slightly reduced cognitive scores, perhaps indicating a greater frequency of concomitant head injuries in this group. Table 9–5 presents total FIM raw scores, but total FIM Rasch measures are not presented since the addition of Rasch measures across two separate dimensions is viewed as inappropriate.

Table 9–6 summarizes an analysis of FIM gain scores and measures among four groupings of level and extent of SCI: (1) persons with high tetraplegia (C1 to C4) and Frankel grade A, B, or C; (2) persons with low tetraplegia (C5 to C6) and Frankel grade A, B, or C; (3) persons with paraplegia and Frankel grade A, B, or C; and (4) all individuals with Frankel grade D.

Both raw score and Rasch measure means are presented at admission and discharge along with the FIM gain (change score) and length of stay efficiency (gain per day length of stay). Gains among FIM motor items range from high tetraplegia, with a raw score gain of 8.9 and a Rasch measure gain of 21.4, to the Frankel D group, with a raw score gain of 39.3 and a Rasch measure gain of 32.1. Efficiency in terms of FIM motor item gains per day are lowest for the high tetraplegia group and highest for those with Frankel grade D. While FIM cognitive gains are less than FIM motor gains, as would be expected among individuals with spinal cord injury, the gains that do occur are somewhat larger

Table 9–6 Analysis of FIM Gain Scores and Measures by Level and Extent of Spinal Cord Injury

Item	*Frankel Grades A, B, or C*			*Frankel Grade D*	*Total*
	High Tetraplegia	*Low Tetraplegia*	*Paraplegia*		
No. of Patients	201	418	813	647	2079
Mean Rehabilitation Length of Stay (Days)	93.4	99.8	54.9	50.3	66.2
FIM Motor Items					
Admission					
Raw Score Mean	13.4	16.3	33.3	35.3	28.6
Measure Mean	1.8	9.7	35.6	33.3	26.4
Discharge					
Raw Score Mean	22.4	41.2	72.7	74.6	62.1
Measure Mean	23.2	40.9	61.5	65.5	54.9
Gain					
Raw Score Mean	8.9	24.9	39.4	39.3	33.5
Measure Mean	21.4	31.2	25.8	32.1	28.5
Efficiency (Gain/Day)					
Raw Score Mean	0.10	0.25	0.72	0.78	0.51
Measure Mean	0.23	0.31	0.47	0.64	0.43
FIM Cognitive Items					
Admission					
Raw Score Mean	28.8	29.4	31.3	31.4	30.7
Measure Mean	71.7	73.9	80.8	80.6	78.5
Discharge					
Raw Score Mean	31.9	32.8	33.5	33.4	33.2
Measure Mean	84.3	86.5	90.0	89.7	88.7
Gain					
Raw Score Mean	3.2	3.4	2.2	1.9	2.4
Measure Mean	12.6	12.7	9.2	9.1	10.2
Efficiency (Gain/Day)					
Raw Score Mean	0.03	0.03	0.04	0.04	0.04
Measure Mean	0.13	0.13	0.17	0.19	0.16
FIM Total (All Items)					
Admission, Raw Score Mean	42.1	45.9	64.8	66.8	59.5
Discharge, Raw Score Mean	54.5	73.6	106.2	107.9	95.3
Gain, Raw Score Mean	12.4	27.8	41.5	41.2	35.9
Efficiency, Raw Score Mean	0.13	0.28	0.76	0.84	0.55

in the high tetraplegia group and decrease with less severe levels of injury. While raw score FIM totals are presented in Table 9–6, the Rasch measure motor and cognitive dimensions are more appropriate for interpretation.

CONCLUSION

The use of impairment and disability measures to determine clinical outcomes in SCI is necessary for accurate prognosis, for determination of the effects of interventions, and for cost justifications for hospital care. This chapter has shown that there is an improvement from admission to discharge in impairment measures, as demonstrated by changes in Frankel grades, neurologic levels, and motor scores. Within the classification of Frankel grades and neurologic levels, these changes appear to be greater for those patients admitted to the System within 24 hours of injury. Data on ASIA motor index scores suggest that those patients admitted with Frankel grades C and D (motor incomplete injuries) will show greater improvement than those classified on admission as Frankel grade A or B (motor complete injuries). The FIM data demonstrated a relationship between disability and impairment as categorized by neurologic level and Frankel grade. This relationship extends to FIM gain scores from admission to discharge. Those gains in FIM scores from admission to discharge from rehabilitation are related to extent and severity of injury.

REFERENCES

1. Young JS, Burns PE, Bowen AM, McCutchen R. *Spinal Cord Injury Statistics: Experience of Regional Model Spinal Cord Injury Systems.* Phoenix, Ariz: Good Samaritan Medical Center; 1982.

2. Frankel HL, Hancock DO, Hyslop G, et al. Value of postural reduction in the initial management of closed injuries of the spine with paraplegia and tetraplegia. *Paraplegia.* 1969;7:179–192.

3. Stover SL, Fine PR, eds. *Spinal Cord Injury: The Facts and Figures.* Birmingham, Ala: University of Alabama at Birmingham; 1986.

4. *International Standards for Neurological and Functional Classification of Spinal Cord Injury—Revised 1992.* Chicago: American Spinal Injury Association; 1992.

5. American Spinal Injury Association. *Standards for Neurological Classification of Injury.* Chicago: American Spinal Injury Association; 1982.

6. American Spinal Injury Association. *Standards for Neurological Classification of Injury.* Chicago: American Spinal Injury Association; 1989.

7. Michaelis LS. International inquiry on neurological terminology and prognosis in paraplegia and tetraplegia. *Paraplegia.* 1969;7:1–5.

8. Stover SL. Benefits of the model spinal cord injury system of care. In: Apple DF, Hudson LM, eds. *Spinal Cord Injury: The Model. Proceedings of the National Consensus Conference on*

Catastrophic Illness and Injury, December, 1989. Atlanta: Georgia Regional Spinal Cord Injury Care System; 1990.

9. Geisler FJ, Dorsey FC, Coleman WP. Recovery of motor function after spinal-cord injury: A randomized, placebo-controlled trial with gm-1 ganglioside. *N Engl J Med.* 1991;324:1829–1838.

10. Ditunno JF Jr, Sipski ML, Posuniak EA, Chen YT, Staas WE Jr, Herbison GJ. Wrist extensor recovery in traumatic quadriplegia. *Arch Phys Med Rehabil.* 1987;68:287–290.

11. Waters RL, Adkins RH, Yakura JS, Sie I. Motor and sensory recovery following complete tetraplegia. *Arch Phys Med Rehabil.* 1993;74:242–247.

12. Rider-Foster D, Marino R, Segal M, Ditunno JF Jr. Superiority of motor level over single neurologic level in motor complete quadriplegics. *J Am Paraplegia Soc.* 1993;16:103.

13. Freed MM. Traumatic and congenital lesions of the spinal cord. In: Kottke FJ, Lehmann JF, eds. *Krusen's Handbook of Physical Medicine and Rehabilitation.* 4th ed. Philadelphia: WB Saunders; 1990.

14. Yarkony GM, Roth EJ, Meyer PR, Lovell LL, Heinemann AW. Rehabilitation outcomes in complete C5 quadriplegia. *Am J Phys Med Rehabil.* 1988;67:73–76.

15. Ditunno JF, Graziani V. Motor recovery and functional prognosis in spinal cord injury. *Rehabil Rep.* 1989;5:no 5.

16. Mange KC, Ditunno JF Jr, Herbison GJ, Jaweed MM. Recovery of strength at the zone of injury in motor complete and motor incomplete cervical spinal cord injured patients. *Arch Phys Med Rehabil.* 1990;71:562–565.

17. Mange KC, Marino RJ, Gregory PC, Herbison GJ, Ditunno JF Jr. Course of motor recovery in the zone of partial preservation in spinal cord injury. *Arch Phys Med Rehabil.* 1992;73:437–441.

18. Stauffer ES. Neurologic recovery following injuries to the cervical spinal cord and nerve roots. *Spine.* 1984;9:532–534.

19. Eschbach KS, Herbison GJ, Ditunno JF Jr. Sensory root level recovery in patients with Frankel A quadriplegia. *Arch Phys Med Rehabil.* 1992;73:618–622.

20. Ditunno JF Jr, Stover SL, Freed MM, Ahn JH. Motor recovery of the upper extremities in traumatic quadriplegia: A multicenter study. *Arch Phys Med Rehabil.* 1992;73:431–436.

21. Bracken MB, Shepard MJ, Collins WF, et al. A randomized controlled trial of methylpred-nisolone or naloxone in the treatment of acute spinal-cord injury. *N Engl J Med.* 1990;322:1405–1411.

22. Bracken MB, Shepard MJ, Collins WF, et al. Methylprednisolone or naloxone treatment after acute spinal cord injury: 1-year follow-up data. *J Neurosurg.* 1992;76:23–31.

23. Blaustein DM, Zafonte R, Thomas D, Herbison GJ, Ditunno JF Jr. Predicting recovery of motor complete quadriplegic patients: 24 hour vs. 72 hour motor index scores. *Am J Phys Med Rehabil.* 1993;72:306–311.

24. Herbison GJ, Zerby SA, Cohen ME, Marino RJ, Ditunno JF Jr. Motor power differences within the first two weeks post-SCI in cervical spinal cord injured quadriplegia. *J Neurotrauma.* 1992;9:373–380.

25. Hamilton BB, Granger CV, Sherwin FS, Zielezny M, Tashman JS. A uniform national data system for medical rehabilitation. In: Fuhrer MJ, ed. *Rehabilitation Outcomes Analysis and Measurement.* Baltimore: Paul H. Brookes; 1987:137–147.

26. *Guide for the Use of the Uniform Data Set for Medical Rehabilitation.* Buffalo, NY: Center for Functional Assessment Research, State University of New York at Buffalo; 1990.

27. Linacre JM, Heinemann AW, Wright BD, Granger CV, Hamilton BB. *The Functional Independence Measure as a Measure of Disability: Research Report 9-01*. Chicago: Rehabilitation Services Evaluation Unit, Rehabilitation Institute of Chicago; 1991.

28. Heinemann AW, Linacre JM, Wright BD, Hamilton BB, Granger CV. Relationships between impairment and physical disability as measured by the Functional Independence Measure. *Arch Phys Med Rehabil.* 1993;74:566–573.

10

The Aftermath of Spinal Cord Injury

Marcel P. Dijkers, Michelle Buda Abela, Bruce M. Gans,
and Wayne A. Gordon

INTRODUCTION

In its consequences, a spinal cord injury (SCI) is like a stone thrown in a pond: increasingly wider areas of the lives of the persons involved, and those around them, are affected. The impairment that is immediately obvious (mostly sensory and muscle control deficits) results in the limitation or even total loss of the ability to perform common tasks such as self-care and walking (see Chapter 9). These abilities, in turn, commonly result in restrictions of role fulfillment as a worker, student, parent, citizen, or other status. Sometimes these disadvantages are due not so much to disability as to societal reactions: negative attitudes and discrimination toward people with a disability, which may be triggered by the mere fact of impairment. The person with SCI has to cope not just with a changed body image, new ways of doing things, and increased reliance on others for the performance of common tasks, but also with changes in his or her social roles and interactions.

Family and friends become involved in this, as caregivers or providers of emotional, spiritual, or monetary support. But sometimes the social network fails to provide support or, even worse, falls away. Failure of a marriage and the dwindling of relationships with friends at work or in recreational pursuits add to the burden, thus making adjustment all the more difficult.

This chapter provides information on various aspects of disadvantage due to impairment and disability—the effects of SCI on place of residence, employment, educational opportunities, and marital status. While there are other areas of disadvantage as a result of SCI, for instance access to (public) transportation

The authors gratefully acknowledge the contribution of Dr. Michael DeVivo, who supplied the numbers on which Figures 10–8 and 10–9 are based.

185

and recreational activities, the ones examined here are among the most important ones and are better documented. This chapter also deals with how the person with SCI "adjusts" to the injury and comes to accept it, or, to the contrary, has trouble living with a changed body and in changed circumstances to the degree that suicide is seen as the only way out. Issues of adaptation and adjustment have had much attention in the SCI literature, discussed under such concepts as depression,[1-3] acceptance of disability,[4] self-concept,[5] and coping.[6] Medical and vocational rehabilitation, including the efforts of social workers and psychologists, aim to minimize disability and disadvantage and assist the person in attaining independence, adjustment, and quality of life. The information presented here on Model System outcomes indicates that in a number of aspects, and for most cases, rehabilitation efforts have been successful.

RESIDENCE

One of the major differences rehabilitation has made in the lives of persons with SCI over the last 50 years is keeping them out of chronic disease hospitals and other types of institutions by making it possible for them to live in the community. Community living is the basis for many other changes in opportunities, activities, and behaviors that have occurred over the last half century.

The data in the National SCI Database show that upon discharge from initial rehabilitation, the vast majority of persons with SCI (92.3%) are discharged to private residences in the community. A very small percentage are admitted to hospitals (including mental hospitals) (1.4%) or nursing homes (including custodial care hospitals) (4.0%). Some of the others go to group living facilities (e.g., dormitories, camps, correctional institutions), usually for reasons other than medical or personal care needs (1.9%).

Nowadays, persons with SCI are admitted to a nursing home or other institutional setting (either after completing rehabilitation or later on during the postinjury years) for one of two reasons: their self-care and health care needs exceed that which they and their family, friends, or employee caregivers can provide, or they lack a social support system (family or personal care attendants) altogether. Once they enter the institution, they have assured access to medical, nursing, and other care. Institutionalization, however, almost always imposes restrictions over and above those due to the impairment or disability itself, including restricted access to community settings; limitations on the number and variety of social interactions (including those with potential romantic/sexual partners); impoverishment of the number and/or quality of social roles played; and decreased self-determination, independence, and privacy.

The literature on nursing homes as discharge destinations for persons with SCI is limited. Most authors stress how existing nursing homes, designed and staffed for care of the elderly with multiple chronic debilitating problems, are less suitable for persons with SCI, who tend to be young, relatively healthy, and in need of ongoing rehabilitative services.[7,8] Even for elderly SCI persons, nursing homes have been considered "unfavorable discharge placements."[9]

According to National Database information, the percentage of individuals discharged to a nursing home or hospital is higher in the older age groups: it rises steadily from 2.1% of those under age 20 to 28.6% for those over age 70 at injury. This may reflect both greater personal care needs due to other health problems and disabilities, and lack of a support system. Higher rates of nursing home placement for elderly persons with SCI have been reported previously.[9,10]

Because of both age and the availability of a family caregiver, institutionalization rates are higher among divorced (9.0%), separated (10.6%), and especially widowed (24.3%) persons than among single (4.4%) or married (4.1%) ones. Care needs result in higher rates of institutionalization for those with tetraplegia (7.5%) than for those with paraplegia (3.3%), and higher rates for persons with complete injuries than for those with incomplete ones. In earlier studies, absence of a wife or parent as caregiver and level of injury (C6 or above) had been identified as determinants of nursing home placement.[9,11] Fuhrer et al.[12] reported that tetraplegic individuals who were dependent on a ventilator were more likely to live in a nursing home or hospital.

Over the years the percentage of persons with SCI discharged to a hospital has declined (from 2.3% in 1972–1976 to 0.8% in 1987–1992). Nursing home discharges, however, have remained relatively constant, the National Database information indicates.

Changes in economic, medical, and social circumstances in the years following discharge may result in changes in residence. Of those initially discharged to a hospital, four out of six (66.4%) move to a community residence (including private residence, group facility, and "other"), and one out of six (16.8%) moves to a nursing home by 1 year after injury. Of those initially discharged to a nursing home, one out of three (31.8%) moves to a community residence, and one out of twenty (4.5%) is admitted to a long-stay hospital. A very small group of those initially discharged to the community changes residence to either a hospital (0.6%) or a nursing home (0.8%) within that first year. The same pattern occurs in each subsequent year, although on a somewhat smaller scale. On the whole, the percentage of persons residing in nursing homes and hospitals declines over successive anniversaries of the injury, and the percentage living in a private residence or other community setting increases (Figure 10–1). A rough estimate of the total percentage of all persons with SCI living in a medical setting would be 2.6 (average over the percentages from discharge through year 15). This is

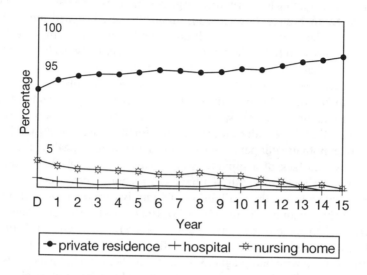

Figure 10–1 Percentage of Persons Living in Each Type of Residence, by Anniversary Year

similar to the finding of a 1988 study conducted for the Paralyzed Veterans of America.[13]

The National Database contains additional information suggesting that nursing home residence often is a temporary status. Based on the reported number of nursing home days in the preceding year, the percentage of persons who had been full-year or part-year nursing home residents was calculated for each year of follow-up (Figure 10–2). During the first few years, part-year stays in a nursing home were more common than full-year stays; in years 4 and later, each year about the same number of stays are full-year as are part-year. Over the years, the total percentage of persons spending *any* time in a nursing home declines from 4.4% (at the first anniversary) to 1.0% (at the 15th anniversary).

EMPLOYMENT

Few studies have evaluated comprehensively to what degree persons with SCI performed productive roles preinjury, and when and to what degree they reestablished them after injury. Family roles (other than the facts of marriage and divorce) and volunteer activities have been largely neglected in previous studies. There are a few investigations of educational accomplishments and recreational

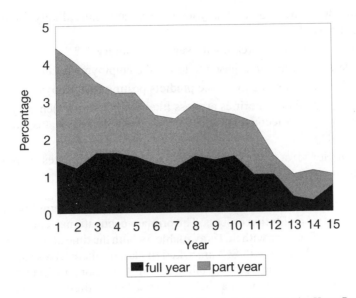

Figure 10–2 Percentage of Persons Who Were Part-Year or Full-Year Nursing Home Residents, by Anniversary Year

---

pursuits. However, based on a narrow definition of productivity, most research has concentrated on vocational issues.

Return to work is often used as an indicator of overall recovery from illness or injury. At one time, employment was even equated with rehabilitation success.[14] Re-employment figures reported in the literature vary tremendously (by when the study was done, sample composition in terms of age, time since injury, and neurologic category, and by definition of employment, etc.). Trieschmann cites a range from 13% to 48%.[15] There is also much variation in the factors, both preinjury (education, employment) and postinjury (neurologic category, receipt of vocational rehabilitation services, etc.), reported to be associated with employment. Small samples, self-selection of subjects, retrospective designs, and other methodologic problems make it difficult to compare results. However, a few generalizations may be made, based on more recent studies:

- Paraplegics have higher (re)employment rates than tetraplegics; and within both categories, those with incomplete injuries are more likely to be employed.[16,17]

- Those who incur SCI at a younger age are more likely to become (re)employed.[16-19]
- Employment rates increase with years after injury.[19,20]
- The less education preinjury, the lower the employment rate.[16,19,20]
- Preinjury vocational experience predicts postinjury employment.[20]
- Blacks and other minorities are less likely to become (re)employed,[16,18,20] even taking into account age, education, gender, marital status, and neurologic category.[16]
- Completion of a vocational rehabilitation program makes employment more likely.[16]

The National SCI Database contains limited information on employment and the vocational rehabilitation process. The primary occupational, educational, or training status of persons with SCI is available for both the time of injury and each follow-up year. Persons with SCI are asked to classify themselves as: working in the competitive labor market (including the military), homemaking, receiving on-the-job training, working in a sheltered workshop, retired, studying, unemployed, or "other" (including volunteering, on disability or medical leave, etc). It should be noted that these categories are not mutually exclusive, and that the primary status is selected by the person involved on the basis of his or her *judgment* as to what is primary.

Primary status at injury, for males and females of various ages, is reflected in Table 10–1. Overall, close to two thirds of the males were working, as were slightly less than half the females. In addition, one out of ten females was a homemaker. It is noteworthy that among both males and females, close to one out of six persons considered himself or herself unemployed.

For those who are working, homemaking, or attending school, an SCI generally forces at least temporary discontinuation of these productive activities. This major change in primary status occurring from injury to the first anniversary of injury is reflected in Table 10–2. Whereas preinjury over 60% were working, afterward the most frequently reported status is unemployed (61.9%). By the first anniversary of injury only 16.0% of those working at the time of injury have returned to work. About 8% of them have entered school, and more than 71% consider themselves unemployed. In contrast, almost half of those who were homemakers at the time of injury resumed that role (48.9%), and over 70% of those who were students have resumed their education or at least consider themselves students.

Some of the major determinants of primary vocational status at the first anniversary confirm the findings of earlier studies. (Re)employment declines with age at injury (excluding some of the younger-age categories, where return to school is common) from 15.8% for the 30- to 39-year-old group to 4.9% for

Table 10-1 Primary Vocational Status at Injury, by Gender and Age at Injury

Age at Injury	Primary Vocational Status						No. of Cases
	Working	Homemaker	Retired	Student	Unemployed	Other	
Total	60.1	2.3	3.4	18.8	14.4	1.0	14,244
Males							
0–15	1.1	0.0	0.0	90.8	6.6	1.5	458
16–30	59.9	0.1	0.0	23.7	15.6	0.7	7,165
31–45	83.4	0.2	0.2	0.4	14.7	1.2	2,488
46–60	82.1	0.1	4.8	0.0	11.6	1.4	1,073
61–75	37.6	0.2	56.3	0.0	5.2	0.7	442
76+	7.3	1.2	87.8	0.0	1.2	2.4	82
Total	63.4	0.1	3.3	18.1	14.2	0.9	11,708
Females							
0–15	0.5	0.0	0.5	88.0	5.8	5.2	191
16–30	46.6	8.0	0.0	27.9	17.0	0.4	1,355
31–45	64.1	16.8	0.0	1.5	16.4	1.2	518
46–60	52.5	23.3	5.2	0.4	15.9	3.0	270
61–75	17.9	29.8	43.5	0.0	7.7	1.2	168
76+	2.9	38.2	55.9	0.0	2.9	0.0	34
Total	44.8	12.7	4.2	21.9	15.1	1.3	2,536

the 70+ group. Males are as likely as females to be employed (10.9% and 10.0%, respectively). About one out of ten females describes herself as a homemaker; males are not likely to claim that as their primary status (0.2%), and instead opt for unemployed more often (64.3%, versus 50.2% for females). Members of minorities are less likely to be employed.

Persons with paraplegia are slightly more likely to be employed (13.2%) or to be a homemaker (2.8%) than those with tetraplegia (8.6% and 1.6%, respectively). Similarly, those with incomplete injuries work more often than those whose injury is incomplete. However, these differences are surprisingly small.

Education level makes more of a difference in primary status at the first anniversary than any other factor. Among those over 25 years of age (a group that presumably has completed its education), the percentage working at the first anniversary ranges from 3.9% for those with less than a ninth-grade education to 52.9% among those with a doctoral degree. (Age may have a minor effect on these numbers, as the elder persons are more likely to have received a limited education and are less likely to return to work.) This finding suggests that better-

Table 10–2   Primary Vocational Status at 1 Year Postinjury by Vocational Status
Preinjury

Preinjury Primary Status	First Anniversary Primary Status						
	Working	Home-maker	Retired	Student	Unem-ployed	Other	No. of Cases
Working	16.0	1.4	1.7	8.2	71.3	1.4	6,432
Homemaker	2.2	48.9	3.5	1.7	43.7	0.0	231
Retired	0.6	0.6	87.7	0.3	10.3	0.6	349
Student	3.2	0.3	0.0	70.7	25.3	0.4	2,065
Unemployed	2.6	1.2	0.8	6.9	87.5	0.9	1,451
Other	3.8	0.0	1.3	15.0	53.8	26.3	80
Total	10.8	2.2	4.1	19.8	61.9	1.2	10,608

educated persons may have vocational roles that provide them with either more support or more environmental flexibility to facilitate their return to work.

Changes in primary vocational status occur continuously after the first anniversary of injury. Of those who at any anniversary describe themselves as working, the next year about 1% will retire, 4% to 6% (in the early years after injury) to 1% (later on) will become students, and 9% to 12% will become unemployed. Of those selecting "student" as primary vocational status, a year later 5% to 10% (in the early years) to 15% (in years 6 onward) will describe themselves as working, and 15% as unemployed. Of those considering "unemployed" the proper label for their status, a year later 1% will select homemaker, 5% to 6% working, 1% retired, and 5% to 11% (in the first 5 years) to 2% (in later years) student. However, after the major changes occurring from preinjury to the first anniversary, stability is more common: from 1 year to the next, at least 79% of those selecting working do so again; for "student," the percentage is at least 58%; and for "unemployed," 80%.

Thus, changes in vocational status appear to be most common in the earlier years after injury, with the exception of leaving the student status. The end results, for both males and females, are employment rates that increase steadily to reach a peak of 32% at about 10 years after injury for males and of 33% at year 11 for females (Figures 10–3 and 10–4).

For those who are interested in and a likely candidate for becoming productive after an SCI (whether working, homemaking, going to school, or just living independently), testing, counseling, and other services are available through each state's Department of Vocational Rehabilitation (DVR), with funds supplied (in part) by the federal Rehabilitation Services Administration (RSA). Information on services from DVR is included in the National SCI Databank, but

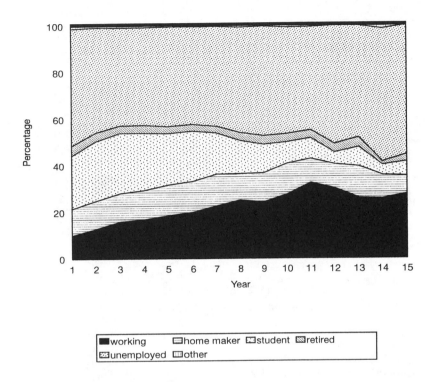

Figure 10–3 Primary Status at Each Anniversary Year, Females

it is limited to whether or not at each point in time the person was evaluated for and/or actually did receive services. On admission to the Model System, 7.5% of all cases are DVR clients. Except for those who were admitted after receiving longer-duration acute and rehabilitation medical services in "pre-System" hospital(s), these services must have been unrelated to the SCI (e.g., for re-employment after mental illness), and as such this figure constitutes a baseline. At the time they enter the rehabilitation care component of the Model System, 13.2% of all cases are DVR clients. As a realistic evaluation of potential for productive roles is most often not possible until the person has entered the rehabilitation phase, it is not surprising that the percentage of DVR clients jumps to 45.9% of all cases by discharge from inpatient rehabilitation. Thereafter, the percentage classified as DVR client is somewhat smaller at the first anniversary of injury, and declines steadily after that (see Figure 10–5).

Table 10–3 reflects the association between receiving DVR services (at the time of discharge from inpatient rehabilitation) and other factors. Males are clients slightly more often than females (possibly reflecting the higher mean age

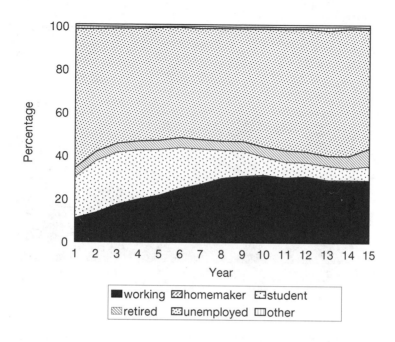

Figure 10–4 Primary Status at Each Anniversary Year, Males

at injury for females). Those in the prime years for return to employment (16 to 30 and 31 to 45) receive services more often. Whites receive services somewhat more often than any other racial or ethnic group. Those with an incomplete injury are clients less often than those with a complete injury, but there is very little difference between those with paraplegia and those with tetraplegia. Persons who were employed or unemployed before injury, or were students, are more likely to receive services than homemakers and retired persons. Finally, only those with an associate's degree at injury (a small group) and those with an eighth-grade education or less stood out as being clients at this time less often than others. The latter group includes many elderly people and youngsters still in school at the time of injury. Both are less likely to be accepted as DVR clients.

Of those who at the time of system discharge were *not* clients, 14.6% became so by the first anniversary. The percentage becoming a client (whether for the first time or returning for assistance) declines at each anniversary thereafter, from 11.1% in year 2 to 3.5% in year 15. On the other hand, of those who were

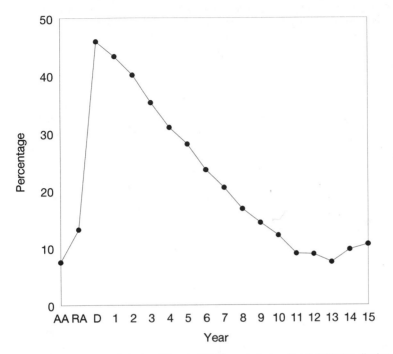

Note: AA, acute care admission; RA, rehabilitation admission; D, rehabilitation discharge.

Figure 10–5 Percentage of Persons Who Are DVR Clients, by Anniversary Year

---

clients at discharge, one fifth (22.2%) completes services (or drops out) by the first anniversary. Terminations as a percentage of the active caseload slowly increase each year thereafter, to peak at about 39% in years 11 to 13. A very small percentage of persons receive DVR services for the first time many years after injury: 1% between the sixth and tenth anniversary of injury, and one tenth of that after the tenth anniversary. Fully 41% have never availed themselves of DVR services at the time of their last follow-up.

EDUCATION

Educational accomplishments postinjury have generally been considered by researchers as part of vocational activities, and as such the focus has been on whether the person with SCI was in school, not on what educational level he or

Table 10–3 Percentages of Persons Who Were DVR Clients at Discharge from Inpatient Rehabilitation, by Age, Gender, Race/Ethnic Group, Preinjury Education, Neurologic Category, and Preinjury Primary Status

	DVR Status		
	Not a Client	Client	No. of Cases
Total	54.1	45.9	11,917
Age Category			
0–15	88.4	11.6	606
16–30	43.7	56.3	7,045
31–45	56.9	43.1	2,476
46–60	70.9	29.1	1,138
61–75	93.6	6.4	548
76+	99.0	1.0	104
Gender			
Male	53.3	46.7	9,735
Female	57.4	42.6	2,183
Race/Ethnic Group			
White	50.8	49.2	8,501
Nonwhite	62.2	37.8	3,401
Education			
8th Grade or Less	72.1	27.9	1,457
9th–11th Grade	54.9	45.1	3,284
High School/GED	46.6	53.4	5,694
Associate's Degree	69.4	30.6	147
Bachelor's Degree	52.3	47.7	639
Master's or Doctorate Degree	58.5	41.5	229
Other	57.8	42.2	45
Neurologic Category			
Paraplegia, Incomplete	58.7	41.3	2,418
Paraplegia, Complete	49.6	50.4	3,147
Tetraplegia, Incomplete	56.0	44.0	3,800
Tetraplegia, Complete	51.4	48.6	2,455
Preinjury Primary Status			
Working	49.2	50.8	7,050
Homemaker	70.1	29.9	298
Retired	97.3	2.7	437
Student	54.1	45.9	2,323
Unemployed	58.5	41.5	1,653
Other	73.3	26.7	116

she started at, nor on what was the highest level attained.[15,16] (One prior report based on the National SCI Database constitutes an exception.[21]) At best, preinjury education level is considered a predictor of success of return to work.[20,22] As shown above, level of education accomplished is a very significant factor for return to work (or first employment, for those who never held a full-time job preinjury), because the disabilities generally resulting from SCI make it highly unlikely, if not impossible, for the person to have a job that requires mobility (e.g., mail carrier), physical strength (e.g., stonecutter), or both. Those occupations that require the least manipulation of objects and least mobility (generally, selected clerical and technical jobs, and most managerial and professional positions) require the highest level of education. Thus it is to be expected that persons with a higher level of education preinjury are more likely to return to work, and that those with a limited education preinjury return to school more often than their peers without SCI. Finally, it would be expected that those in school at the time of injury achieve a higher educational level (after an interruption) than their peers or than they themselves planned preinjury.

For the time of injury and each anniversary thereafter, the SCI Database has information on the highest level of education accomplished at that time. This information is classified as 8th grade or less, 9th through 11th grades, high school diploma or GED, associate's degree, bachelor's degree, master's degree, doctoral degree, or other. Of all cases entered into the National Database, at the time of their latest follow-up 15.1% had improved their education from the level at injury (Table 10–4). As expected, the change is most pronounced for those under age 17 at the time of injury (in most states the age compulsory education ends). Of those who were 17 through 25 years old at injury, 19.3% improve their grade level, as do 6.2% of those who were at least 26 at the time they incurred their SCI. Gender makes little difference in educational improvement for any age group. Race does make a difference: whites more frequently than nonwhites improve their grade level. Except in the highest age group, tetraplegics achieve a higher level of education more often than do paraplegics, and those with complete injuries do so more often than those with incomplete injuries. This presumably reflects their *need* to obtain a higher level of education, rather than ability or other factors.

The cumulative effect of education level changes after injury is reflected in Figure 10–6. The average education level attained at each anniversary year increases gradually. The education level of those for whom 15th anniversary data are available is better than that of the U.S. population as a whole.[23] Selective dropout from the study due to mortality or other factors may contribute to the picture of continued educational change. However, analysis of education level change for those for whom fifth and tenth anniversary data are available confirms this. At 5 years after injury, the education level of individuals with SCI is

Table 10–4 Percentages of Persons with Postdischarge Improvement in Education, by Age at Injury and Gender, Race/Ethnic Group, Education at Injury, and Neurologic Impairment Category

	Age at Injury							
	Under 17		17–25		26 or Over		Total	
	%	No. of Cases	%	No. of Cases	%	No. of Cases	%	No. of Cases
Total	49.3	1,153	19.3	6,008	6.2	7,151	15.1	14,312
Gender								
Males	49.6	856	19.3	5,117	6.2	5,792	15.0	11,765
Females	48.5	297	19.4	891	6.0	1,359	15.7	2,547
Race/Ethnic Group								
White	54.4	857	22.0	4,401	6.8	4,782	17.5	10,040
Nonwhite	35.3	292	11.9	1,605	5.0	2,351	9.7	4,248
Education Level at Injury								
8th Grade or Less	50.6	425	11.9	278	6.3	982	18.4	1,685
9th–11th Grades	49.6	708	33.0	1,916	10.2	1,281	28.6	3,905
High School/GED	*	5	13.0	3,438	4.5	3,405	8.8	6,848
Associate's Degree	—	0	12.5	56	13.3	120	13.1	176
Bachelor's Degree	—	0	11.5	182	6.6	606	7.7	788
Master's Degree	—	0	*	8	6.2	162	5.9	170
Doctoral Degree	—	0	*	2	3.3	92	3.2	94
Other	*	4	60.0	20	44.9	49	47.9	73
Neurologic Impairment Category								
Paraplegia, Incomplete	38.8	196	14.5	1,162	5.5	1,558	11.3	2,916
Paraplegia, Complete	44.3	291	18.6	1,657	7.4	1,845	15.1	3,793
Tetraplegia, Incomplete	53.7	367	21.0	1,666	5.2	2,451	15.1	4,484
Tetraplegia, Complete	56.6	288	22.5	1,468	7.3	1,247	19.4	3,003

*Less than 10 cases.

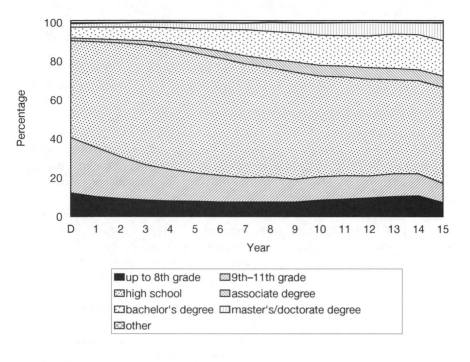

Figure 10–6 Education Level Completed, by Anniversary Year

somewhat less than that of the U.S. population as a whole (which is much older, on average); at 10 years, it is somewhat higher. Thus, these data suggest a delay and prolongation of the education process.

MARITAL STATUS

It is natural to assume that if one of the partners incurs an SCI, a tremendous strain will be placed on a marriage. A number of the direct or indirect consequences of SCI are known to be stressors for both spouses and for marriage, and may result in increased chances of separation and divorce. These include the injured partner's limited capacity to fulfill household and child care tasks; his or her care needs; reduced mobility, resulting in reduction of outings and social contacts; loss of social supports; financial pressures and a lowered standard of living; changes in sexual functioning; job loss (and the resulting loss of social status); assumption of the stigmatized disabled status; and last but not least, psychologic adjustment problems.

Abrams[24] concluded that there is no evidence that SCI has a devastating effect on marriages. Studies that compare the divorce rate of marriages in which one partner had incurred an SCI with the U.S. population divorce rate seem to confirm this.[25,26] Two authors even claimed that the divorce rate is lower for the SCI population.[27,28] However, these studies may be criticized for methodologic weaknesses. An earlier analysis of National SCI Database information concluded that in the first 3 years after injury, divorce was at least 2.3 times as frequent as would have been expected on the basis of U.S. population statistics.[29] The slight increase this study reported in the number of divorces each year after injury suggests that these are *not* divorces that would have occurred anyway, but were "delayed" because of the injury.

In previous research several factors have been found to be associated with SCI divorce: age at injury[30] (young persons were more likely to divorce), gender[30,31] and race (females and blacks more frequently get divorced), prior divorce,[25] childlessness,[32] and a more severe injury.[32] The influence of age, race, prior divorce, and childlessness on SCI divorce rates is similar to their effects for the general population.

It is likely that SCI plays a role in the chances single or divorced persons have in marrying after injury. The state of poverty many persons with SCI live in is only one factor in this. More important are the impoverishment of their social life due to mobility problems and abandonment by old friends; the prejudice and stigma existing vis-à-vis persons with a disability, which culminates in rejection of those with SCI as a marriage prospect; and psychologic adjustment problems in the early years after injury, which may distract one from matters of romance.

Research on marriage rates after SCI is limited to one study based on National SCI Database information.[29] It found that among persons who were single at the time of injury, significantly fewer marriages occurred in the first 3 years postinjury than would have been expected based on age- and sex-specific first-marriage rates for the U.S. population. The decreasing frequency of marriages over these 3 years suggests that some of the marriages were planned preinjury and the wedding took place without much delay. Research on remarriage among those who were separated, divorced, or widowed at the time of injury is lacking altogether.

A number of studies have compared preinjury marriages of SCI persons with those occurring postinjury and have found that the latter tend to be better[32,33] and less likely to result in divorce.[32–34] While the spinal injury and its consequences may constitute the same type of challenge or burden in postinjury marriages, it is one that is not *imposed* on the noninjured partner, but freely chosen. In addition, it would appear that those who get married post-SCI are a select group, more motivated for independence and better adjusted psychologically with more inner-directedness,[31] higher educational achievement, and more likely to be working.[35] There is evidence to suggest that it is not marriage that enhances the

SCI person, but that "only individuals who are especially likable, active and well adjusted succeed in attracting partners."[33] As a consequence, postinjury marriages are happier,[31] and the injured partners report more satisfaction with their sex lives, living arrangements, health, emotional adjustment, and social lives.[33,35]

As expected, the divorce rate for postinjury marriages has been reported in one study to be not different from the overall U.S. divorce rate.[32] However, a previous analysis of National SCI Database information indicated that in 8 years of follow-up, postinjury marriages were more likely to result in divorce than expected, given age and sex-specific US rates (44% vs. 23%). Males and those marrying a second time were more likely to see their postinjury marriage end in divorce.[32]

The National SCI Database contains information on the marital status at injury, at discharge from rehabilitation, and at each anniversary of injury. Given the young age at which SCI typically occurs, it is not surprising that the majority of cases (54.2%) were single at the time of rehabilitation discharge. In addition, 30.1% were married, 9.0% divorced, 4.4% separated, and 2.1% widowed. Marital status changes occurring each year after injury can be determined from the National Database information. During the first 6 years, from one anniversary to the next, about 2% to 2.5% of those who were single (never married) become married. This trend peaks in year 8, when 4.0% of all single persons get married; thereafter the rate goes down to 0% in year 15. Depending on the assumptions one is willing to make with respect to selective loss to follow-up, from 10% to 30% of all those single at injury marry by the 15th anniversary.

Of those who are married, in any year a small percentage gets separated or divorced. The separation rate declines from 4.2% in year 1 after injury to close to 1% in year 15. Similarly, the divorce rate varies between 2.2% and 3.1% in years 1 through 8, and thereafter quickly declines to almost 0%. In addition to these marriage dissolutions, each year from 0.2% to 0.7% of all married persons become widowed.

Those SCI persons who are separated at the beginning of each year are very likely to become divorced (at a rate ranging from 11.5% to 28.0%). A smaller number each year becomes married (3.9% to 11.5%). Those who are divorced at any anniversary are most likely to remain so. However, a minority (varying from 0.8% to 7.1%) get married. (This is a higher percentage marrying than among the never-married, which includes a large number too young to get married). Finally, of those who are widowed, an increasingly small group (3.2% to 0%) gets married.

All rates of change in marital status tend to be highest in the early years after injury, indicating that the disturbances of marital relationships that SCI brings about decline in importance over the years—as do the opportunities or incentives to marry. The net result of all these status changes is reflected in Figure 10–7. The total percentage divorced increases over the years, as does the percentage married. The percentage who are single declines correspondingly, while the separated, widowed, and "other" groups stay about the same size.

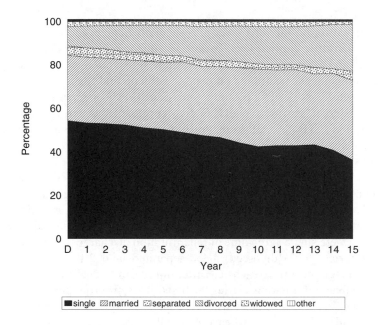

Figure 10–7 Percentages of Persons in Each Marital Status, by Anniversary Year

Of those who were not married (single, separated, divorced, or widowed) on discharge, 883 are known to have become married in any of the follow-up years. (A few [23] did so twice, and two persons even three times.) The marriage rate was highest for the 16 to 30 and 31 to 45 years of age groups, and declined with increasing age at injury (Table 10–5). Females were somewhat more likely to marry than males; paraplegics were somewhat more likely to marry than tetraplegics.

Of those who were married on discharge, 8.7% separated at some point in time during the years they were followed (Table 10–5). As separation is in most instances followed by divorce, also tabulated is the percentage that was separated and/or divorced, a total of 15.0% of the entire group of those who were married on discharge. Marriage failures were most common in the youngest age groups and declined to zero in the oldest group, confirming results of earlier studies. As in the reports by others, neurologic category made a large difference in rates of divorce and separation. Gender, however, did not, and contrary to expectations males divorced or separated somewhat *more* frequently than did females. It is possible that the married females in this sample are older, and older SCI persons have fewer divorces in preinjury marriages.

Table 10–5 Percentages of Persons Changing Marital Status in Any Follow-Up Year from Marital Status at Discharge

	Not Married on Discharge		Married on Discharge		
	% Married after Discharge	No. Not Married on Discharge	% Separated after Discharge	% Separated or Divorced	No. Married on Discharge
Total	8.8	10,018	8.7	15.0	4,347
Age at Injury (y)					
0–15	3.8	651	0.0	0.0	1
16–30	9.5	7,138	14.4	24.7	1,448
31–45	9.4	1,453	9.1	15.1	1,580
46–60	6.0	480	3.1	6.2	876
61–75	5.0	242	0.3	1.1	379
76+	3.7	54	0.0	0.0	63
Gender					
Male	8.6	8,173	8.9	15.2	3,638
Female	9.5	1,846	7.9	14.2	710
Race/Ethnic Group					
White	9.9	6,876	9.1	15.9	3,196
Nonwhite	6.5	3,127	7.8	12.9	1,143
Neurologic Impairment Category					
Paraplegia Incomplete	9.9	1,974	7.3	12.6	950
Paraplegia Complete	10.4	2,665	10.5	18.5	1,139
Tetraplegia Incomplete	8.3	3,058	6.8	11.8	1,444
Tetraplegia Complete	7.0	2,241	11.9	19.7	772

Figure 10–8 depicts the proportion of single (never married) persons at injury who were still single in each of the first 5 postinjury years. Only persons with known marital status at injury who had 5 consecutive complete years of follow-up were included in this analysis. Also provided are the expected marriage rates. The expected number of marriages among these persons was calculated using 1982 age- and sex-specific first-marriage rates for the United States. Substantially fewer marriages occurred than were expected during each postinjury year.

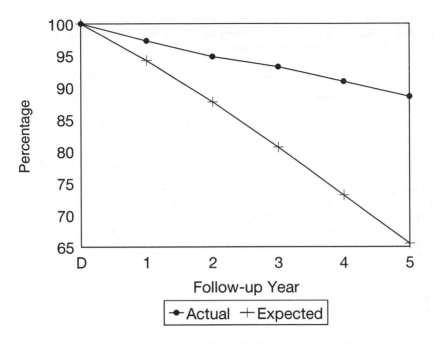

Figure 10–8 Percentage of Persons Remaining Single, by Anniversary Year

---

Overall, 88.5% of all persons single at injury were still single 5 years postinjury, compared with an expected value (in the absence of SCI) of 65.4%.

Figure 10–9 depicts the proportion (of persons with intact marriages at injury) who were still married in each of the first 5 postinjury years. The expected number of divorces among these persons was calculated using the 1982 age- and sex-specific divorce rates for the United States. Of 1128 married persons at injury meeting these criteria, 916 (81.2%) were still married 5 years postinjury, compared with an expected value in the absence of SCI of 88.7%. It should be noted that an additional 55 persons (4.9%) were legally separated but not yet divorced 5 years postinjury. Therefore, the marriages of only 76.3% of persons married at injury were still intact 5 years postinjury.

Of all those who divorced after discharge from rehabilitation, 15.9% are known to have remarried (4 cases remarried more than once). Remarriage rates are about equally high for all age groups. Females are slightly more likely to have remarried than males (19.8% vs. 15.2%). Those with paraplegia more often remarry (20.2%) than persons with tetraplegia (11.5%).

Quite a few of the postinjury marriages resulted in separation or divorce—21.7%, which is higher than the 15.0% for preinjury marriages. (The percentage is very much the same for both genders, all age groups, and the various neurologic

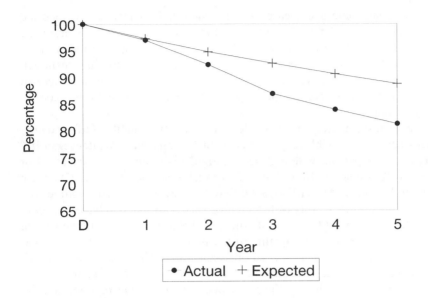

Figure 10–9 Percentage of Persons Remaining Married, by Anniversary Year

---

categories.) This contradicts the findings reported by others of greater strength and stability of postinjury marriages. A possible explanation is that those in the preinjury marriages were older (on average, age 40 years at the time of injury) than those in the postinjury marriages (on average, age 27 years at the time of injury, and an estimated age 31 years at the time of marriage). Further analysis, controlling for age at injury and age at time of divorce, is necessary.

Trieschmann[15] eloquently states that, like those without a spinal injury, persons with a spinal cord injury are continuously learning to adapt to their (ever-changing) environment in better and more satisfying ways. Consequently, adjustment should be considered a process, not an end point, and *coping* may be a better term to use than *adjustment*. It is not unreasonable, however, to consider the basic requirement of incorporating into one's life all the changes (physical, financial, social, vocational, etc.) created by or necessitated by the injury as the first stage of adjustment. This first stage has an end point, the time when a basic level of equilibrium has been regained. Specialists disagree on the duration of this period, quoting "several" to 7 years. Longitudinal studies of change and adjustment after SCI are rare; most information available on these processes is derived from cross-sectional studies. There is some agreement among researchers that time elapsed since injury is related to acceptance of the disability and to life satisfaction. For instance, a longitudinal study that focused on the first year after discharge found a decrease in depression and an increase in reported adjustment in personal, familial, social, and vocational areas.[36] However, in one study, quality-of-life ratings were not related to time since injury,[37] and in an 11-year longitudinal study, Crewe and Krause[38] detected no increases in adjustment. Small sample sizes, differences in research designs, and use of a variety of specific adjustment or coping measures may explain these and other contradictory findings.

However, it seems clear that a high level of subjective quality of life and high life satisfaction are possible for persons with SCI. For instance, Whiteneck et al.[39] reported on 128 persons with high-level tetraplegia (complete injury at C4 or higher level) discharged from three SCI Model Systems, of whom 23% were respirator dependent. Most (93%) specified that they were glad to be alive, and only 10% called their quality of life poor or very poor. Such judgments would be a better indicator of the level of adjustment that is possible if comparable information on the subjective quality of life preinjury were available. Alternatively, others may be used as a comparison group. Cushman and Hassett[37] reported that of their subjects, most saw their quality of life as comparable to or somewhat better than that of their age peers. Others have reported similar findings.[40] A Swedish study found that quality-of-life ratings by persons with SCI, especially those injured over 4 years, did not differ much from those by a control population.[41]

Most significant is that various studies[37,41,42] have indicated that life satisfaction, quality-of-life ratings, or depression and other indicators of mental well-being and coping are *not* or minimally related to level or completeness of injury. This would suggest that it is the quality of rehabilitation, the social support system, and possibly the personality and mind-set of persons with SCI themselves that determine coping and ultimately satisfaction with life after injury.

SUICIDE

Attending school, going to work, fulfilling family roles, volunteering: for most persons with SCI these and other forms of productivity provide the challenges and the rewards that make life worth living. Many may consider suicide[39] soon after injury or at some later point when setbacks disturb the delicate balance of costs and benefits of living with so serious an impairment. And some persons continue to find the gap between what had been (or could have been) and the present unacceptable, and either commit suicide or bring about death through systematic and prolonged self-neglect (e.g., inattention to skin care) or refusal of necessary care (e.g., operative or rehabilitative interventions). The frequency of deaths due to such "indirect suicide" or "physiologic suicide" is difficult to estimate.

Obvious suicides have been investigated in a number of studies. Suicide as a percentage of all deaths in follow-up years has been reported at rates typically varying from 5% to 10%,[43-45] although higher rates have been found, especially in the earlier studies and in groups with high risk factors (e.g., substance abuse).[46] In comparison, for the U.S. population as a whole, 1.4% of all deaths are due to suicide. One study suggests that many of the risk factors for postdischarge suicide are similar to those found for the population at large, and can be identified during rehabilitation admission, including alcohol and drug abuse, a psychiatric and/or criminal history, a history of family fragmentation, and attempts at suicide preinjury or during hospitalization.[47]

In the U.S. population, suicide is much more common among males than among females (by a factor of 5), and within both genders more common among whites than among blacks (by a factor of 2). For males, suicide rates are highest among the 25- to 34-year-old age group; among females, those 45 to 54 years old are most likely to end their lives.

Among cases entered into the National SCI Database, a total of 923 deaths has been reported, of which 55 (6.0%) can reliably be attributed to suicide. This number is almost certainly an underestimate; quite likely some of the deaths classified as having an accidental or unknown cause were suicides. Also, among the persons who are lost to follow-up, deaths may have occurred that were due to suicide as well as other causes. The percentage that suicides constitute of all deaths varies somewhat by age, gender, race/ethnic group, and neurologic category. Deaths among young adults, males, whites, and those with complete paraplegia were somewhat more likely to have resulted from suicide.

The rate of suicide (and of other deaths) reported cannot be directly compared with cause-specific mortality rates for the U.S. population as a whole. United States rates are given for 1-year periods, while the deaths reported for the SCI group are cumulated for a period that varies from 1 year to 19 years. (The average number of years of follow-up is 4.4.) However, a previous study of causes of death in SCI used largely the same population of National SCI Database cases, but because of a different methodology (separate data collection, with reporting of date of death) *could* compare actual deaths (by cause) with expected deaths (based on age, sex, and race-adjusted cause-specific death rates). Suicides among this group of persons who sustained SCI between 1973 and 1984, and who were followed through 1985, were five times as frequent as would have been expected.[48,49] Suicides were also higher than expected for various subgroups, including persons less than age 25 years, persons aged 25 through 54 years, and persons over 54 years (although not significantly). Persons in all four neurologic categories (complete or incomplete paraplegia or tetraplegia) committed suicide more often than expected based on population rates. Finally, both whites and blacks and males and females committed suicide more often than expected, although for blacks and females the difference was not statistically significant.[48,49]

In the current study, comparisons of suicide rates *between* SCI subgroups are valid (assuming that the average years of follow-up are similar) (Table 10–6). Suicide rates are highest for young adults (with the exception of a high incidence of 0.65 suicide death per 100 persons in the 61- to 75-year-old group), for males, and for whites, confirming the results of the earlier study and following general population trends. Suicide rates are higher for persons with complete (compared with incomplete) paraplegia, similar to the earlier study. However, in contrast with the earlier study, persons with complete tetraplegia committed suicide *less* often than those with incomplete tetraplegia. Suicide is most common during the first few years after injury, with a rate of about 0.1% per year. Of the 55 suicides reported, 44 (80%) occurred in the first 5 years after injury; an additional 9 (16%) occurred in the next 5 years. A decreasing trend is also shown by the rate per year. This suggests that those who fail to learn how to cope

Table 10–6 Number of Suicides and of Deaths in Follow-Up Years, per 100 Persons at Risk, by Age at Injury, Gender, Race/Ethnic Group, and Neurologic Category

| | Deaths per 100 Persons Discharged Alive | | | No. of Cases |
	Suicide	Other	Total	
Total	0.38	6.06	6.45	14,312
Age at Injury (y)				
0–15	0.00	3.37	3.37	652
16–30	0.40	3.31	3.70	8,562
31–45	0.43	6.43	6.87	3,015
46–60	0.30	13.05	13.34	1,349
61–75	0.65	23.82	24.47	617
76+	0.00	39.32	39.32	117
Gender				
Male	0.41	6.17	6.58	11,766
Female	0.27	5.58	5.85	2,547
Race/Ethnic Group				
White	0.48	5.86	6.33	10,040
Nonwhite	0.16	6.59	6.75	4,249
Neurologic Category				
Paraplegia, Incomplete	0.27	4.12	4.39	2,916
Paraplegia, Complete	0.66	4.35	5.01	3,793
Tetraplegia, Incomplete	0.36	6.22	6.58	4,484
Tetraplegia, Complete	0.20	10.05	10.25	3,004

with SCI will commit suicide in the early years. For those who "tough it out" for the first 5 to 10 years, suicide rates are very similar to those for the population at large.

CONCLUSION

An SCI is not any longer the almost-certain threat to life it once was, before the invention of antibiotics and the development of medical technology. It also is not the catastrophe many still consider it to be. The majority of persons survive, as is indicated in Chapter 14, and go back to living. The data in this chapter indicate that, due in no small measure to the interventions of medical, social, and vocational rehabilitation, many are successful. The vast majority lives in the community, not an institution. Most of those who were in school at the time of injury go back, and some of those who had completed schooling or dropped out return, with the end result that persons with a spinal injury tend to be as well-educated as, if not better educated than, the population as a whole. However, in spite of educational efforts, work is still an elusive goal for many. The present study does not allow determining the specific reasons; others have pointed to physical and social barriers, as well as disincentives built into the U.S. Social Security system. These data may also indicate a need for changes in vocational rehabilitation programs—and possibly the psychologic support services available as part of and after rehabilitation.

The various consequences of SCI do have an effect on family life and a person's chances of becoming married; compared with their peers, persons with a spinal injury are more likely to become divorced and less likely to get married. The data also show that postinjury marriages of persons with spinal cord injury are *not* more stable than preinjury marriages, as previously had been thought.

These various forced and other changes in social roles, added to health problems and issues of psychologic adjustment to a changed body, together constitute formidable challenges. A variety of studies have indicated that, after a stormy initial 2 to 5 years, most persons learn how to cope. Some, however, fail to do so and see suicide as the only way out. The rates of suicide are clearly higher among persons with SCI, especially in the early years after injury, than for the U.S. population as a whole.

Advances in rehabilitative processes in recent years have resulted in shorter rehabilitation stays and increased functional abilities upon discharge. This was due to a focus on care and management immediately postinjury. However, the data in this chapter point to the need for long-term interventions to enhance social functioning, coping, and adjustment over the long term.

Rather than focusing on where persons with SCI fail (or where medical care, rehabilitation, and society fail), it is beneficial to focus on where they succeed;

most become well-adjusted, productive citizens who enjoy a high quality of life. Further study may be helpful in determining how professionals can help persons with SCI to reach that status faster, and in exploring social and political structures that contribute to a full and satisfying life for all persons with a spinal injury.

REFERENCES

1. Cushman L, Dijkers M. Depressed mood during rehabilitation of persons with spinal injury. *J Rehabil.* 1991;57:35–38.

2. Davidoff G, Roth E, Thomas P, et al. Depression among acute spinal cord injury patients: A study utilizing the Zung Self-Rating Depression Scale. *Rehabil Psych.* 1990;35:171–180.

3. Woodbury B, Redd C. Psychosocial issues and approaches. In: Buchanan LE, Nawoczenski DA, eds. *Spinal Cord Injury: Concepts and Management Approaches.* Baltimore, Md: Williams & Wilkins; 1987:187–217.

4. Woodrich F, Patterson JB. Variables related to acceptance of disability in persons with spinal cord injuries. *J Rehabil.* 1983;49:26–30.

5. Green BC, Pratt CC, Grigsby TE. Self-concept among persons with long-term spinal cord injury. *Arch Phys Med Rehabil.* 1984;65:751–754.

6. Frank RG, Umlauf RL, Wonderlich SA, et al. Differences in coping styles among persons with a spinal cord injury: A cluster-analytic approach. *J Consult Clin Psychol.* 1987;55:727–731.

7. Ulmer DB. Special needs of the young spinal cord injured patient in a nursing home. *SCI Nursing.* 1990;7:27–30.

8. Graham P. Bridge building: Linking a spinal cord injury unit to a skilled nursing facility. *J Rehabil Nursing.* 1985;10:22–25.

9. Roth EJ, Lovell L, Heinemann AW, et al. The older adult with a spinal cord injury. *Paraplegia.* 1992;30:520–526.

10. Stover SL, Kartus PL, Rutt RD, et al. Outcomes of the older patient with spinal cord injury. *Arch Phys Med Rehabil.* 1987;68:672.

11. Woolsey RM. Rehabilitation outcome following spinal cord injury. *Arch Neurol.* 1985; 42:116–119.

12. Fuhrer MJ, Carter RE, Donovan WH, et al. Post-discharge outcomes for ventilator-dependent quadriplegics. *Arch Phys Med Rehabil.* 1987;68:353–356.

13. Paralysis Society of America. *Research briefs: Estimates of SCI prevalence.* Washington, DC; 1990: issue 4.

14. Neff W. Rehabilitation and work. In: Neff W, ed. *Rehabilitation Psychology.* Washington, DC: American Psychological Association; 1971:109–142.

15. Trieschmann RB. *Spinal Cord Injuries. Psychological, Social and Vocational Rehabilitation.* 2nd ed. New York: Demos; 1988.

16. DeVivo MJ, Rutt RD, Stover SL, Fine PR. Employment after spinal cord injury. *Arch Phys Med Rehabil.* 1987;68:494–498.

17. MacKenzie EJ, Shapiro S, Smith RT, et al. Factors influencing return to work following hospitalization for traumatic injury. *Am J Public Health.* 1987;77:329–334.

18. DeVivo MJ, Fine PR. Employment status of spinal cord injured patients 3 years after injury. *Arch Phys Med Rehabil.* 1982;63:200–203.

19. Krause JS. Employment after spinal cord injury. *Arch Phys Med. Rehabil.* 1992;73:163–169.

20. Wilson WC, Hensley BS, Owens JR. Vocational outcomes of spinal cord injured clients in Virginia: A ten-year study. Fishersville, Va: Woodrow Wilson Rehabilitation Center; 1984.

21. DeVivo MJ, Richards JS, Stover SL, Go BK. Spinal cord injury: Rehabilitation adds life to years. *West J Med.* 1991;154:602–606.

22. Goldberg RT, Freed MM. Vocational development of spinal cord injury patients: An 8-year follow-up. *Arch Phys Med Rehabil.* 1982;63:207–210.

23. U.S. Bureau of the Census. *Statistical Abstract of the United States 1991.* Washington, DC; 1991.

24. Abrams KS. Impact on marriage of adult-onset paraplegia. *Paraplegia.* 1981;19:253–259.

25. El Ghatit AZ, Hanson RW. Outcomes of marriages existing at time of a male's spinal cord injury. *J Chronic Dis.* 1975;28:383–388.

26. Pinkerton AC, Griffin ML. Rehabilitation outcomes in females with spinal cord injury: Follow-up study. *Paraplegia.* 1983;21:166–175.

27. Comarr AE. Marriage and divorce among patients with spinal cord injury. *J Indian Med Assoc.* 1962;9:4353–4359.

28. Guttmann L. Married life of paraplegics and tetraplegics. *Paraplegia.* 1964-1965;2: 182–188.

29. DeVivo MJ, Fine PR. Spinal cord injury: Its short-term impact on marital status. *Arch Phys Med Rehabil.* 1985;66:501–504.

30. Brown JS, Giesy B. Marital status of persons with spinal cord injury. *Soc Sci Med.* 1986;23:313–322.

31. Crewe NM, Athelstan GT, Krumberger BA. Spinal cord injury: A comparison of pre-injury and post-injury marriages. *Arch Phys Med Rehabil.* 1979;60:252–256.

32. El Ghatit AZ, Hanson RW. Marriage and divorce after spinal cord injury. *Arch Phys Med Rehabil.* 1976;57:470–472.

33. Crewe NM, Krause JS. Marital status and adjustment to spinal cord injury. *J Am Paraplegia Soc.* 1992;15:14–18.

34. Deyoe F. Marriage and family patterns with long-term spinal cord injury. *Paraplegia.* 1972;10:219–224.

35. Crewe NM, Krause JS. Marital relationships and spinal cord injury. *Arch Phys Med Rehabil.* 1988;69:435–438.

36. Richards JS. Psychologic adjustment to spinal cord injury during first post discharge year. *Arch Phys Med Rehabil.* 1986;67:362–365.

37. Cushman LA, Hassett J. Spinal cord injury: 10 and 15 years after. *Paraplegia.* 1992;30:690–696.

38. Crewe NM, Krause JS. An eleven-year follow-up of adjustment to spinal cord injury. *Rehabil Psychol.* 1990;35:205–210.

39. Whiteneck G, Charlifue S, Hall K, Menter R, Wilkerson M, Wilmot C. *A Collaborative Study of High Quadriplegia.* Englewood, Colo: Craig Hospital; 1985.

40. Cook DW. Dimensions and correlates of post-service adjustment to spinal cord injury: A longitudinal inquiry. *Int J Rehabil Res.* 1982;65:373–375.

41. Lundquist C, Siosteen A, Blomstrand C, et al. Spinal cord injuries: Clinical, functional and emotional status. *Spine.* 1991;16:78–83.

42. MacDonald MR, Nielson WR, Cameron MGP. Depression and activity patterns of spinal cord injured persons living in the community. *Arch Phys Med Rehabil.* 1987;68:339–343.

43. Nyquist R, Bors E. Mortality and survival in traumatic myelopathy during 19 years from 1946–1965. *Paraplegia.* 1967;5:22–48.

44. Geisler W, Jousse A, Wynne-Jones M, Breithaupt D. Survival in traumatic spinal cord injury. *Paraplegia.* 1983;21:364–373.

45. DeVivo MJ, Kartus PL, Stover SL, et al. Cause of death in patients with spinal cord injuries. *Arch Intern Med.* 1989;149:1761–1766.

46. Wilcox NE, Stauffer ES. Follow-up of 423 consecutive patients admitted to the spinal cord centre, Rancho Los Amigos Hospital, 1 January to 31 December, 1967. *Paraplegia.* 1972;10:115–122.

47. Charlifue SW, Gerhart KA. Behavioral and demographic predictors of suicide after traumatic spinal cord injury. *Paraplegia.* 1991;72:488–492.

48. DeVivo MJ, Black KJ, Richards JS, Stover SL. Suicide following spinal cord injury. *Paraplegia.* 1991;29:620–627.

49. DeVivo MJ, Black KJ, Stover SL. Causes of death during the first twelve years after spinal cord injury. *Arch Phys Med Rehabil.* 1993;74:248–254.

11

Consumer Involvement in Research: Inclusion and Impact

Barry Corbet

INTRODUCTION

In what might seem like an abrupt change to some, consumer direction has become the passion of federal agencies funding disability and rehabilitation research and service delivery.

In 1991, William Graves, former director of the National Institute on Disability and Rehabilitation Research (NIDRR), introduced a model then known as Participatory Action Research (PAR), based on the insights of William Foot Whyte.[1] The goals, he said, were better science and improved relevance to people with disabilities.

In 1992, in amending and reauthorizing the Rehabilitation Act of 1973, Congress stipulated that research and training supported by NIDRR must be relevant and responsive to the self-identified needs of people with disabilities.

President Clinton, lest any doubt remained, said his administration's policy is to "shift disability policy in America away from exclusion toward inclusion; away from dependence toward independence; away from paternalism and towards empowerment."[2] He underlined his commitment by appointing Judith Heumann, who has a disability, Assistant Secretary of Special Education and Rehabilitation Services.

And in 1993, NIDRR issued a Proposed Policy Statement: In order to assure that NIDRR-funded research and training initiatives are scientifically sound and relevant to the issues of its constituencies and beneficiaries (such as individuals with disabilities, their families or guardians, researchers, trainers and/or service providers), it is recommended that NIDRR implement this policy of Constituency-Oriented Research and Dissemination (CORD).[3]

CORD, like PAR, prescribes consumer involvement in all phases of research. Not surprisingly, this new direction—with quibbles—has been welcomed by

213

people with disabilities. For researchers and practitioners, however, it raises thorny questions about its effects on the quality of science and service delivery, the conditions of new funding, academic freedom, and their own roles in research. Will untrained constituents decide what projects need funding, tinker with methodology, and divert scarce resources on whim? Consumer orientation clearly demands some rethinking of the status quo.

But this move toward consumer direction did not evolve in a social or political vacuum. Its roots are entirely familiar.

NATIONWIDE TRENDS

Since the turn of the century, America has been evolving a consumer-driven society. Democracy itself, it might be argued, insists on the individual's right to influence society, and consumerism is one of its legitimate children.

Another trend, not unconnected, is what Zola and Vash call the self/mutual-help movement. They credit Alcoholics Anonymous, the seminal program of the 1930s, for the proliferation of self-help groups that eventually found their way into most aspects of American life by the late 1960s.[4]

A third and related trend is the civil rights movement. It has enriched the first two with righteous fervor and moral imperatives, and brought attention to disadvantaged groups.

And in the 1980s, American business, struggling to compete in global service and manufacturing markets, embraced a fourth trend in the form of total quality management (TQM). TQM, say Zola and Vash, relies on the consumer of services or products to help identify what does or does not work—using customer surveys, focus groups, consumer councils, complaint-tracking systems, and test marketing.[4] These are familiar practices to any social scientist.

Given the nationwide confluence of consumerism, self-help, civil rights, and TQM, consumer-driven research is center track. Much the same can be said about its position in the specialized field of disability and rehabilitation research.

CONSUMER DIRECTION IN REHABILITATION

During the 1970s, notes Joseph Fenton, one of the authors of the CORD Proposed Policy Statement, and in varying forms since, NIDRR-funded research projects have been advised by and reported to Regional Advisory Councils, an early form of the multistakeholder approach to decision making. Since 1975, the Institute on Rehabilitation Issues has offered specific guidance on how to increase consumer involvement and empowerment. It has become common practice for researchers to gather consumer panels to add focus and diversity of perspective.

Although it was consumers who first identified and brought attention to the late effects of poliomyelitis, it was rehabilitation that had the sense to pay attention. Together, consumers, researchers, and practitioners organized conferences, published findings, and forged a genuine partnership. The study of aging with SCI followed a similar course.

The CORD Proposed Policy Statement is itself a demonstration of its own principles at work. A large steering committee, representing a multitude of constituencies, canvassed the field for opinions and brought them to the planning process. According to medical sociologist Margaret Campbell, PAR founder William Foot Whyte—whose principles inform CORD—was himself a poliomyelitis survivor who was denied tenure at Harvard because of his disability before settling in at Cornell.

Rehabilitation medicine itself has discovered the need to include consumers as active participants. Just as survivors were once conditioned toward helplessness, practitioners were once conditioned toward paternalism. Now much of medicine, and research by association, is moving away from paternalistic models in favor of more active partnerships between provider and client. Rehabilitation uniquely demonstrates both the trailing and leading edges of this shift—patients with acute SCI invite paternalistic attention, yet they are soon expected to go forth into the world and stay healthy. Consequently, rehabilitation has been long aware of the need for patient education and participation in treatment. In order to keep its patients out of the hospital, it has had to make a working assumption of survivor responsibility.

And if the expectation that the patient will act in his or her own enlightened self-interest is valid, then the survivor must be seen as competent in other fields as well. Why, then, should survivors not participate in research decisions that affect them?

Virtually every Model System and Rehabilitation Research and Training Center (RRTC), many unaffiliated centers, and thousands of researchers and practitioners have long histories of learning from consumers and including their input. The ways, means, and degree of commitment vary greatly—specifics are discussed later in this chapter—but the beginnings have been made.

SURVIVORS—FROM PASSIVITY TO EMPOWERMENT

In the past, no one was less able to consume goods, contribute to decision making, benefit from self-help principles, or exercise civil rights than a person with a new SCI. He or she was a defining image of physical helplessness.

By the time medical treatment had improved enough to allow SCI survivors to leave institutions and family homes, they found that their helplessness was extended into society by ignorance, exclusive attitudes, and inaccessible environments. Poverty, lack of education, and the virtual absence of social opportunity became the norm.

Passivity, consequently, was a given. Disenfranchised people—especially those hidden away from sight—seldom make waves, so who is to blame if the early survivors were not asked to assist in solving the dilemmas of their own lives? And how, after all, could they be effective consumers? Consumers need capital, either fiscal or political.

Times and circumstances have changed. Education, employment, physical access, transportation, recreation, and media exposure are available for most survivors who seek them. Without saying that discrimination and disadvantage have ended—they haven't—an age of empowerment for people with disabilities is at hand. This empowerment is the new given and the disability rights movement is its offspring. National and local organizations were formed, peer support was legitimized, and advocacy groups emerged. The growing mental health and disability movement started looking very much like civil rights movements among ethnic minorities, women, and gays and lesbians.

Independent living centers, catalytic since the late 1960s, demanded that people with disabilities participate in the decisions that affect their lives. Their charters routinely specified significant or total control by people with disabilities, and a measure of influence soon followed. It was no longer acceptable for social services to be delivered according to protocols designed by nondisabled providers; they were to be delivered in the manner deemed by recipients to be most useful.

While it was undoubtedly a rude shock for the bureaucrats first confronted by assertive survivors, the results of this movement have been almost uniformly beneficial. Survivors have moved out of institutions, their quality of life has improved, and costs to the public are down.

By the 1980s, says researcher Jean Campbell, people with mental retardation had begun People First chapters and were starting their own research projects using oral histories and transcripts of meetings. The Well-Being Project, funded in 1986, utilized mental health survivors in developing research instruments and interviewing respondents.[5]

The advent of consumer-driven research projects, such as those funded by the World Institute on Disability, Paralyzed Veterans of America, the American Paralysis Association, and the Spinal Cord Society, underlines another realization—survivors can and do seize the research initiative.

This empowerment reached its current zenith with the 1990 Americans with Disabilities Act, which granted full civil rights protection to people with disabilities. Capital has accrued. For the first time in U.S. history, there is a viable disability movement. It may be young and fragmented, but it has potency.

Viewed in this context, it should be apparent that the trend toward consumer direction is not a passing fad in governmental circles, nor an annoying exercise in compliance, but a logical continuation of the history of rehabilitation, research, and disability in the United States.

PAR/CORD/CONSUMER INVOLVEMENT: WHAT DO THEY MEAN?

The terms *PAR* and *CORD*, nuances notwithstanding, are used almost inter-changeably. PAR was changed by NIDRR to CORD to avoid confusion with another agency with the same acronym, but the principles remain unchanged and PAR remains the defining philosophy behind CORD. Some see PAR as the broader term because it includes methodology. In this chapter, PAR and CORD are used in direct quotes or descriptions of specific documents or programs, but the more generic term *consumer involvement* or *consumer direction* is used where specificity is not required. And it should be recognized that CORD, as of this writing, is still proposed policy, not official practice. NIDRR's incoming administration may see fit to rename, change, or drop it. In the meantime, it is hoped that the reader can sort through the multitude of terms.

CORD's directives, as presently stated by the Proposed Policy Statement, are formulaic. But like most calls for change, CORD stems from a problem perceived with the status quo. The essence of that problem, says researcher Fredrick Menz,[6] is the charge that "Rehabilitation research produces minimal new practices or solutions to current problems because consumers are not integral to the research effort."

"The utility of rehabilitation research for rehabilitation practice must be dramatically increased," Menz continues. "The time gap between research and practice must be narrowed. . . . The objective is to produce better science and better application."[6]

Some of the apparent vagueness of the CORD Proposed Policy Statement is in response to the need for enough flexibility to accommodate dissimilar programs: "PAR," writes researcher Esther Lee Pederson, "is one vehicle for change that does not define a specific strategy for research or planning, but, instead, defines an attitude toward the development of research and planning."[7]

That attitude, says Whyte, challenges the detachment from subject that has traditionally characterized science. "In general," he wrote, "social scientists have refrained from linking research directly with action. We have been afraid that our involvement in action will contaminate the scientific basis of our research."[8] "Science," Whyte and colleagues elaborated, "is not achieved by distancing oneself from the world. . . . The greatest conceptual and methodological challenges come from engagement with the world."[9]

Researcher Rodney Adkins sees consumer involvement as a partnership in which people with disabilities identify research questions: "I can have all the research tools I want, but if I don't have the questions, it's not going to do me any good."

J. Campbell offers a particularly pithy understanding: "The primary focus of NIDRR and of CORD is to meet the self-defined needs of people with disabilities."

Exhibit 11–1 compares traditional research with PAR.[10]

Exhibit 11–1 A Comparison of Conventional Research and Participatory Action Research

	Conventional Research	Participatory Action Research
Goals	Advance academic knowledge. Evaluate services.	Advance practical knowledge. —Solve problems. —Legitimatize group claims. Service group goals. Strengthen service capacity and empower members. Generate new knowledge.
Methods	Linear from theory to data to results to use Standardized measurement Replicability Positivist and deductive	Reflexive and cyclic from data to use and action to theory Measures generated in and responsive to local situation Interpretive and deductive
Relationships with participants/ groups	Researcher control Researcher apart from the field Objectivity through detachment	Participant and researcher co-control or participant control Researcher a part of the field Objectivity through reflexivity Reduce professional monopoly
Products and actions	Take few or no actions. File research reports. Contribute to scientific literature. Test or advance theory.	Participate in group improvement or service system changes. Generate lay and scientific theory. Write reports for public/ academic audiences.

Source: Adapted from Chesler MA, Participatory Action Research with Self-Help Groups: An Alternative Paradigm for Inquiry and Action, *American Journal of Community Psychology,* Vol. 19, No. 5, p. 757, with permission of Plenum Press, © 1991.

For many, Exhibit 11–1 may offer too much policy and too little process. A possible touchstone is that it looks like nothing so much as a similar exhibit comparing traditional quality assurance with TQM (Exhibit 11–2).[11] The TQM model must have looked equally unmanageable to its first users, but it has accomplished a revolution. It remains to be seen whether consumer direction can do as well in disability and rehabilitation research.

In either consumer-driven research or TQM, the assurance of quality resides in an alliance of providers and consumers of goods, services, and skills. From the CORD Proposed Policy Statement: "CORD is an approach through which appropriate members of constituencies and beneficiaries participate in all stages of the NIDRR research and training process. Members are actively involved in defining problems; carrying out the research; evaluating the validity, relevancy and impact of the outcomes; disseminating the findings; and supporting training and the utilization of the results."[1]

Exhibit 11–2 A Comparison of Traditional Quality Assurance with Total Quality Management

Traditional Quality Assurance	Total Quality Management
Management centered	Consumer/customer centered
Quality intangible	Quality definition
Product focus	Process focus
Reactive	Preventive
Acceptable quality level	Error-free attitude
Management by intuition	Management by fact
Consumer and employee control	Consumer and employee empowerment
Quality department	Total organization
Status quo	Continuous improvement
We/they relationships	Supplier/provider relationships
Individual	Team
Rigid/hierarchical	Flexible/flat
Client identification, client tracking, vertically integrated information, mass inspection	Sampling, customer and community surveys, focus groups, concept mapping, longitudinal follow-up
Management defines quality, determines if quality is provided	Consumers define quality; measures developed to determine if consumer requirements are met

Source: Adapted from *Humanizing Decision Support Systems* by J Campbell and DF Frey, p. 4, with permission of the Maine Department of Mental Health and Mental Retardation, © 1993.

In a nutshell, CORD requires constituent participation in *all* NIDRR research and training activities. But the mechanics of implementation are not so easy to grasp, and hard questions leap to mind. The Proposed Policy Statement addresses some of them, and offers tentative solutions (see Exhibit 11–3).

CONCERNS OF PROFESSIONALS

The problem universally cited by researchers and practitioners is money. NIDRR has acknowledged that CORD will require additional funding, but the fiercely competitive quest for research dollars has so far discouraged applicants from writing significant expenses for consumer involvement into grant applica-

Exhibit 11–3 Anticipated Problems and Their Solutions

Anticipated Problem	Solution/Position
Identifying relevant constituencies	Will vary from project to project; flexibility to suit project is seen as essential.
Conflicts between ensuring social relevance and scientific competency	Specific roles will be assigned to ensure that constituencies operate within their areas of expertise.
Large well-funded constituencies over-riding small underfunded ones	NIDRR will seek broad input, including constituencies that do not receive the *Federal Register*.
Tokenism, such as advisory committees with no real influence	NIDRR requires meaningful participation from the earliest planning stages onward.
Constituency definition of research areas causing "errors of omission" in research	Academic freedom will be respected as long as it meets the needs of NIDRR's constituencies.
Economic and bureaucratic inefficiency caused by constituency partnership	CORD will have costs, but its benefits must exceed the costs of implementation. Grant applicants will have flexibility in how to best implement CORD.
Inadequate resources	NIDRR recognizes that additional funding, time, and training are required.

Source: Adapted from *Proposed Policy Statement for NIDRR on Constituency-Oriented Research and Dissemination* by J Fenton, A Batavia, and DS Roody, National Institute on Disability and Rehabilitation Research, 1993.

tions. Furthermore, there is uncertainty about how much to budget if and when the funds become available.

Menz[6] has compiled a list of primary concerns he sees among his peers. The first questions the motivation behind the initiative: "It comes across as an imposition from the federal government, and as in any good academic group, that just isn't tolerable." Another concern is implementation: "If it's part of the research process, how will it work? Will it add something, or is it something that will look good, add nothing and cost more?" A paramount concern is research quality: "As you move more and more toward the individual as the basis for the researcher, and more and more toward what public opinion might be about what good research looks like, what happens to the quality of the research itself?"

A closely related point, and something of a Pandora's box, is this question: Is research an inherently democratic—or democratizable—process? What will all that input do to methodology? Most consumers are ignorant about research, and consumers with disabilities—historically deprived of education—compound the problem. They may be asked to contribute expertise they don't have. Must researchers summon a sense of collegiality with the scientifically unanointed? Will the beneficial serendipities outweigh the inevitable errors? And, suggests researcher Karen Hart, "People are afraid that the most obnoxious patient you ever had will show up on your doorstep to give input."

Consumers, it is said, will not have a researcher's perspective on the issues. Some say that is precisely the point. The real question, say others, is what effect that diversity of perspective will have on credibility. Given constituent emphasis on relevancy, will it usurp methodology?

The doubts are not limited to any one professional field. There is vague agreement that consumer direction is less welcome in the basic sciences, among bench scientists, and in university settings, but hard lines are not evident. Some feel that researchers with a background in counseling find consumer involvement more workable. Opinions tend to become more fixed when it comes to basic versus applied science, and some researchers want consumers to keep hands off the holy grail of basic science. The customer may always be right, they imply, but in basic science the only customer is truth.

Menz[6] feels that the crusade for relevance has given NIDRR research an emphasis on qualitative and applied research: "Research which provides improvements of apparent or immediate value and qualitative contributions to individuals is considered of greater importance. Research for science, for knowledge building or of conceptual and individual interest to the researcher is of lesser value. What we end up doing sometimes is to give face validity to a process that may not have much relevance when it comes, in particular, to replicability."

Menz catalogues additional areas of concern: the lack of guidance from NIDRR on standards of implementation and practice, the challenge of involving consumers with limited communication skills, and the incorporation of consumers into the peer review process.[6]

But to almost all researchers, always and ever, it is the edifice of quality science that is most jealously guarded. It is the bottom line. This excerpt from the CORD Proposed Policy Statement may be reassuring: "Researchers will continue to have the authority to determine the research design, conduct the research methodology and ensure that the research is conducted objectively and with scientific rigor. Other constituencies will be responsible for ensuring that the research is relevant to their needs and that alternative interpretations of results are presented."[3]

Fenton confirms that consumer involvement will not force consumers and researchers into an adversarial position: "Are consumers going to tell us how to do research? The concept is that each one has a role in the development and execution and dissemination of research, and it's a partnership, not an activity dominated by one constituent. The essence is opening up a dialog and understanding between people with disabilities and researchers."

"It has nothing to do with telling people what to do," agrees Campbell.[5] "It has to do with focus, with goals, with aims. How you do the research, what questions you ask, what demonstration projects are set up—that's the scientific rigor we talk so much about." Yet Campbell points out that scientific rigor is frequently compromised by samples too small for analysis, for example, or by studies that cannot be reliably replicated. Consumers are hardly the only compromising influence. Nor are they the only people untrained in research methodology, notes Adkins. Physicians—and many other professionals—have the same shortcoming.

Vash, a researcher who has a disability, disputes the wisdom of mixing lay consumers and scientists on review panels. She favors the separation of social value review and scientific merit review, and wants them performed in that order. It's a waste of time and money, she says, to design research and then decide, "This is methodologically perfect, but signifies nothing."

Menz frames an attitudinal challenge for researchers:

> We may need to more often choose not to chase the "elusive hypothesis" (keeping in mind that doing so is what we as researchers-in-the-guise-of-scientists do if we want to achieve image, publications, tenure and promotions), but instead choose to work with real people in real settings. . . . Probably among the greatest challenges . . . will be to responsibly reconcile our professional needs to look into the unknown . . . and, perhaps, a responsibility to join such curiosity to solving some of the broader social issues to which our skills may add the new critical value."[6]

CONCERNS OF CONSUMERS

Survivors have long recognized that there is, as Campbell says, "an incongruence of perspective between how consumers and providers see the world."[5] Most see consumer direction as a laudable effort to narrow the gap.

Yet some contest CORD's particulars. They object to the use of the term *relevant constituency*. It includes not only people with disabilities and their families, guardians, and others directly affected by research, but also researchers, trainers, service providers, policymakers, and unspecified others. There is an attempt to subdivide constituencies into ultimate beneficiaries and intermediate beneficiaries, but the definitions are overlapping and obscure. *Constituent,* however, is far from synonymous with *consumer.*

The involvement of people with disabilities, runs the criticism, should not be equated with that of others affected more tangentially. It is illogical to weight them equally, and to do so flies in the face of congressional and presidential mandates. People with disabilities do not want to exclude other constituents, but they do want primary control.

A second objection has to do with CORD's definition of *meaningful participation* as "partnership by members of the relevant constituencies in a purposeful and promising set of activities that will affect the research, dissemination and training process." If people with disabilities only "affect" research, then what has been accomplished? In their historic role as mere objects of NIDRR research, survivors affected research. It is general dissatisfaction with that limitation, the argument concludes, that has resulted in the current statutory orientation toward empowerment.

FIELD EXPERIENCE

The SCI Model Systems have gathered a lot of experience in working cooperatively with consumers. RRTCs, in particular, have enabled the Model Systems to expand that experience rapidly. But those looking for a how-to manual will be disappointed. It does not exist. Should it? There was strong pressure on the CORD steering committee to recommend what became known as "the cook book," but it chose to avoid prescriptive methodology. The consensus was that there are innumerable creative ways to bring consumers into decision making, and no single right way. In fact, the Proposed Policy Statement's most telling sentence may be this: "NIDRR maintains that the best way to learn how to implement CORD is by doing it."

The National Association of RRTCs in 1991 and 1992 convened study groups to catalogue examples of consumer involvement, identify consumer roles, and voice questions about the new policy. Their conclusions can be found in a very helpful monograph by Menz.[6] This document also provides an excellent hypothetical example of how a research question might successfully involve consumers in each of the traditional steps of research. But the larger body of information remains in the experience of those researchers, consumers, and centers already applying one or another concept of participation by people with disabilities.

Virtually every RRTC in the country utilizes some form of consumer involvement, although virtually none, says Menz, manage it in all stages of the research process as CORD unequivocally requires. The great variety of programs makes procedural generalizations difficult, but it is possible to get a feel for how the process works anecdotally.

CONSUMER INVOLVEMENT: MAKING IT WORK

Recruitment

Most members of consumer advisory boards, focus panels, and oversight committees are recruited from the client base of the institution conducting the research. The evident advantages are convenience and proximity. The disadvantages are that selection is biased and the same people recycle through successive projects. Consequently, many researchers augment their pool of candidates by contacting independent living centers, service delivery agencies, and disability organizations. Some have identified larger population-based samples from which they can draw participants at random. Most have sought diversity in type of disability, ethnicity, gender, and discipline. Yet most advisory boards, it should be said, do not claim to represent all survivors. The goal, rather, is eclecticism.

Credentials

There is wide disagreement on what qualifications a consumer advisor should have. Some feel that often simply having a disability, the interest, and availability is enough. Most want additional credentials such as representing a constituency, having experience in working with groups, and being articulate and capable of analytic thinking. Even so, several projects have successfully brought people with mental retardation or who are nonverbal or nonreading onto advisory boards.

Requirements are likely to change according to what the advisory board is asked to do. Priority setting is one thing, says researcher Roberta Trieschmann, but methodology, execution, and peer review require training. If consumer direction is to apply to all phases of research, clearly there will be an enhanced demand for consumers who are also researchers. While the number of researchers with disabilities presently is low, new consumer involvement should cause that number to climb.

Facilitation

A range of supports may be needed by consumers participating in research. Transportation (including an attendant if necessary), an accessible meeting place (bathroom, too), and expenses are basic. Clerical and telephone help are also common. The goal is to assist and support, not to manipulate. Less basic are issues of attitude.

Jeffrey Cressy, a community liaison expert, says the person facilitating meetings must actively want input to make the project better. Pederson feels that the researcher acts more as a coach for team building than as a disciplinary expert, and needs to relinquish the power of decision making to all members of the group. Values guiding all stakeholders, she advises, should be respect, equality, and trust.[7]

With or without credentials, notes Deborah Roody, a co-author of the CORD Proposed Policy Statement, consumers need training in research just as researchers need training in disability issues. There is uniform agreement on the need to expend time and energy tutoring participants about goals, missions, and effective board membership. This need exists for new members of any decision-making body, Congress included. Pederson recommends *Representing the Consumer: Strategies for Effective Board Participation,* by R.A. Cohen,[12] as a teaching resource.

Power and Consensus

Hart says that the advisory boards she has worked with have decision-making power and can often make changes "on the spot." What about larger projects? "If you've got a collaborative project all over the country and promises have been made," she says, "it's hard to change things on the spot. But if you're really doing CORD right, you don't make those promises until you get some consumer input."

The amount of decision-making power conferred is a matter of planning, says Hart. "There's nobody saying you must give them control. You usually put pretty clearly into your grant application what the role of the consumer will be, so NIDRR knows and accepts the role you specify. It could be an advisory role, a reviewing role or a decision-making role. Then you feel you have license to do that."

M. Campbell says she strives to run her advisory committee "as a working board of directors, not just a titular advisory group." But Hart and Campbell agree that the heart of the process is consensus building. Hart: "You and they are looking at a big picture together and come to conclusions about what will be good science and what will be useful and relevant to people out there." Campbell: "What has evolved in practice is that we really work as a group of colleagues." She cautions that you cannot use a consensus model if you only meet once a year: "It just doesn't work. There has to be enough exposure and interaction to let the consensus evolve."

Roles Consumers Play

The experience of the Model Systems and RRTCs suggests that consumers have been utilized in an extremely broad array of roles (see Exhibit 11–4).[4] As

Exhibit 11–4 Consumer Roles

As Information Resource	Needs assessment, surveys, focus groups, subject in research study, sensitivity issues
As Functional Resource	Research advisory boards, liaison with community, constituencies, advocacy and policy sectors, promotion of research aims, training relevant constituencies, encouraging involvement among others
In Research Operations	Collaborator, co-author of research projects, co-designer of methodologies, interviewer, research assistant, crossover roles
In Application and Research Utilization	Reviewer and interpreter of products, applications, research documents, program development, identification of new applications
In Dissemination and Marketing	Co-presenting, co-authoring, direct promotion, creating awareness within relevant markets, technical assistance
In Advocacy	Preparing community, organizations, and consumers for utilization; advancing new considerations and solutions, liaison with other relevant advocates, programs and policy sectors for adoption of research solutions

Source: Excerpted with permission from *Strengthening Applications from Research through Involvement of Consumers and Practitioners* by FE Menz, unpublished paper, University of Wisconsin-Stout, 1992.

researchers are exposed to more and more input from the people their research aims to help, and as consumers learn to make those contributions, these roles will expand.

Payment for Consumers

Researchers differ sharply on this point, but budget realities may beg the question until change occurs. Even given funding changes, the division would remain. Those who feel that consumer advisors should not be paid have a list of reasons:

- Consumers contribute their expertise to make life better for themselves and other survivors, and do not want to be paid.
- Since researchers operate in an academic climate and frequently sacrifice their weekends for conferences and other duties, consumers should be inspired to do the same.
- The government does not have enough money to pay consumers without slighting research.
- Once consumers are paid they lose their status as advisors and become hired staff.
- Participation is an opportunity for the light of volunteerism to shine brightly.

These points are easy to respond to, if difficult to resolve:

- Most researchers and practitioners justify their work on the basis of helping people, yet it does not prevent them from accepting salaries.
- Those salaries continue through weekends and other time "contributed," and professional perks are a bonus.
- It may be true that government does not have enough money to pay for consumers' time plus all things researchers want. If hard choices ensue, someone's ox will probably be gored.
- How easily consumers are thought to lose their innocence, and how quickly we accuse others of prostitution.
- And it hardly needs saying, does it, that other people's time is not ours to volunteer?

Slightly in the majority are researchers who more or less agree with the above tirade, who feel that consumers with disabilities are experts, that living with a disability is high-level training, and that paid staff cannot equitably ask consumers to volunteer. Roody frames the rudiments: "If you invite the unpaid participation of someone, it has to be because you invite the unpaid participation of everyone for that particular purpose. It can not have to do with whether a person has a disability or not. That should be fundamental."

PROBLEMS ENCOUNTERED IN PRACTICE

Money and Time

The two most commonly cited problems in implementing consumer participation are money and time. Until funds are routinely written into grants, researchers are improvising.

Time is money, and involving consumers can be extremely time consuming. M. Campbell, a CORD enthusiast, has had to go into the community—with help from consumers—to raise money to pay expenses and honoraria. She has found the going slow. It takes time, she finds, to recruit, train, meet, listen, exchange information, encourage consensus, and maintain community liaison. Efficiencies are lost.

Some researchers feel that if NIDRR continues to fund whichever entity promises to do the most programmatically, there may never be enough dollars for CORD. If consumer involvement is to survive, they imply, it needs to become a primary expense of research rather than a dip in the petty cash drawer.

Tokenism

Tokenism, at least temporarily, is a pervasive problem. If disability and rehabilitation research is in transit from minimum consumer input to maximum input, it is not surprising that many advisory boards are poorly selected, underutilized, and denied significant power. Much of the poor management is caused by inexperience.

Attitudinal barriers are more insidious. Not all researchers and institutions are hungry for consumer input, and some do posture for funding. Andrew Batavia, one of the CORD Proposed Policy Statement's authors, feels that there are remedies: "From NIDRR's perspective, in evaluating proposals and peer reviews, they have to look at the quality of consumer input as well as the fact that it exists."

Physiatrist Frederick Maynard notes that CORD is not the only coercion being experienced by researchers and institutions. The Commission for Accreditation of Rehabilitation Facilities now requires meaningful involvement from consumers as a condition of accreditation. "Unless you're very committed to pick good people who have the time and interest to donate their input," Maynard says, "it's probably more image than it is substance." He applauds the initiative, but feels that early compliance may be cosmetic.

Tokenism, Pederson notes, can be found in both the number of consumers involved and the level of responsibility assigned.[7] Or it can take the form of ethnic exclusion. Weaving cultural diversity into CORD, says M. Campbell, is a problem that has not been meaningfully addressed.

People Problems

There is no guarantee that interactions with boards will be smooth. Not all consumers are equally ready for advisory positions, and most facilitators have encountered survivors who are resume builders, loose cannons, or single-issue zealots. They may lack leadership skills, fail to grasp the group's mission, misunderstand methodology, or interact insensitively with staff. And, as physiatrist Theodore Cole notes, "A consumer's opinion has the same fundamental weakness as a provider's opinion: it's based on personal experience."

Pederson, who works often with people with mental retardation, finds that board members can be "hesitant to offer an opinion, even more hesitant to criticize an opinion expressed by a professional, and certainly hesitant to criticize a research hypothesis."[7] People with SCI—and those with concurrent head injuries—may not differ in dealing with what has colorfully, if unfairly, been called the "M.D.eity."

Today's insistence on political correctness is seen as a barrier by most players—"If you say the wrong thing, you're likely to be ostracized permanently," says one. And being against consumer involvement, or wanting to modify it, can be an attack on Mom and apple pie. The result is a reluctance to express opinions or differences.

These are real people and real problems. While diligent selection and training are usually successful countermeasures, the key obstacle is that someone has to be available and willing to put them into practice.

PROBLEMS IDENTIFIED BY CONSUMERS

The most common complaint of consumers serving on research boards is insincerity on the part of professionals. While the recruitment process is usually a process of mutual respect and goodwill—it precedes the grant approval, after all—consumers are often confronted later by staff members who have no use for their experience, disparage their expertise, scorn their education, and resent their input. Meaningful participation is not satisfied by quotas.

Survivors have advice and caveats for prospective consumer advisors. Ask questions, they say, before joining any research project: Is it a figurehead position, or does the advisory group control anything? Will advisors be paid? How much time will be required, and will it be used efficiently? There is some accord that when wine and cheese gatherings outlast meetings, the participation has been squandered.

Ed Roberts, President of the World Institute on Disability, counsels wariness of exploitation: "We should not consume our time and energy being ripped off to rubber stamp somebody's project. It's flattering to be asked, but people should look at how they're contributing their valuable time and energy. Make sure it's something you believe in.

"If we can be involved from the beginning," Roberts continues, "I think it makes sense for us to contribute more to it. But a lot of times people have an agenda they've made up without us and want us to buy into later. We want to promote our own agenda." A ubiquitous shortcoming, he says, is the failure to see the core of that agenda: "People don't understand the civil rights perspective. They have no idea what people with disabilities are trying to do. I really believe in the civil rights perspective, and I really believe in the ADA. If they don't care about the ADA, and they're doing research, then they've missed the boat and they're using people. If discrimination is against the law, then I think we ought to act that way."

Expressly, consumers offer this imperative to researchers: *Use the advice given*. More than any other offense, disregarding input is prima facie evidence of tokenism. It is grounds for resignation.

BETTER DISSEMINATION

"It's an important consideration that we have," says NIDRR's Fenton, "that research is not done, put on the shelf and the researcher goes on to the next project. This process will bring about greater utilization of whatever the findings are." One of the driving forces behind consumer-oriented research is the view that research that is not used is research that has failed.

CORD suggests that peer review scoring points should reflect a high priority for effective dissemination to constituencies. But improved dissemination, says Hart, is also a reliable product of consumer involvement: "One of the ways you disseminate is by involving people from the very beginning so they own the project and therefore get the word out. We've been doing that in our RRTCs from the beginning."

Roody urges planning dissemination from start-up: "It's a lot harder to take something that's been done and then disseminate it. It's a lot easier and more effective if dissemination is one of the threads that carries through the whole process. So now we need not only consumers who are trained researchers, but also consumers who are trained disseminators."

A journal article, in the era of consumer-oriented research, is not the pinnacle and end point of dissemination. Consumers—both those with credentials in science and those without—can share results with the community, promote acceptance of change, conduct demonstration projects, author publications, present at conferences, and provide technical assistance.

CORD, THE MODEL SCI SYSTEMS, AND THE FUTURE

For consumer involvement to flourish within the Model SCI Systems and beyond, it is widely agreed that funding must be provided and standardized. Budgeting will give it the accountability it needs. What is said less often is that some of that funding must go to consumers.

M. Campbell puts a finer, tougher point on the problem: "The real implications of supporting CORD, in terms of reducing the scope of our projects to allow for these costs, haven't been fully recognized. I think it's a matter of not seeing how it all is connected—to truly satisfy CORD, and make it more than just a new buzzword or simple tokenism, something is going to have to go."

There are sentiments that consumers can be used more in peer review, and also in the Model Systems SCI Database. This is the tip of the iceberg, perhaps, but it is a direction for growth. It also demonstrates what has not been accomplished.

While CORD is gaining a strong foothold in NIDRR-based research, the Model Systems have been slower to involve consumers in their operations. When most applied for Model Systems designation, NIDRR had no such requirement and grant planners, consequently, made no effort to include it. "We have the relationship (with consumers) for specific projects," says Cole, "but we don't have it for the Model System. We should." Most Model Systems centers are just now starting to involve consumers effectively.

Health care reform may speed acceptance and implementation. Whatever variant is ultimately adopted, it is likely to encourage institutions to deal with consumer satisfaction and dissatisfaction. For those with solid consumer input, their involvement will provide a ready avenue for two-way information flow.

Efficient management of that information is critical. The information super-highway is here and now, and electronic networking technologies will facilitate the management of data from diverse sources. It will no longer be necessary to ask why we should try to accommodate so many inputs from so many sources. The answer is that now we *can*.

Menz, who has probed the possibilities and liabilities of consumer involvement more than most, remains an optimistic skeptic: "It may be a major opportunity to improve the way we do research, or it may not be. And if it isn't,

I hope we are wise enough to draw back and redefine it so that it supports the scientific process."

Roody, on the other hand, reminds us that while consumer direction may be on the cutting edge, it is also the continuation of a venerable social evolution: "We're talking about how we can learn to live together well and respect one another's differences. The world's been struggling with this for a very long time, and this is just what it looks like in our generation. I think we need clarity and understanding around the issues in order to move people a step further, as opposed to so staunchly advocating one side or another that we just create conflict. We need to understand where the emotion and the ardency come from on both sides, because it's real. If we don't get beyond that, we're not going to get anywhere."

And the consumer perspective? There has been enough speculation and imputation about what people with disabilities need and want. A promising alternative is to ask them. With the help of all players, it will enrich disability and rehabilitation research.

Unreferenced quotes and glosses all derive from personal communications with the following people, who are acknowledged with gratitude. They are responsible for most of this chapter's insights, and none of its shortcomings: Rodney Adkins, PhD, Co-Director, Regional SCI Care System of Southern California, Rancho Los Amigos, Downey, California; Andrew Batavia, JD, MS, Abt Associates, Washington, DC; Jean Campbell, PhD, Director of Research Quality Assurance and Information Services, Department of Mental Health and Mental Retardation, State of Maine; Margaret Campbell, PhD, Research Director, RRTC on Aging with Disability, Downey, California; Theodore M. Cole, MD, Chairman, Department of Physical Medicine and Rehabilitation, University of Michigan, Ann Arbor; Jeffrey M. Cressy, Community Liaison, Rancho Los Amigos, Downey, California; Alfred H. DeGraff, President, Saratoga Access and Fitness, Inc., Fort Collins, Colorado; Joseph Fenton, EdD, Special Assistant to the Director, NIDRR, Washington, DC; Karen Hart, PhD, Vice President for Education, The Institute for Rehabilitation and Research, Houston, Texas; Julie M. Madorsky, MD, President, California Society of PM&R, Casa Colina Hospital for Rehabilitative Medicine, Pomona, California; Frederick M. Maynard, MD, Medical Director, The Center for Rehabilitation at Metro Health, Cleveland, Ohio; Fredrick E. Menz, PhD, Associate Director/Research Director, RRTC on Improving Community-Based Rehabilitation, Menomonie, Wisconsin; Esther Lee Pederson, MEd, University-Affiliated Cincinnati Center for Developmental Disorders, Cincinnati, Ohio; Ed Roberts, President, World Institute on Disability, Oakland, California; Deborah Roody, The Network, Inc., Andover, Massachusetts; Roberta Trieschmann, PhD, President, RBT Associates, Scottsdale, Arizona; Carolyn L. Vash, PhD, Senior Researcher, Conwal, Inc., Falls Church, Virginia; Gale G. Whiteneck, PhD, Craig Hospital, Englewood, Colorado; Irving K. Zola, PhD, Department of Sociology, Brandeis University, Waltham, Massachusetts.

REFERENCES

1. Whyte WF, ed. *Participatory Action Research*. Newbury Park, Calif: Sage Publications, Inc; 1991.

2. Clinton WJ. Statements to the National Council on Disability, April 16, 1993, Washington, DC.

3. Fenton J, Batavia A, Roody DS. *Proposed Policy Statement for NIDRR on Constituency-Oriented Research and Dissemination*. Washington, DC: National Institute on Disability and Rehabilitation Research; 1993.

4. Zola IK, Vash CL. *Consumers*. New York, NY: Macmillan; in press.

5. Campbell J. *The Well-Being Project: Mental Health Clients Speak for Themselves*. Sacramento, Calif: California Department of Mental Health; 1989:23.

6. Menz FE. *Strengthening Applications from Research through Involvement of Consumers and Practitioners*. Menomonie, Wis: University of Wisconsin-Stout; 1992. Unpublished paper.

7. Pederson EL, et al. Strategies that close the gap between research, planning and advocacy. In: *Older Adults with Developmental Disabilities: Optimizing Choice and Change*. Baltimore, Md: Paul H. Brookes; 1993.

8. Whyte WF. On the uses of social science research. *Am Sociol Rev.* 1986;51:551–563.

9. Whyte WF, Greenwood D, Lazes P. Participatory action research. *Am Behavioral Scientist.* 1989;32:513–551.

10. Chesler MA. Participatory action research with self-help groups: An alternative paradigm for inquiry and action. *Am J Community Psychol.* 1991;19:757.

11. Campbell J, Frey DF. *Humanizing Decision Support Systems*. Augusta, Me: Maine Department of Mental Health and Mental Retardation; 1993:4.

12. Cohen RA. *Representing the Consumer: Strategies for Effective Board Participation*. Washington, DC: American Association for Retired Persons; 1982.

12

The Economic Impact of Spinal Cord Injury

Michael J. DeVivo, Gale G. Whiteneck, and Edgar D. Charles, Jr.

INTRODUCTION

Although SCI does not occur as often as many other types of injuries and debilitating diseases, its costs to both individuals and society are staggering. In fact, with advancing medical technology and increasing life expectancies, the direct costs of SCI are increasing at a rapid pace. Moreover, unlike most chronic diseases that usually occur among older persons, SCI is predominantly a scourge of youth. As a result, despite its low incidence, the indirect costs of SCI are very high and frequently exceed its direct costs.

The severity of both the physical and economic consequences of SCI and the uncertainty over who will sustain these injuries should prompt public concern. With exceedingly high federal budget deficits and public unwillingness to support tax increases, however, both the administration and Congress are vigorously searching for ways to reduce federal spending on a variety of social, health, and welfare programs. Therefore, it is essential to have rigorous estimates of the aggregate costs of SCI to society to ensure that adequate funds are allocated to prevention activities, appropriate research initiatives aimed at improving the quality of life for these individuals, and the medical management of persons for whom the government serves as the responsible third-party payer. Information on average costs to individuals is also extremely valuable to persons with SCI, life care planners, case managers, lawyers, and insurance companies, who must ensure that adequate resources are set aside to meet the needs of an individual with SCI over the remainder of his or her lifetime.

Although many studies have addressed individual components of overall costs, such as lengths of stay and hospital charges for acute care, rehabilitation, and rehospitalizations, these studies are generally inadequate to determine either the total costs to individuals with SCI or the total aggregate costs to society.[1-15]

Until recently, only one study, published in 1981, attempted to estimate the present value of lifetime direct and indirect costs of persons with SCI.[16] Rather than acquiring new data upon which to project these costs (a difficult and extremely expensive task), however, this study relied primarily on the inadequate data reported by previous investigators. Therefore, although the analytic approach used was impeccable, the results could only be treated as gross approximations of the actual costs. Moreover, given the age of the data used in these analyses, as well as rapid changes in technology and increasing life expectancies, these projections are now clearly out of date.

The National SCI Database of the Model Systems initially included many variables aimed at documenting both initial and long-term direct and indirect costs for persons with SCI. These variables included pre-System days hospitalized and associated charges; length of stay and charges for acute care and rehabilitation within the Model System; number of days and associated charges for rehospitalizations and nursing home stays; charges for emergency medical services, physician services, equipment, environmental modifications, attendant care, outpatient therapy, medications, supplies, and vocational rehabilitation; and information on third-party sponsor of care, employment status, type of job, whether employment was full-time or part-time at time of injury and annual follow-up, and gross annual income from numerous sources at time of injury and annual follow-up visit. Results of this early data collection activity were published in 1982.[10]

Not surprisingly, this information proved extremely difficult, time consuming, and expensive to collect on a routine basis. As a result, given the rather limited resources of the Model System data collection activity, most of these items were deleted from the Database in 1983. Only the information on pre-System days hospitalized and associated charges, acute care and rehabilitation length of stay and charges within the Model System, number of days rehospitalized and spent in nursing homes, sponsors of care, and employment status at injury and annual follow-up was retained. Information on these items continues to be collected, but no additional variables have been added in the area of economics.

To fill this void, two new comprehensive cost studies were initiated. Building on their own previous work, as well as that of others, Berkowitz and colleagues recently published the results of a detailed investigation of the economic consequences of SCI.[17-19] At the same time, a collaborative study of the long-term costs of SCI incurred by persons initially treated at Model Systems was undertaken. Both of these studies amassed extensive cost data from several hundred persons with SCI. The study by Berkowitz et al. utilized a population-based sample augmented by persons from membership lists of organizations representing the disabled population, from independent living centers, and from referrals by persons already included in the study. The Model System study included a random sample of persons from the National SCI Database. Berkowitz et al. used standard cost estimates for each service, whereas the Model System study used actual charges incurred by the study participant. The detailed methodology and results of the Model System study are presented in this chapter, and are compared with those of Berkowitz et al. [17-19] where appropriate.

DIRECT COSTS

For purposes of the Model System study, direct costs were defined as the charges incurred by either persons with SCI or their responsible third parties that are the direct result of the injury. Charges pertaining to medical conditions that are not directly related to SCI are not included. Therefore, the figures reported herein represent incremental charges for health care and living expenses. Although methods differ, the study by Berkowitz et al. was also based on incremental costs of SCI.[17-19]

The study population included a random sample of 508 persons originally treated since 1973 at a Model System and enrolled in the National SCI Database. A 1-year cross-section of data was collected prospectively between 1989 and 1990. These data included all charges incurred during the year as a direct result of the injury. Initial data collection was by periodic telephone interviews and diaries kept by study subjects. In most instances, charges were verified by either the provider or the third-party payer. All National SCI Database information was also collected at this time for use in explaining variation in reported charges among individuals and in developing predictive models for lifetime charges.

In addition, 227 newly injured persons were randomly enrolled to assess, prospectively, the unique expenses for emergency medical services, acute care, and rehabilitation that occur during the first year after injury. Data collection methods were identical to those used to document charges after the first postinjury year. Therefore, the total study population was 735 persons.

It should be emphasized that the Model System study was based on charges rather than the actual costs incurred by vendors to deliver health services and supplies. Often, charges and costs are not highly correlated.[20] Since the main purpose of the Model System study was to estimate lifetime expenses incurred by individuals with SCI and their responsible third parties, however, charge data served as a reasonable proxy. No attempt was made to determine the amounts of charges that were actually reimbursed, or the proportion of charges that constituted actual out-of-pocket expenses for the person with SCI.

A technique known as shadow pricing was utilized in instances when free items or services were provided to estimate and include their fair-market value in the cost analysis. However, no attempt was made to adjust for needed items or services that were not received because of the limited resources of the study participant.

Total Annual Charges

Mean itemized first-year charges appear in Table 12–1, while mean itemized charges that recur annually appear in Table 12–2. Mean and median total charges are also shown. All charges are adjusted to 1992 dollars using the medical care component of the U.S. Consumer Price Index.

Because charges varied greatly from person to person primarily as a function of injury severity, all individuals were divided into four neurologic groups: (1) injury level between C1 and C4 with Frankel grade A, B, or C; (2) injury level between C5 and C8 with Frankel grade A, B, or C; (3) thoracic, lumbar, or sacral injury with Frankel grade A, B, or C; and (4) Frankel grade D regardless of injury level.[21] During preliminary analyses, this categorization scheme produced the

Table 12–1 Mean First-Year Postinjury Charges (1992 Dollars) Incurred by Persons with SCIs, by Neurologic Category

| | Frankel Grade A, B, or C | | | | |
	Group 1 (C1–C4)	Group 2 (C5–C8)	Group 3 (T1–S5)	Group 4, Frankel Grade D	Total
No. of Patients	26	50	73	78	227
Emergency Medical Services	$ 1,229	$ 974	$ 992	$ 810	$ 953
Acute Care	160,567	73,867	51,742	47,437	67,601
Rehabilitation	178,110	144,028	72,676	59,118	95,810
Rehospitalizations	21,895	5,653	7,459	4,669	7,756
Nursing Home Care	0	5,893	243	149	1,428
Outpatient Services	3,462	2,887	2,559	2,626	2,758
Outpatient Physician Fees	627	462	548	512	526
Durable Equipment	14,170	10,279	3,511	1,795	5,633
Environmental Modifications	7,988	7,568	6,175	304	4,672
Medications	1,374	1,224	887	475	875
Supplies	1,183	1,220	1,310	330	939
Attendant Care	25,358	14,622	2,879	3,686	8,317
Household Assistance	0	157	41	501	220
Vocational Rehabilitation	877	152	583	157	375
Miscellaneous Charges	227	338	791	345	472
Total Mean	417,067	269,324	152,396	122,914	198,335
Total Median	404,033	249,264	137,756	116,694	161,110

Table 12-2 Mean Charges (1992 Dollars) Incurred Annually after the First Year Postinjury by Persons with SCIs, by Neurologic Category

	Frankel Grade A, B, or C			Group 4, Frankel Grade D	Total
	Group 1 (C1–C4)	Group 2 (C5–C8)	Group 3 (T1–S5)		
No. of Patients	55	131	200	122	508
Rehospitalizations	$14,296	$ 5,064	$ 4,828	$ 2,082	$ 5,255
Nursing Home Care	1,666	578	1,064	0	748
Outpatient Services	2,027	1,168	909	640	1,032
Outpatient Physician Fees	368	401	332	200	322
Durable Equipment	3,421	1,660	1,132	486	1,361
Environmental Modifications	616	1,048	1,115	58	790
Medications	1,467	1,393	887	581	1,007
Supplies	1,556	1,508	1,309	547	1,204
Attendant Care	47,563	16,527	3,106	3,390	11,448
Household Assistance	655	364	368	369	398
Vocational Rehabilitation	408	421	184	98	249
Miscellaneous Charges	664	470	273	163	340
Total Mean	74,707	30,602	15,507	8,614	24,154
Total Median	36,794	21,967	7,235	2,281	10,417

most homogeneous groups and explained a greater proportion of variance in charges than other injury severity combinations.

Mean and median first-year charges were $198,335 and $161,110, respectively. Mean first-year charges ranged from $417,067 for persons in neurologic group 1 to $122,914 for persons in neurologic group 4. Median charges were slightly lower than mean charges for each neurologic group. Overall, dividing all persons into the four neurologic groups explained 55.6% of the variance in total first-year charges. Nonetheless, Figure 12–1 reveals that considerable variation exists among individuals within each neurologic group.

Mean total charges that recurred annually were $24,154, while median total annual charges were only $10,417. The sizable difference between mean and median total annual charges indicates a highly skewed distribution in which most individuals have relatively low charges and several persons have very high charges. Mean total annual charges ranged from $74,707 for persons in neurologic group 1 to $8,614 for persons in neurologic group 4. Again, median charges were substantially lower than mean charges for each neurologic group. Overall, dividing all persons into the four neurologic groups explained only 22.8% of the variance in total annual charges. Therefore, there is still

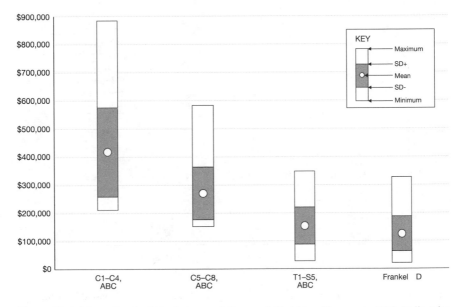

Figure 12–1 Mean, Standard Deviation, and Range of First-Year Charges in 1992 Dollars by Neurologic Group

---

substantial variability in total annual charges within each neurologic group (Figure 12–2).

Interestingly, after adjusting for inflation, these new estimates of total annual charges are not substantially different from estimates derived as long ago as 1968.[22] At that time, mean annual expenses for a person with traumatic paraplegia were estimated to be $2,270. In 1992 dollars, this figure would be $13,824, which is very similar to both the new estimate of $15,507 appearing in Table 12–2 and the new estimate by Harvey et al.[18] of $13,705 (also in 1992 dollars). However, average charges for individual items were substantially different, with almost two thirds of those charges in 1968 resulting from rehospitalizations.[22]

Emergency Medical Services

Charges for emergency medical services include those services performed at the site of injury, emergency transportation to the first acute care facility, and transportation between hospitals up to the first definitive discharge from the Model System. These charges averaged $953 per person, with only slight variation among the neurologic groups.

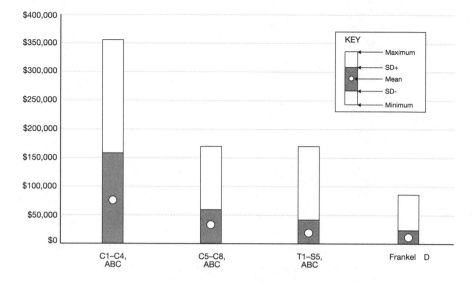

Figure 12–2 Mean, Standard Deviation, and Range of Annual Charges Incurred after the First Postinjury Year in 1992 Dollars by Neurologic Group

Acute Care

Overall mean length of stay in acute care was 24.9 days (median = 19 days). Mean length of stay in acute care for each neurologic group was 45.8 days for group 1, 30.6 days for group 2, 18.3 days for group 3, and 20.3 days for group 4. These lengths of stay are substantially reduced from those reported in previous years.[23]

Figure 12–3 depicts the acute care length of stay for all persons enrolled in the National SCI Database who were admitted to a Model System within 24 hours of injury. Since 1973, mean length of acute care stay has declined from 38 to 33 days for group 1, 39 to 29 days for group 2, 28 to 20 days for group 3, and 27 to 17 days for group 4. These decreased lengths of stay, coupled with improved treatment outcomes documented elsewhere in this book, represent a significant achievement of the Model Systems.

Acute care charges included emergency room fees, charges for room and board, X-ray, laboratory, pharmacy, central supply, intensive care unit, operating room, recovery room, anesthesia, nuclear medicine, respiratory therapy, inpatient physician fees, and other miscellaneous inpatient charges occurring prior to transfer to the rehabilitation service. These charges averaged $67,601, and ranged from $160,567 for persons in neurologic group 1 to $47,437 for persons in neurologic group 4.

Figure 12–3 also depicts the acute care charges (exclusive of inpatient physician fees) for all persons enrolled in the National SCI Database who were admitted to a Model System within 24 hours of injury. Despite reduced lengths of stay, acute care charges have risen (in constant 1992 dollars) even after adjusting for medical care cost inflation, particularly for neurologic group 1. This is most likely due to the increasing percentage of ventilator-dependent persons in this group over time.[23] Increasing intensity of service provided during acute care is undoubtedly also responsible for much of the increase in inflation-adjusted charges for all groups.

Rehabilitation

Overall mean length of stay in rehabilitation was 77.5 days (median = 74.0 days). Mean length of stay in rehabilitation for each neurologic group was 111.0 days for group 1, 116.0 days for group 2, 62.4 days for group 3, and 55.8 days for group 4. Therefore, when combined with acute care, the mean total length of stay from injury to completion of rehabilitation was 156.8 days for group 1, 146.6 days for group 2, 80.7 days for group 3, and 76.1 days for group 4.

Mean rehabilitation length of stay for all persons enrolled in the National SCI Database who were admitted to a Model System within 24 hours of injury has declined substantially since 1973 for all neurologic groups (Figure 12–3). For group 1, mean rehabilitation length of stay decreased from 134 to only 99 days. Decreases in mean rehabilitation length of stay for the remaining groups were from 171 to 102 days for group 2, 100 to 65 days for group 3, and 87 to 54 days for group 4. Once again, these declines in length of stay, coupled with improved treatment outcomes, represent a significant achievement of the Model Systems.

Rehabilitation charges included all charges for room and board, X-ray, laboratory, pharmacy, central supply, nuclear medicine, rehabilitation medicine, respiratory therapy, physical therapy, occupational therapy, recreational therapy, speech therapy, psychologic services, physician services, and other miscellaneous items occurring during inpatient rehabilitation. These charges averaged $95,810, and ranged from $178,110 for persons in neurologic group 1 to $59,118 for persons in neurologic group 4. Therefore, when combined with emergency medical services and acute care, mean total charges from injury to completion of rehabilitation were $339,906 for group 1, $218,869 for group 2, $125,410 for group 3, and $107,365 for group 4. Mean total charges for emergency medical services, acute care, and rehabilitation for all persons combined was $164,364.

By comparison, after adjusting the findings of Harvey et al. to 1992 dollars, average hospitalization charges were $126,715.[18] Their figure is lower in part

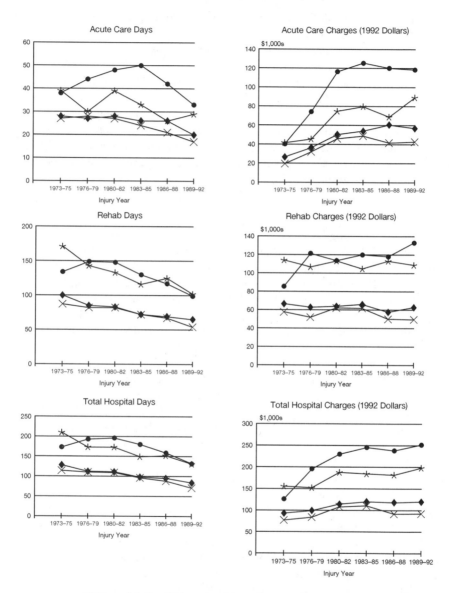

Figure 12–3 Acute Care, Rehabilitation, and Total Length of Stay and Associated Charges for All Persons Admitted to a Model System within 24 Hours of Injury by Neurologic Group and Injury Year

because it does not include charges for emergency medical services and inpatient physician fees. It does, however, include rehospitalizations during the first 2 years after injury. Their figure is also lower because their study population includes relatively few persons with neurologically complete injuries or high-level tetraplegia. Moreover, because their hospitalization data were collected retrospectively, their results are biased slightly by the exclusion of more severely injured persons who died prior to initiation of the study. Taking all these factors into consideration, the results of the two studies seem reasonably comparable.

Interestingly, for all persons enrolled in the National SCI Database who were admitted to a Model System within 24 hours of injury, mean charges for inpatient rehabilitation have decreased slightly since 1973 in constant 1992 dollars for all neurologic groups except group 1 (Figure 12–3). Once again, the increased charges for inpatient rehabilitation in group 1 are probably due to the increase in the percentage of ventilator-dependent persons in that group.

Rehospitalizations

Charges for rehospitalizations appearing in Tables 12–1 and 12–2 include all of the types of charges listed previously for inpatient acute care and rehabilitation, as well as charges for emergency room visits when no hospitalization occurred. These charges averaged $7756 during the remainder of the first postinjury year and $5255 annually thereafter. Given study population differences in injury severity levels, the latter figure is consistent with that reported by Harvey et al. ($3937 in 1992 dollars).[18] Both studies revealed considerable variability in these charges by neurologic group.

Additional information from the National SCI Database on days rehospitalized appears in Tables 12–3 and 12–4. Initially, each person with SCI is rehospitalized on average once every 2 years. As time postinjury increases, rehospitalizations become less frequent and appear to occur about once every 3 years. Average length of stay per rehospitalization is approximately 17 days (Table 12–3).

The frequency of rehospitalizations has declined significantly since the inception of the Model System program. For example, during the fifth postinjury year, the frequency of rehospitalizations has decreased by 43% (Table 12–4). This has led to a corresponding decline in average number of days rehospitalized from 11.64 to only 4.78. Average length of stay per rehospitalization has also declined. Similar declines in number of rehospitalizations and associated lengths of stay during the second postinjury year for persons treated at Model Systems have been reported previously.[23]

Nursing Home Care

Only 7 of 227 persons (3.1%) required nursing home care during the first postinjury year, while only 10 of 508 persons (2.0%) required nursing home care

Table 12–3　Rehospitalization Data by Postinjury Year for All Persons Enrolled in the National SCI Database since 1973

Postinjury Year	Average Days Rehospitalized per Year	Average Rehospitalizations per Year	Average Days per Rehospitalization
1–5	9.60	0.55	17.5
6–10	6.97	0.44	15.8
11–15	7.31	0.39	18.7
16–18	5.74	0.32	17.9

during a subsequent study year. As a result, estimates of average nursing home charges are somewhat unstable. Average nursing home charges for all individuals were $1428 during the first postinjury year and $748 annually thereafter. These charges include physician fees associated with nursing home visits. Among those few individuals who actually spent time in nursing homes or extended care facilities, mean charges were $46,294 (median = $14,528) during the remainder of the first postinjury year and $38,018 (median = $23,399) in other postinjury years.

These figures are somewhat higher than those reported by Harvey et al. for postinjury institutional care.[18] Adjusted to 1992 dollars, they reported average annual charges for institutional care of $252 for all persons and $10,593 for persons who were actually institutionalized. Their estimates are based on per-diem charges and do not include physician fees. They also reported 2.6% of all persons with SCI alive in 1988 resided in long-term care facilities, a figure that is consistent with Model System data.[24]

Table 12–4　Rehospitalization Data for Fifth Postinjury Year by Date of Injury for All Persons Enrolled in the National SCI Database since 1973

Injury Year	Average Days Rehospitalized	Average Rehospitalizations	Average Days per Rehospitalization
1973–1975	11.64	0.61	19.1
1976–1979	8.64	0.52	16.6
1980–1982	6.65	0.48	13.9
1983–1985	5.20	0.32	16.3
1986–1987	4.78	0.35	13.7

Outpatient Services and Physician Fees

Outpatient services include physical therapy (even when conducted in the home), occupational therapy, speech therapy, psychology, laboratory, X-ray, and other miscellaneous charges associated with outpatient visits. Charges for time spent in transitional living units are also included. Physician visits and associated charges are considered separately.

Mean charges for outpatient services were $2758 during the remainder of the first postinjury year and $1032 annually thereafter. After the first postinjury year, mean annual charges for outpatient services ranged from $2027 for neurologic group 1 to $640 for neurologic group 4.

Mean outpatient physician fees were $526 during the remainder of the first postinjury year and $322 annually thereafter. Physician charges did not vary much by neurologic group.

Somewhat higher charges were reported by Harvey et al.[18] Adjusted to 1992 dollars, they reported average charges for practitioner visits (physician and nonphysician) of $2992 per year. Moreover, their figure does not include laboratory and X-ray charges. Therefore, the reason their reported charges in this category are higher than those of the Model System population is unclear.

Durable Equipment

Durable equipment charges included all charges for purchase, rental, or repair of equipment such as hospital beds, special mattresses, commodes, wheelchairs, wheelchair cushions, wheelchair backpacks, cushion covers, caliper straps, crutches, braces, splints, orthoses, ventilators, ventilator parts, and environmental control units. The purchase or lease price of a new car or van was specifically excluded, since individuals in the general population presumably purchase new cars at the same pace as persons with SCI.

Average charges for durable equipment were $5633 during the remainder of the first postinjury year and $1361 annually thereafter. These charges increased substantially as injury severity increased, particularly during the first postinjury year.

Harvey et al. did not estimate equipment charges specifically for the first postinjury year.[18] Instead, they spread equipment charges over the expected lifetime of the equipment. Adjusted to 1992 dollars, they found average annual equipment charges of $1146. However, unlike the Model System study, their study did not include equipment repair and maintenance charges. Taking this into consideration, results of the two studies appear to be comparable.

Environmental Modifications

Environmental charges include all charges for modifications to residences and work sites. The purchase or lease price of a new car or van is once again specifically excluded. However, if a car or van the person already owns or newly purchases is appropriately modified during the year (hand controls, lift, etc.), then charges for these modifications are included.

Average charges for environmental modifications were $4672 during the remainder of the first postinjury year and $790 annually thereafter. Persons in neurologic group 4 (many of whom are ambulatory) had substantially lower charges for environmental modifications than persons in the other three neurologic groups.

Harvey et al. assumed that all home modification charges occurred during the second postinjury year and did not include charges for work site or vehicle modifications.[18] Using a slightly less precise method than that of the Model System study, they found that average charges for home modifications adjusted to 1992 dollars were $9546, a figure that is somewhat higher than the combined charges for all environmental modifications found for the Model System study population during the first 2 years after injury.

Medications and Supplies

Charges for medications and supplies included those for both prescription and nonprescription drugs and supplies. Typical medications include muscle relaxers, urine acidifiers, antacids, laxatives, analgesics, and antibiotics. Typical supplies include catheters, tubing, leg and bed bags, disposable gloves, adhesive tape, cement, detergent, skin lotions, powder, bed pads, bandages, and diapers.

Average charges for medications were $875 during the remainder of the first year after injury and $1007 annually thereafter. Average medication charges increased significantly as injury severity increased, ranging from $475 (group 4) to $1374 (group 1) during the remainder of the first postinjury year, and from $581 to $1467 annually thereafter for those same neurologic groups.

Average charges for supplies were $939 during the remainder of the first postinjury year and $1204 annually thereafter. Persons in neurologic group 4 (many of whom have normal bladder function) had significantly lower charges for supplies than persons in the other three neurologic groups.

Harvey et al. reported average charges for prescription drugs adjusted to 1992 dollars of $150 per year, and average charges for nonprescription medications and supplies of $2244 per year.[18] These figures are almost identical to the combined average annual medication and supply charges of $2211 after the first postinjury year for persons in the Model System study.

Attendant Care and Household Assistance

Charges for attendant care included those for unskilled services provided by paid family members, friends, neighbors, aides, and orderlies, as well as skilled services provided by registered nurses or licensed practical nurses. House-hold assistance charges included those for any additional help required for such activities as cleaning the residence, cooking, laundry, shopping, and yardwork. For this category of expenses, shadow pricing was used to include the cost of unpaid attendant care, but not the cost of unpaid household assistance.

On average, annual charges for attendant care are higher than for anything else for persons in neurologic groups 1, 2, and 4, and rank second only to charges for rehospitalizations for persons in neurologic group 3. Average attendant care charges were $8317 during the remainder of the first postinjury year and $11,448 annually thereafter. However, these charges varied substantially by neurologic group. Because neurologic group 4 includes some persons with cervical injuries, average attendant care charges for that group are slightly higher than those for neurologic group 3. Average attendant care charges for persons in neurologic group 1 were $25,358 during the remainder of the first postinjury year and $47,563 annually thereafter.

Most persons with SCI did not incur additional charges for paid household assistance other than what may have been provided by their attendants. Average charges for household assistance were $220 during the remainder of the first postinjury year and $398 annually thereafter.

Harvey et al. estimated costs for all forms of personal assistance by applying a standard wage for each hour of paid or unpaid assistance received.[18] Fringe benefits and other agency fees were not included. Adjusted to 1992 dollars, they reported average annual charges for personal assistance of $8092. Again, these charges varied substantially by neurologic group. This figure is lower than the average charges for attendant care found for persons treated at Model Systems ($11,448) because the Model System population was on average more severely injured than the population studied by Harvey et al., and because fringe benefits and agency fees were included in the Model System study as a portion of the charges to the person with SCI. Given these methodologic differences, results of the two studies with respect to attendant care should be viewed as reasonably consistent.

Vocational Rehabilitation

Vocational rehabilitation charges included all charges for vocational and educational preparation and vocational counseling purchased either by the person with SCI or a third party (such as a vocational rehabilitation agency). Most persons with SCI did not incur any charges for vocational rehabilitation. As a result, these charges averaged $375 during the remainder of the first postinjury year and only $249 annually thereafter. Harvey et al. did not include charges for vocational rehabilitation in their study.[18]

Miscellaneous Charges

Miscellaneous charges included all items not reported under any other category, such as transportation to and from medical service providers (after discharge from rehabilitation), appropriate long-distance phone calls, and care and maintenance of helper animals (excluding pets). Average miscellaneous charges were $472 during the remainder of the first year after injury and $340 annually thereafter. After the first postinjury year, average annual miscellaneous charges increased significantly as injury severity increased, ranging from $163 for persons in neurologic group 4 to $664 for persons in neurologic group 1. These charges were not included in the study by Harvey et al.[18]

Predictive Models for Total Charges

Because there is considerable variability in charges among individuals with SCI (Figures 12–1 and 12–2), the averages shown in Tables 12–1 and 12–2 are not that useful in projecting future charges for any particular person. Therefore, stepwise multiple linear regression analysis was used to develop separate predictive models that could produce more precise estimates of first-year and annual recurring charges. Only variables making a statistically significant contribution to explained variance in charges were included in the final models.

The predictive model for charges incurred during the first year after injury appears in Table 12–5. In addition to neurologic group, variables that had a

---

Table 12–5 Predictive Model for Charges (1992 Dollars) Incurred during the First Postinjury Year by Persons with SCIs (n = 227)

Predictor	1992 Dollars
C1–C4, Frankel Grade A, B, C	$173,475
C5–C8, Frankel Grade A, B, C	90,627
T1–S5, Frankel Grade A, B, C	20,085
Ventilator Dependent	194,471
Nursing Home	63,957
Each Rehospitalization	12,503
Each Complication	13,926
Spinal Surgery	17,094
Northeast U.S. Residence	43,443
Attendant Care	
Each Skilled Hour per Day	4,382
Each Unskilled Hour per Day	1,672
Constant	73,238

statistically significant effect on first-year postinjury charges were ventilator dependency, nursing home stay, number of rehospitalizations, number of secondary medical complications (as defined in Appendix A), whether spinal surgery was performed, residence in the Northeastern United States (New England plus New York, Pennsylvania, New Jersey, and Delaware), and number of skilled and unskilled hours of attendant care per day (whether paid or unpaid). Each variable is coded zero if absent or one if present, except for number of rehospitalizations, number of secondary medical complications, and number of hours per day of skilled and unskilled attendant care. Episodes of secondary medical complications that were counted included scoliosis, contractures, heterotopic ossification, spasticity, pressure sores, postoperative wound infections, gastrointestinal hemorrhages, aspiration, atelectasis, autonomic dysreflexia, pneumonia, pulmonary embolus, deep vein thrombosis, ventilatory failure, heart attack, orchitis, and kidney stones. Other complications were not considered. Adding these variables to group membership increased the explained proportion of variance in first-year charges from 55.6% to 71.6%.

To use the model in Table 12–5, multiply the value of each variable by the appropriate charge estimate and sum the results, including the constant. The constant represents the average basic cost for persons in the Frankel grade D group who have no complications, surgery, rehospitalizations, attendant care, or nursing home stays. The values for the other neurologic groups represent the average incremental basic costs for those groups over and above the average costs for the Frankel grade D group. For example, assume that a person has a C4 injury level of Frankel grade A (neurologic group 1), is not ventilator dependent, does not need to spend time in a nursing home after discharge, does not need to be rehospitalized during the remainder of the first postinjury year, has two secondary medical complications during acute care and one during rehabilitation, has spinal fusion performed during acute care, does not reside in the Northeast, and needs 16 hours per day of unskilled attendant care but no skilled attendant care postdischarge. Then, by using the model, this person's predicted charges for the first postinjury year in 1992 dollars would be:

\$173,475	C1–C4, Frankel Grade A, B, C
+ 3(\$13,926)	Complications
+ \$17,094	Spine Surgery
+ 16(\$1,672)	Unskilled Attendant
+ \$73,238	Constant
\$332,337	Total

Additional variables that were included in the analysis but not in the final model because their effect on first-year postinjury charges was statistically insignificant were age, sex, race, method of bladder management, and sponsor of care. No statistically significant interactive effects were identified.

The model contained in Table 12–5 provides at least a partial explanation of differences in first-year postinjury charges between individuals. Its use is often not necessary for projecting lifetime charges for persons with SCI, however, because by the time one usually begins this process, actual first-year charges will already be known.

The predictive model for recurring charges incurred annually over the remaining lifetime of the person with SCI appears in Table 12–6. In addition to neurologic group, variables that had a statistically significant effect on recurring annual charges were ventilator dependency, nursing home stay, number of rehospitalizations, and number of skilled and unskilled hours of attendant care per day (whether paid or unpaid). Unlike first-year postinjury charges, there was no overall effect on recurring annual charges of living in the Northeastern United States. There was, however, a significant interaction between Northeast residence and attendant care charges that were substantially higher, on average, in that part of the country. Adding these variables to group membership increased the explained proportion of variance in recurring annual charges from 22.8% to 73.8%.

The model in Table 12–6 can be used in the same way as the one in Table 12–5. Continuing the previous example used for Table 12–5, assume that the same person is anticipated to be rehospitalized once every other year. The predicted recurring annual charges for that person in constant 1992 dollars would be:

$13,503	C1–C4, Frankel Grade A, B, C
+ $15,868/2	Rehospitalization
+ 16 ($1,799)	Unskilled Attendant
+ $2,067	Constant
$52,288	Total

Additional variables that were included in the analysis but not in the final model because their effect on recurring annual charges was statistically insignificant were age, sex, race, method of bladder management, and sponsor of care. No other statistically significant interactive effects were identified.

The trend in recurring annual charges over time was also not statistically significant, perhaps because the study was limited to 18 years of follow-up with an average of 8.5 years. In fact, when using the model contained in Table 12–6, it is not necessary to assume that the recurring annual charges are constant. For example, it could be assumed that when the person reaches a certain age, attendant care needs, the rehospitalization rate, or the need for nursing home services will change. To accommodate this change in needs, one can recalculate the predicted recurring annual charges beginning at that time.

In developing an individual life care plan, because of the extreme variability in attendant care and nursing home charges, a more precise estimate of recurring

Table 12-6 Predictive Model for Charges (1992 Dollars) Incurred Annually after the First Postinjury Year by Persons with SCIs (n = 508)

Predictor	1992 Dollars
C1–C4, Frankel Grade A, B, C	$ 13,503
C5–C8, Frankel Grade A, B, C	5,573
T1–S5, Frankel Grade A, B, C	4,791
Ventilator Dependent	115,866
Nursing Home	23,389
Each Rehospitalization	15,868
Attendant Care in Northeastern U.S.	
Each Skilled Hour per Day	11,048
Each Unskilled Hour per Day	3,770
Attendant Care Elsewhere in U.S.	
Each Skilled Hour per Day	3,735
Each Unskilled Hour per Day	1,799
Constant	2,067

annual charges would be obtained if the actual charges to provide the needed level of service in the person's community could be determined. For example, consider the same person that has been used in the previous examples. Assume further that the potential provider of attendant care services indicates that these 16 hours of unskilled services will cost $35,000 per year (slightly higher than predicted by the model). Then using the predictive model for items other than attendant care and substituting the actual attendant care charges, the predicted recurring annual charges for this person in constant 1992 dollars would be:

$13,503	C1–C4, Frankel Grade A, B, C
+ $15,868/2	Rehospitalization
+ $35,000	Attendant Care
+ $2,067	Constant
$58,504	Total

In this way, when actual data for items other than attendant care and nursing home stays are difficult to obtain, the values appearing in the predictive model for each neurologic group plus the constant (plus ventilator dependency if appropriate) can be used to represent annual anticipated incidental expenses in constant 1992 dollars for supplies, medications, equipment, environmental modifications, outpatient therapy, laboratory fees, physician visits, household assistance, and other miscellaneous charges incurred on average by these persons. For persons in neurologic group 4, only the constant would be used to represent these anticipated charges.

As expected, the regression model shown in Table 12–6 suggests that rehospitalizations among persons with SCIs are, on average, considerably more expensive than rehospitalizations among the general population. Based on the model, the average charge for each rehospitalization among persons with SCIs is $15,868. However, adjusting 1987 data from the National Medical Expenditure Survey to 1992 dollars, the average charge per hospitalization for persons from the general population is only $8,763.[25] Both figures include in-patient physician fees. These data are consistent with length of hospitalization stays: rehospitalizations for persons with SCIs average approximately 17 days (Table 12–3), while hospitalizations for persons in the general population average approximately 7 days but frequently include surgery.[26]

Lifetime Direct Costs

Once the first-year postinjury and recurring annual charges have been either determined from actual data or estimated from the predictive models, this information can be combined with future annual survival probabilities to estimate total charges over the remaining lifetime of an individual. This is done by calculating the "present value" (PV) of future charges as follows:

$$\text{PV Lifetime Charges} = \Sigma \ (DC_t) \ (PS_t)/(1 + d)^{t-1}$$

where:

t = the number of years postinjury
DC_t = direct charges in postinjury year t
PS_t = probability of surviving to postinjury year t given survival to the year of injury
d = the discount rate

For these purposes, PS_t was determined by applying the standardized mortality ratios appearing in Chapter 14 to standard life tables published by the federal government for the most recent year available (1988).[27] Beyond the first postinjury year, DC was based on 1992 price levels and assumed to be constant over time. However, apart from changing price level, one dollar today is worth more than one dollar in the future because of the interest it could earn between now and then. Since charges were assumed to be constant over time, the discount rate used in the model represents the real rate of return on investments over and above inflation.

Based on the average charges during the first postinjury year appearing in Table 12–1 and the average recurring annual charges appearing in Table 12–2, the present value of average lifetime direct costs in constant 1992 dollars by neurologic group for persons who are either 25 or 50 years of age at time of injury appears in Table 12–7. Because the choice of an appropriate discount rate is never entirely clear, and because this selection has such a huge impact on the estimation of lifetime costs, results are provided using several different discount rates.

Using a 4% discount rate, the present value of average lifetime direct costs for a person injured at 25 years of age ranged from $1,349,029 for persons in neurologic group 1 to $287,001 for persons in neurologic group 4. For someone injured at 50 years of age, the comparable average lifetime direct costs would be reduced to $876,287 and $231,018, respectively, because of the reduced life expectancies for persons injured at this age compared with those injured at 25 years of age.

It is difficult to compare these estimates of average lifetime direct costs with those of Berkowitz et al. because they are based on different ages and different injury severity groupings.[17] Adjusting their estimate to 1992 dollars, they found average lifetime direct costs discounted at 4% for a 27-year-old person with neurologically complete (Frankel grade A) tetraplegia of $591,128. Most of these individuals would probably be in neurologic group 2 of the Model System study with average lifetime direct charges at 25 years of age of $748,234 using the same discount rate. This difference is partially accounted for by the 2-year age difference, since the Model System study estimate would be almost $60,000 lower at 27 years of age. As discussed previously, much of the remaining difference may be accounted for by inclusion of charges in the Model System study that were omitted from the study by Berkowitz et al.[17–19] After adjusting for age differences and inflation, their estimates of lifetime direct costs for other

---

Table 12–7 Present Value of Average Lifetime Direct Costs (1992 Dollars) for Persons with SCIs by Age at Injury, Neurologic Category, and Assumed Discount Rate

| Age at Injury | Discount Rate | Frankel Grade A, B, or C | | | Group 4, Frankel Grade D |
		Group 1 (C1–C4)	Group 2 (C5–C8)	Group 3 (T1–S5)	
25	0	$1,962,586	$1,147,026	$714,289	$479,150
	2	1,593,157	900,818	532,307	355,089
	4	1,349,029	748,234	427,733	287,001
	6	1,179,425	648,395	363,410	246,537
50	0	1,013,940	625,227	413,901	295,570
	2	937,900	570,466	363,067	257,340
	4	876,287	528,021	326,272	231,018
	6	825,680	495,291	298,919	212,114

neurologic categories also appear slightly lower than those of the Model System study.

It would be possible to build an adjustment into the model for potential changes in real values over time to reflect the fact that medical sector prices have risen more rapidly than prices in other sectors of the economy. However, although this trend has existed for several years, it is unlikely that it will continue, particularly as the federal government is anticipated to initiate additional efforts to curtail the spiraling costs of health care. Therefore, no adjustment was made. Previous investigators have also argued against such an adjustment.[16,17] If this trend were to continue, then an anticipated real increase in medical sector prices could be accommodated by choosing an appropriately smaller discount rate. For example, assume that the normal rate of return on investments is 10% and the overall rate of inflation is 4%. In this case, use of a 6% discount rate (the real rate of return on investments) would be appropriate for future expenditures. However, if medical sector prices were rising at 8% per year (a 4% real differential above overall inflation), then use of a 2% rather than a 6% discount rate would reflect the real increase in medical sector prices.

The use of no discount rate (0%) reflects the assumption that health care inflation will exactly equal future real investment potential, implying that health care prices will continue to rise considerably faster than the overall rate of inflation. As previously indicated, this is unlikely over the long term. Therefore, this column is included in Table 12–7 for illustration purposes only.

In fact, all of the estimates shown in Table 12–7 are meant only for illustration purposes. These estimates are of necessity extrapolations of present data into the future. Changes in future medical care and management as well as technologic advances may have a significant effect on future direct costs. Moreover, these estimates are based on the average values provided in Tables 12–1 and 12–2 rather than the more precise predictive models appearing in Tables 12–5 and 12–6 or the actual needs and experiences of the individual up to the time the projection is made.

These estimates are conservative because some persons undoubtedly have unmet needs that were not included. Moreover, there is at least anecdotal evidence that charges rise substantially during the last few years of life for persons with SCIs.[28] Although these extra charges are not included in the present study, the bias toward conservative results that this causes is relatively small because these charges occur many years after injury and are therefore subject to considerable discounting over time.

Sponsors of Care

No discussion of the direct costs of SCI would be complete without considering the financial burden these extraordinary charges place on responsible third parties and individuals with SCI. Given these high costs, it is not surprising that the type of third-party coverage each person has influences at least to some extent the rehabilitation outcomes that are achieved. For persons with SCI, length of initial hospital stay, likelihood of nursing home placement and length of nursing home stay, likelihood and length of rehospitalization, likelihood of acquiring professional attendant care services and returning to work, and overall quality of life are all affected in part by type and amount of third-party coverage.[29,30] Coverage by public or private insurance is also associated with greater use of health care services and higher average expenditures in the general population.[25,31] Interestingly, however, sponsor of care was not included in the final predictive models for first-year and annual charges (Tables 12–5 and 12–6) because it did not add significantly to explained variance after controlling for the other items in the models.

Fortunately, most persons have at least partial third-party coverage of their expenses. Information on sponsors of care for the initial admission and the fifth postinjury year taken from the entire National SCI Database appears in Table 12–8. The percentages shown in Table 12–8 do not sum to 100 because many persons have more than one sponsor sharing responsibility for their care. Although each sponsor is identified in the Database, the coding scheme precludes determination of the percentage of charges for which each is responsible.

Table 12–8 Percentages of Persons with SCIs Having Each Sponsor of Care at Initial Admission and 5 Years Postinjury*

Sponsor	Initial Admission	5 Years Postinjury
Private Insurance	55.5	44.6
Medicaid	18.1	21.5
Vocational Rehabilitation	14.0	11.6
Workers' Compensation	11.9	11.5
Medicare	5.0	38.8
CHAMPUS or Other Insurance	3.8	3.0
Crippled Children's Service	2.9	0.7
Health Maintenance Organization	1.4	0.8
Self-Pay	1.1	2.1
Indigent	1.0	0.1
SCI System Funds	1.0	0.8
County Medical	0.7	0.6
Public Health Service	0.6	1.7
Veterans Administration	0.2	1.4
Other Private Funds	0.1	0.1

*Percentages do not sum to 100 because many individuals had more than one sponsor.

Approximately half of these persons have private insurance to cover at least part of their bills. Approximately one fifth are covered by Medicaid, state vocational rehabilitation agencies, or workers' compensation. Given the young age at which these injuries typically occur, it is not surprising that Medicare initially covers only 5% of these persons. However, by the fifth postinjury year, 38.8% of these individuals are receiving Medicare benefits, due to a combination of aging plus a provision that allows some persons below age 65 to qualify for Medicare benefits after a period of permanent disability.

Interestingly, this pattern of coverage is quite different from that of the general population. Among persons in the general population, 36% of health care expenses are paid by private insurance, 18% by Medicare, 8% by Medicaid, 9% by other public programs, 5% by other sources (such as workers' compensation, private charity, etc.), and 24% by the individual.[25]

These SCI sponsorship data should be interpreted cautiously because some sponsors such as the Veterans Administration and health maintenance organizations are undoubtedly under-represented in the National SCI Database. Also, the indigent category was added to the Database only a few years ago. Many persons listed in the self-pay category are in fact indigent.

INDIRECT COSTS

The indirect costs of SCI are predominantly those that result from losses in wages, fringe benefits, and productivity. These indirect costs are typically assessed by using either a human-capital or a willingness-to-pay approach.[16,32,33] The human-capital approach is based on using the value of expected postinjury lifetime earnings and fringe benefits losses discounted back to the year of injury as a surrogate of future productive worth in the absence of that injury. The limitations of this approach are relatively straightforward. For example, the discounted future earnings projections are based on current earnings data, current survival rates, and uncertain estimates of future changes in productivity. As a result, because of current inequities in the marketplace, working-age white men are consistently valued at higher levels than women and minorities.[16,33] Moreover, the value of other factors, such as lost leisure time activities, is not considered.[32] Nonetheless, with its inherent limitations, the discounted value of future earnings and fringe benefits is relatively easy both to measure and understand.

The willingness-to-pay approach attempts to measure the value of reduced quality (and quantity) of life by asking what one would be willing to pay to eliminate the risk of SCI and its consequences.[16,32,33] This information would be obtained from surveys of persons without SCI. However, this approach also has severe limitations. Willingness to pay is not easy to quantify. It is conceptually difficult for most healthy persons to evaluate either the probability of injury (and possibly death) or the severity of its consequences. Stated preferences often differ from actual behavior. As a result, most economists continue to use the human-capital approach to determine indirect costs.

To use the human-capital approach, one must estimate what the person's earnings would have been had he or she not sustained an SCI, and what his or her earnings are after the injury. One way to estimate expected earnings in the absence of SCI is to use information from the Bureau of Labor Statistics on average earnings for full-time and part-time workers. This information is differentiated by age, gender, race, and education. General-population employment rates can also be obtained from the Bureau of Labor Statistics. Therefore, average expected earnings can be obtained by multiplying the appropriate average earnings for workers in the general population by the corresponding probability of employment. A percentage increase can be applied to reflect the value of fringe benefits. Annual loss is then calculated as the difference between expected and actual earnings and fringe benefits. This was the approach used by Berkowitz et al.[17]

In addition to the limitations of the human-capital approach already discussed, one limitation that is particularly troublesome for studies of SCI is that estimates of future earnings are based on educational attainment at the time of injury. Yet, given the typical age when these injuries occur, educational plans are often interrupted and not subsequently completed. Berkowitz et al. reported that the educational plans of over 41% of persons in their study were altered as a result of injury.[17] Therefore, future earnings potential will be underestimated. Moreover, there may be other differences between persons with SCI and the general population on variables other than age, gender, race, or education that would affect earnings potential. If so, this would cause a potential bias when using general-population averages as a surrogate for the expected experiences of persons with SCI.

The Model System collaborative study of long-term costs used a slightly different approach. All persons from the study of direct costs who were between the ages of 15 and 57 years at injury and were either employed in the competitive labor market or unemployed at injury were included in the study of indirect costs. Students, homemakers, and retired persons at injury were excluded. Persons who were currently of retirement age or who had been injured for less than 3 years were also excluded. Overall, 332 persons met these criteria.

Each person was asked about his or her current wage as well as that at the time of injury. Disability benefits and income not related to employment were excluded. Reported preinjury and postinjury wages were adjusted for inflation to 1992 dollars using the Employment Cost Index. In accordance with data from the Bureau of Labor Statistics, wages from part-time employment were increased by 12.2% and wages from full-time employment were increased by 36.7% to reflect the value of fringe benefits.[34] Moreover, in accordance with historic trends, wages were increased by an additional 1.7% per year to reflect increased productivity. These are the same figures used by Berkowitz et al.[17] Inflation- and productivity-adjusted preinjury wages and benefits were then assumed to equal the expected postinjury wages and benefits, and annual losses were calculated as the actual postinjury wages and benefits minus the expected postinjury wages and benefits.

Annual Lost Wages and Fringe Benefits

Estimates of annual lost wages and fringe benefits in 1992 dollars for each of the four neurologic groups appear in Table 12–9. Mean annual forgone earnings and fringe benefits ranged from $50,470 in group 1 to $34,375 in group 4. However, the medians were considerably below the means for each group, indicating the presence of several high-loss outliers, particularly in group 1. Moreover, these groups were not very homogeneous with respect to forgone earnings, as seen in Figure 12–4. In fact, given the considerable overlap between groups shown in Figure 12–4, it is not surprising that neurologic group explained only 1.3% of the variance in annual forgone earnings and fringe benefits. As is seen later, there are more effective ways to group persons with respect to annual forgone earnings that would explain a considerably greater proportion of the variance; however, the present neurologic grouping was retained for consistency with the discussion of direct costs, thereby facilitating calculation of total direct and indirect costs. Given the sampling methodology used to derive the figures in Table 12–9, these estimates should be interpreted as annual losses from the time of injury (or the anticipated time of entry into the labor force for young

---

Table 12–9 Annual Forgone Earnings, Including Fringe Benefits (1992 Dollars), for Persons with SCIs by Neurologic Category

	Frankel Grade A, B, or C				
	Group 1 (C1–C4)	Group 2 (C5–C8)	Group 3 (T1–S5)	Group 4, Frankel Grade D	Total
No. of Patients	34	79	135	84	332
Mean	$50,470	$39,753	$35,783	$34,375	$37,876
Median	36,003	32,649	30,538	27,867	31,308

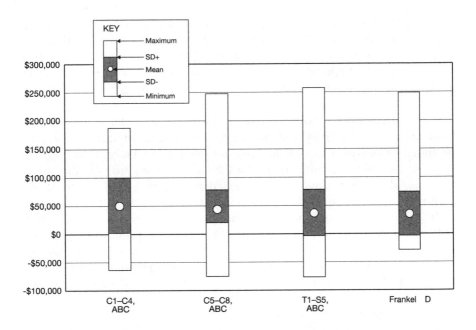

Figure 12–4 Mean, Standard Deviation, and Range of Annual Lost Wages and Fringe Benefits in 1992 Dollars by Neurologic Group

persons who are still students at the time of their injury) until normal retirement at age 65, after which no further losses are assumed.

The differences in annual forgone earnings between groups are primarily a function of differences in the likelihood of returning to work. However, part of the difference in forgone earnings for group 1 also results from a somewhat higher mean earnings level at time of injury that is probably a statistical artifact resulting from the relatively small sample size of that group.

Although most persons do not return to work, losses also occur among some persons who do return to work. Among persons who were employed both before and after injury (n = 109), the mean annual wages plus the value of fringe benefits was 71.4% of inflation- and productivity-adjusted mean preinjury wages plus the value of fringe benefits. These lost earnings occurring among persons who return to work reflect the fact that some individuals switch from full-time to part-time jobs after their injury while others must accept lower-paying and less physically demanding jobs because of their disability.

Adjusting the findings of Berkowitz et al. to 1992 dollars using the Employment Cost Index, the value of average annual lost earnings and benefits was

$14,785.[17] Without going into detail, suffice it to say this figure also includes a nominal amount for the value of lost homemaker services. However, this figure represents an average over all ages, rather than just typical working ages. In a previous study by Berkowitz that was limited to ages 18 to 64, and once again adjusting findings to 1992 dollars, average annual lost earnings and benefits were $25,097.[32]

The annual indirect costs reported by Berkowitz et al. are somewhat lower than those found in the Model System study in large part because of differences in the postinjury employment rate for the two study populations. Only 25% of persons who met the rigid eligibility criteria for the indirect cost portion of the Model System study were employed at the time of data collection. Conversely, 35.3% of all persons at least 16 years of age (including those who were retired) who were in the Berkowitz et al. study population were employed at the time of that study.[17] Differences in injury severity between the two study populations probably account for this difference in postinjury employment rates. There may also be a slight geographic bias in the Model System study population, since most facilities are located in large urban areas where wages tend to exceed the national average.

A final note of caution about these estimates of average annual forgone earnings and fringe benefits: Wages were self-reported and there were no attempts at verification. Therefore, this information is entirely dependent on the recall of the person with SCI and the quality of any records they may have used to form the basis for estimates these individuals provided to the project team. Moreover, it is possible that a very few individuals have not told the complete truth about postinjury income because of fears of losing disability benefits. As a result, this information is probably not as reliable as the information provided on direct costs.

Predictive Model for Return to Work

Once again, because there is considerable variability in lost wages and fringe benefits among individuals (Figure 12–4), the averages shown in Table 12–9 are not useful in projecting future losses for any particular person. Instead, projections for individuals should be based on the likelihood of returning to work and the anticipated difference in earnings that might result from any necessity to change jobs or reduce hours of employment. Several previous studies have identified factors associated with the likelihood of return to work that include, among others, severity of injury, education level, age, gender, race, preinjury employment history, marital status, motivation, and economic disincentives.[17,35–48] A more complete discussion of this topic is contained in Chapter 10.

Given the multitude of factors associated with return to work, a single approach is needed that combines the effects of each of these predictive factors. Therefore, stepwise multiple logistic regression analysis was used to develop a predictive model that could be used to estimate the probability of return to work for persons with SCI.

The results of this analysis appear in Table 12–10. The relationship between each of the variables in the predictive model and return to work is statistically significant except for two items: ability to ambulate independently and postinjury year. Those two items were included in the model because they added meaningfully to predictive accuracy even though their contribution was not quite statistically significant. Other potential predictors that were included in the analysis but deleted from the final model because of lack of statistical significance included gender, geographic region, and whether the person was ever a vocational rehabilitation client.

The odds ratios appearing in Table 12–10 are adjusted estimates of the likelihood of being employed postinjury for persons with that characteristic relative to that of persons who do not have that characteristic. The adjustment is for the possible confounding effects of other predictors contained in the model. For example, all other items in the model being equal, persons with intact marriages and persons who have never been married at the time of injury are 2.9 times more likely to be employed after injury than are divorced, separated, or widowed persons. In the case of education, the comparison group for each education level shown is persons who have not graduated from high school, while

---

Table 12–10 Predictive Model Derived from Logistic Regression for Probability of Return to Work after SCI (n = 332)

Predictor	Coefficient	Odds Ratio
Age at Injury	–0.056	0.9
Education at Injury		
High School Graduate	1.071	2.9
College Graduate	2.559	12.9
Master's/Doctoral Degree	4.219	67.9
White	1.188	3.3
Postinjury Year 4–14	0.793	2.2
Independent in Self-Care Activities	2.526	12.5
Ambulatory	0.615	1.8
Intact Marriage or Never Married at Injury	1.070	2.9
Employed at Injury	2.738	15.5
Constant	–7.680	—

for age at injury, the odds ratio represents the relative likelihood of being employed given a 1-year increase in age.

Based on the results of the logistic regression analysis, the strongest predictors of return to work are education level, being functionally independent in performing self-care, and being employed at the time of injury. Age at injury is also a very strong predictor, with younger persons being much more likely than older persons to return to work. Overall, this model with 80.7% sensitivity and 80.2% specificity has slightly more predictive accuracy than previously published models.[35–37]

To use the model in Table 12–10, multiply the age at injury by its coefficient (−0.056) and sum that product with each of the other applicable coefficients plus the constant. Then exponentiate that sum and divide by one plus the exponentiated sum. The result is the predicted probability of employment. Because of the inclusion of the time factor (postinjury year) in the model, two separate estimates will be calculated. One will be for postinjury years 4 through 14, and the other will be for the remaining years. For example, assume that a person is 25 years of age at injury and is a college graduate, African-American, independent in self-care activities, divorced, employed at injury, and not ambulatory. Then the probability of this individual's being employed during the first 3 years after injury as well as years 15 through retirement would be:

$\exp(-0.056 \times 25)$	Age
+ 2.559	College Graduate
+ 2.526	Independent Self Care
+ 2.738	Employed at Injury
− 7.680	Constant
$\exp(-1.257) = .28$	$.28/1.28 = .22$

Therefore, this person is estimated to have a 22% chance to be employed in each of those postinjury years. The corresponding chance of employment for postinjury years 4 through 14 would be 39%:

$\exp(-0.056 \times 25)$	Age
+ 2.559	College Graduate
+ 0.793	Year 4–14
+ 2.526	Independent Self Care
+ 2.738	Employed at Injury
− 7.680	Constant
$\exp(-0.464) = .63$	$.63/1.63 = .39$

Caution should be exercised when applying this predictive model to individual cases because many potentially important factors are not included. The person's level of motivation to return to work is one such factor previously shown to be strongly associated with return to work.[36] Also, the coefficient for postgraduate education (master's degree/doctorate) is somewhat unstable because of the small sample size of persons in that category in the study population. Moreover, although this model has apparent face validity, it has not been validated by testing its accuracy in another SCI population. Sensitivity and specificity usually decline slightly when predictive models generated from the experiences of study populations are applied in the real world. Nonetheless, given the high degree of precision of this model, it should be a useful adjunct to the process of estimating the probability of individuals returning to work by providing a baseline estimate that might be adjusted slightly to reflect other factors known to influence the likelihood of employment that are not included in the model.

Lifetime Indirect Costs

Using the human-capital approach, perhaps the ideal way to calculate the present value of lifetime forgone earnings and fringe benefits for any individual would be to use the following formula:

$$\text{PV Lost Wages} = \Sigma \, [(NPS_t)(NPE_t)(IWAGE) - (PS_t)(PE_t)(PWAGE)] \, (1+p)^{t-1}/(1+d)^{t-1}$$

where:

t	=	the number of years postinjury
NPS_t	=	the normal probability of surviving to postinjury year t in the absence of SCI given survival to the year of injury
NPE_t	=	the normal probability of being employed in year t in the absence of SCI
$IWAGE$	=	the annual wages plus the value of fringe benefits at the time of injury
p	=	the assumed annual increase in productivity
PS_t	=	the probability of surviving with SCI to postinjury year t given survival to the year of injury
PE_t	=	the probability of being employed in postinjury year t given SCI
$PWAGE$	=	the annual wages plus the value of fringe benefits after SCI
d	=	the discount rate

This is essentially the model used by Berkowitz et al., except that they also added terms representing the lost value of homemaker services to the model.[17] NPS_t can be obtained from life tables published by the federal government.[27] PS_t can be obtained by applying the standardized mortality ratios appearing in Chapter 14 to the general-population life tables, using the methodology discussed in detail in that chapter. Presence at the time of injury of other medical conditions such as cancer that might have a meaningful impact on life expectancy should also be considered whenever possible in estimating both NPS_t and PS_t. NPE_t can be obtained from tables provided by the Bureau of Labor Statistics that are specific for age, gender, race, and education.[49] PE_t might be obtained from the predictive model for return to work described previously (Table 12–10). IWAGE and PWAGE can be obtained from appropriate employment records if available, or if unavailable can be estimated from tables provided by the Bureau of Labor Statistics.[49] The estimate from this study that postinjury wages for persons who return to work are approximately 71.4% of preinjury wages adjusted for inflation and productivity might also be useful in estimating PWAGE when it is unknown.

Because both preinjury and postinjury wages were known for each person, the Model System study used a much simpler approach to estimating the present value of forgone earnings and fringe benefits:

$$PV\ Lost\ Wages\ =\ \Sigma\ (IWAGE - PWAGE)(NPS_t)(1+p)^{t-1}/(1+d)^{t-1}$$

where both IWAGE and PWAGE were adjusted upward to reflect the value of fringe benefits for full-time or part-time employment as described previously. These data were then adjusted to 1992 dollars using the Employment Cost Index. IWAGE was assumed to be zero for unemployed persons at injury, while PWAGE was assumed to be zero for persons who were unemployed at the time of postinjury data collection. Therefore, employment probabilities were built into the wage terms.

This simplified approach has the advantage of using actual data from each person. However, one disadvantage of this approach is that it assumes that postinjury survival rates are normal. Since postinjury survival rates are in fact below normal, postinjury earnings will be overestimated by this model, and as a result, annual losses will be underestimated. Therefore, estimates of lifetime forgone earnings will be conservative. To some extent, this should offset the impact of the high-income outliers in the dataset.

Using this simplified approach, estimates of the present value of average lifetime forgone earnings and fringe benefits in constant 1992 dollars by neurologic group for persons who are either 25 or 50 years of age at time of injury appear in Table 12–11. Once again, results are provided using several different discount rates.

Using a 4% discount rate, the present value of average lifetime forgone earnings and fringe benefits for a person injured at 25 years of age ranged from $1,289,005 for persons in neurologic group 1 to $878,334 for persons in neurologic group 4. For someone injured at 50 years of age, the comparable average lifetime indirect costs would be reduced to $611,872 and $416,249, respectively, because of fewer remaining years of potential employment.

Table 12–11   Present Value of Average Lifetime Indirect Costs (Forgone Earnings and Fringe Benefits) in 1992 Dollars for Persons with SCIs by Age at Injury, Neurologic Category, and Assumed Discount Rate

| Age at Injury | Discount Rate | Frankel Grade A, B, or C | | | Group 4, Frankel Grade D |
		Group 1 (C1–C4)	Group 2 (C5–C8)	Group 3 (T1–S5)	
25	0	$2,670,318	$2,103,234	$1,893,191	$1,818,916
	2	1,803,512	1,420,006	1,278,690	1,228,474
	4	1,289,005	1,015,451	914,312	878,334
	6	970,567	765,274	688,438	661,350
50	0	797,553	628,197	565,461	542,613
	2	695,184	547,008	492,883	472,946
	4	611,872	481,512	433,814	416,249
	6	543,485	427,740	385,328	369,717

Use of the median values from Table 12–9 would produce more conservative estimates of average lifetime forgone earnings and fringe benefits. At age 25, the present value of median lifetime forgone earnings and fringe benefits in constant 1992 dollars discounted at 4% ranged from $920,577 for a person in neurologic group 1 to $712,721 for a person in neurologic group 4.

Once again, these projections are meant only for illustration purposes. These estimates are based on the mean values provided in Table 12–9 rather than the more precise predictive model for return to work appearing in Table 12–10. Limitations of the data contained in Table 12–9 have been discussed previously.

Since differing methodologies were used, it is interesting to compare the results in Table 12–11 with those of Berkowitz et al.[17] The same difficulties are encountered as with the comparison of direct costs, including the use of different ages and injury severity groupings. Nonetheless, adjusting their estimate to 1992 dollars, they found average lifetime indirect costs discounted at 4% for a 27-year-old person with neurologically complete (Frankel grade A) tetraplegia of $911,022. Again, most of these persons would be in group 2 of the Model System study, with average lifetime indirect costs of $1,015,451 at age 25. Part of this difference in average lifetime indirect cost estimates is accounted for by the 2-year age difference, while the rest is probably due to the higher postinjury employment rate found by Berkowitz et al. that was discussed previously. After adjusting for age differences and inflation, their estimates of average lifetime indirect costs for other neurologic categories are also slightly lower than those of the Model System study. Nonetheless, given the understandable differences in postinjury employment rates, the two statistical approaches appear to have produced reasonably comparable results. Accordingly, the credibility of both studies seems enhanced.

Aggregate Costs to Society

The final question to be addressed is how these estimates of average lifetime direct and indirect costs for individuals translate into aggregate costs of SCI to society. Aggregate costs can be calculated by using either an incidence or prevalence approach. The incidence approach involves estimating the present value of costs for all new cases of SCI occurring in a given year. As a result, the incidence-based estimate of aggregate costs is the present value of current and future losses that could be avoided if all new cases occurring in a given year could be prevented.

In 1989, DeVivo used the incidence approach to estimating aggregate costs of SCI to society.[50] An annual incidence rate for hospitalized cases of 32.5 per million persons at risk and an annual incidence rate of 20.9 cases per million persons at risk for persons who die before hospital admission were used to make this projection.[51] These incidence rates were combined with current (at the time) Model System cost data and somewhat outdated information on costs from other sources that was the best available information at the time.[16] Adjusted to 1992 dollars, the aggregate costs of new cases of SCI found by DeVivo would be $7.2 billion annually.[50] Of this total, $3.1 billion is direct costs and $4.1 billion is indirect costs. This estimate was based on a 6% discount rate.

Estimates of aggregate costs of SCI to society were also developed by Berkowitz et al.[17] Using an incidence rate of 30 cases per million persons at risk and excluding costs associated with immediate fatalities, their estimated aggregate costs adjusted to 1992 dollars and using a 6% discount rate would be $6.4 billion annually. Of this total, $2.7 billion are direct costs and $3.7 billion are indirect costs. Using a 4% discount rate, aggregate costs would increase to $7.8 billion, $3.1 billion of which would be direct costs and $4.7 billion of which would be indirect costs. Slightly higher estimates were also provided, assuming an incidence rate of 40 cases per million persons at risk.

The aggregate cost estimates provided by Berkowitz et al.[17] are admittedly conservative because of the exclusion of costs associated with fatalities as well as the exclusion of certain other direct costs discussed previously. While immediate fatalities have on average minimal direct costs, their indirect costs are substantial. In fact, $2.8 billion of the $7.2 billion in aggregate costs estimated by DeVivo resulted from indirect costs associated with immediate fatalities.[50]

Berkowitz et al. also used the prevalence approach to estimate aggregate costs of SCI to society.[17] The prevalence approach involves estimating the economic costs of all cases existing in a given year plus the present value of lost future earnings for persons who die during the given year. Therefore, the prevalence-based estimate represents the value of what could be saved in a given year if all existing cases of SCI could be cured.

Adjusting their estimates to 1992 dollars and not adding anything for the increase in existing cases since that time, the aggregate costs to society of all existing cases of SCI would be $7.1 billion, $4.5 billion of which would be direct costs and $2.6 billion of which would be indirect costs.[17] Since no discount rate was stated, it appears that this estimate excludes lost future output of persons who die during the year. It is expected that the value of lost future output would be only a small fraction of total costs, since annual mortality only slightly exceeds 1% of all persons with SCI (see Chapter 14). Nonetheless, this estimate should also be considered conservative.

At the present time, new estimates of aggregate costs of SCI to society have not been developed using the Model System study population. The information necessary to make such a projection is available, and an estimate will likely be developed in the future. Given the results of the Model System study to date, any resulting estimate of aggregate costs of SCI to society should be slightly higher than those developed by Berkowitz et al.[17]

To put these estimates of aggregate costs of SCI into perspective, it is interesting to compare them with those of other types of injuries that occur much more frequently. Adjusting the findings of Rice, MacKenzie et al. that were developed using a 6% discount rate to 1992 dollars, the annual aggregate costs to society of several other types of injuries are as follows: poisonings—$11.4 billion ($2.6 billion direct and $8.8 billion indirect); burns—$5.1 billion ($1.4 billion direct and $3.7 billion indirect); drownings—$3.2 billion ($0.1 billion direct and $3.1 billion indirect).[52] By comparison, the annual incidence rates (including fatalities) are as follows: SCI—50 per million; poisonings—7182 per million; burns—6172 per million; drownings—159 per million.[52] Therefore, SCI is much more expensive on an individual basis than are other types of injuries.

It is also interesting to compare the aggregate costs of SCI to those of other major disabling conditions. Adjusting the findings of Hartunian et al.[16] that were developed using a 6% discount rate to 1992 dollars, the annual aggregate costs to society of major health impairments are as follows: cancer—$66.6 billion; all motor vehicle–related injuries (including those that result in SCI)—$42.5 billion; coronary heart disease —$37.7 billion; stroke—$19.3 billion. Therefore, despite its extremely low incidence, the aggregate costs of SCI to society are more than one tenth the costs of cancer, one sixth the costs of both motor vehicle–related injuries and coronary heart disease, and one third the costs of stroke.

CONCLUSION

Given the rapidly escalating overall costs of health care in the United States, coupled with large government budget deficits, the extremely high costs of SCI clearly represent a growing national dilemma.[50] As advancing medical technology causes life expectancies to increase further, direct costs of SCI will continue to increase. Nonetheless, these costs are well justified given the relatively good quality of life reported by most persons with SCI.

There are several obvious ways to reduce these enormous costs, and each has an important role to play in the total process. First and foremost is to reduce the incidence of SCI. Although not specifically limited to SCI, Rice, MacKenzie, et al. conservatively estimated the overall costs of injuries in the United States at $158 billion in 1985 dollars.[52] They also estimated the potential savings associated with numerous individual injury-prevention activities, many of which are targeted at the leading causes of SCI such as motor vehicle crashes, gunshot wounds, and diving injuries.[52] A national directory of SCI prevention programs was recently developed and can be obtained from the National Spinal Cord Injury Statistical Center.[53]

The beneficial economic impact of ongoing secondary prevention activities also cannot be overlooked. These activities are well documented, along with recommendations for the future, in *Proceedings of the First Colloquium on Preventing Secondary Disabilities among People with Spinal Cord Injuries.*[54] Advances in the prevention of secondary medical complications among persons with SCI have already led to a substantial reduction in the annual rehospitalization rate.[23]

Improving treatment efficiency is another means of reducing costs. Since 1973, lengths of stay for both acute care and rehabilitation for persons treated at Model SCI Systems have declined dramatically, as have lengths of stay for rehospitalizations caused by secondary medical complications.[23] Unfortunately, many therapeutic modalities used in rehabilitation became common practice before their cost-effectiveness was adequately demonstrated. As a result, it has been difficult for the field of rehabilitation medicine to conduct such cost-effectiveness studies. Nonetheless, there is a need to conduct these studies whenever possible, particularly as new therapeutic modalities are introduced.

Finally, the percentage of persons who return to work after SCI must be increased so that indirect costs can be reduced. Only minimal progress has occurred in this area since the Model SCI System program began.[23] A disturbing trend has occurred in recent years that is undoubtedly at least partially responsible for this lack of progress. As a result of funding cutbacks, the percentage of persons who become clients of the state Departments of Vocational Rehabilitation has declined from 52.4% in 1974 to only 26.4% in 1990.[55] Given that many persons with SCI have low education levels and need job retraining, an attempt must be made to return vocational rehabilitation activities to previous funding levels so that employment rates might increase.

Strong economic disincentives to employment also exist following SCI.[39,40] These disincentives must be eliminated and replaced by financial inducements to return to work.

Other reasons for low employment rates following SCI include discriminatory hiring practices, architectural and attitudinal barriers, and transportation difficulties. The Americans with Disabilities Act (Public Law 101-336) is a step in the right direction, but progress will likely continue at a slow pace.

REFERENCES

1. Charles ED, Fine PR, Stover SL, Wood T, Lott AF, Kronenfeld J. The costs of spinal cord injury. *Paraplegia.* 1978;15:302–310.

2. Charles ED, Van Matre JG, Miller JM. Spinal cord injury—a cost benefit analysis of alternative treatment models. *Paraplegia.* 1974;12:222–231.

3. DeVivo MJ, Potter MY, Stover SL, Fine PR. Costs of acute care and rehabilitation for spinal cord injury patients. *Arch Phys Med Rehabil.* 1987;68:657. Abstract.

4. Fine PR, Stover SL, DeVivo MJ. A methodology for predicting lengths of stay for spinal cord injury patients. *Inquiry.* 1987;24:147–156.

5. Keith RA, Breckenridge K. Characteristics of patients from the hospital utilization project data system: 1980–1982. *Arch Phys Med Rehabil.* 1985;66:768–772.

6. Stover SL, Fine PR, eds. *Spinal Cord Injury: The Facts and Figures.* Birmingham, Ala: University of Alabama at Birmingham; 1986.

7. Webb SB Jr, Berzins E, Wingardner TS, Lorenzi ME. First year hospitalization costs of the spinal cord injury patient. *Paraplegia.* 1978;15:311–318.

8. Webb SB Jr, Berzins E, Wingardner TS, Lorenzi ME. Spinal cord injury: Epidemiologic implications, costs, and patterns of care in 85 patients. *Arch Phys Med Rehabil.* 1979;60:335–340.

9. Whiteneck GG, Carter RE, Charlifue SW, et al. A collaborative study of high quadriplegia. In: *Abstracts Digest.* Chicago: American Spinal Injury Association; 1986;12:148–152.

10. Young JS, Burns PE, Bowen AM, McCutchen R. Spinal cord injury statistics. Phoenix, Ariz: Good Samaritan Medical Center; 1982.

11. Whiteneck GG. The high costs of high-level quadriplegia. In: Apple DF Jr, Hudson LM, eds. *Spinal Cord Injury: The Model.* Atlanta: Georgia Regional Spinal Cord Injury Care System; 1990:114–117.

12. Meyers AR, Branch LG, Cupples LA, Lederman RI, Feltin M, Master RJ. Predictors of medical care utilization by independently living adults with spinal cord injuries. *Arch Phys Med Rehabil.* 1989;70:471–476.

13. Davidoff G, Schultz JS, Lieb T, et al. Rehospitalization after initial rehabilitation for acute spinal cord injury: Incidence and risk factors. *Arch Phys Med Rehabil.* 1990;71:121–124.

14. Meyers AR, Feltin M, Master RJ, et al. Rehospitalization and spinal cord injury: Cross-sectional survey of adults living independently. *Arch Phys Med Rehabil.* 1985;66:704–708.

15. Smart CN, Sanders CR. *The Costs of Motor Vehicle Related SCI.* Washington, DC: Insurance Institute for Highway Safety; 1976.

16. Hartunian NS, Smart CN, Thompson MS. *The Incidence and Economic Costs of Major Health Impairments.* Lexington, Mass: DC Heath and Co; 1981.

17. Berkowitz M, Harvey C, Greene CG, Wilson SE. The economic consequences of traumatic spinal cord injury. Washington, DC: Paralyzed Veterans of America; 1990.

18. Harvey C, Wilson SE, Greene CG, Berkowitz M, Stripling TE. New estimates of the direct costs of traumatic spinal cord injuries: Results of a nationwide survey. *Paraplegia.* 1992;30:34–50.

19. Berkowitz M, Harvey C, Greene CG, Wilson SE. *The Economic Consequences of Traumatic Spinal Cord Injury.* New York: Demos Publications; 1992.

20. Finkler SA. The distinction between costs and charges. *Ann Intern Med.* 1982;96:102–109.

21. Frankel HL, Hancock DO, Hyslop G, et al. The value of postural reduction in the initial management of closed injuries to the spine with paraplegia and tetraplegia. *Paraplegia.* 1969;7:179–192.

22. Miller JM. The role of regional cord injury centers in the rehabilitation of the spinal cord-injured. In: Cull JG, Hardy RE, eds. *Physical Medicine and Rehabilitation Approaches in Spinal Cord Injury.* Springfield, Ill: Charles C Thomas, Publisher; 1977:100–121.

23. DeVivo MJ, Rutt RD, Black KJ, Go BK, Stover SL. Trends in spinal cord injury demographics and treatment outcomes between 1973 and 1986. *Arch Phys Med Rehabil.* 1992;73:424–430.

24. Harvey C, Rothschild BB, Asmann AJ, Stripling T. New estimates of traumatic SCI prevalence: A survey-based approach. *Paraplegia.* 1990;28:537–544.

25. Hahn B, Lefkowitz D. *Annual Expenses and Sources of Payment for Health Care Services.* Rockville, Md: Agency for Health Care Policy and Research, 1992; HHS publication No. (AHCPR) 93-0007 (National Medical Expenditure Survey; Research Findings No. 14).

26. Hogan C. *Urban and Rural Hospital Costs: 1981–1985.* Rockville, Md: National Center for Health Services Research and Health Care Technology Assessment, 1988; HHS Publication No. (PHS) 88-3419 (Hospital Studies Program Research Note 12).

27. *Vital Statistics of the United States, 1988.* Vol. 2: *Mortality.* Hyattsville, Md: National Center for Health Statistics; 1992.

28. Menter RR. Aging and spinal cord injury: Implications for existing model systems and future federal, state, and local health care policy. In: Apple DF Jr, Hudson LM, eds. *Spinal Cord Injury: The Model.* Atlanta: Georgia Regional Spinal Cord Injury Care System; 1990:72–80.

29. DeVivo MJ, Stover SL, Fine PR. The relationship between sponsorship and rehabilitation outcome following spinal cord injury. *Paraplegia.* 1989;27:470–479.

30. Tate DG, Forchheimer M, Daugherty J, Maynard F. Insurance benefits coverage for persons with spinal cord injuries: Determining differences across payors. *J Am Paraplegia Soc.* 1993;16:76–80.

31. Lefkowitz D, Monheit A. Health Insurance, Use of Health Services, and Health Care Expenditures. Rockville, Md: Agency for Health Care Policy and Research, 1991; HHS Publication No. (AHCPR) 92-0017 (National Medical Expenditure Survey; Research Findings No. 12).

32. Berkowitz M. *Economic Consequences of Spinal Cord Injury.* New Brunswick, NJ: Bureau of Economic Research; 1985.

33. Hodgson TA, Meiners MR. Cost-of-illness methodology: A guide to current practices and procedures. *Milbank Mem Fund Q.* 1982;60:429–487.

34. Bureau of Labor Statistics. Employer costs for employee compensation. *BLS News.* 1988;88:298.

35. DeVivo MJ, Fine PR. Employment status of spinal cord injured patients 3 years after injury. *Arch Phys Med Rehabil.* 1982;63:200–203.

36. DeVivo MJ, Rutt RD, Stover SL, Fine PR. Employment after spinal cord injury. *Arch Phys Med Rehabil.* 1987;68:494–498.

37. James M, DeVivo MJ, Richards JS. Postinjury employment outcomes among African-American and white persons with spinal cord injury. *Rehabil Psychol.* 1993;38:151–164.

38. Kraus JS. Employment after spinal cord injury. *Arch Phys Med Rehabil.* 1992;73:163–169.

39. Better SR, Fine PR, Simison D, Doss GH, Walls RT, McLaughlin DE. Disability benefits as disincentives to rehabilitation. *Milbank Mem Fund Q.* 1979;57:412–427.

40. Walls RT, Masson C, Werner TJ. Negative incentives to vocational rehabilitation. *Rehabil Lit.* 1977;38:143–150.

41. Goldberg RT, Freed MM. Vocational development of spinal cord injury patients: 8-year follow-up. *Arch Phys Med Rehabil.* 1982;63:207–210.

42. El Ghatit AZ, Hanson RW. Variables associated with obtaining and sustaining employment among spinal cord injured males: Follow-up of 760 veterans. *J Chronic Dis.* 1978;31:363–369.

43. El Ghatit AZ, Hanson RW. Educational and training levels and employment of the spinal cord injured patient. *Arch Phys Med Rehabil.* 1979;60:405–406.

44. Deyoe FS Jr. Spinal cord injury: Long-term follow-up of veterans. *Arch Phys Med Rehabil.* 1972;53:523–529.

45. Felton JS, Litman M. Study of employment of 222 men with spinal cord injury. *Arch Phys Med Rehabil.* 1965;46:809–814.

46. Geisler WO, Jousse AT, Wynne-Jones M. Vocational re-establishment of patients with spinal cord injury. *Med Serv J Can.* 1966;22:698–709.

47. Weidman CD, Freehafer AA. Vocational outcome in patients with spinal cord injury. *J Rehabil.* 1981;47(2):63–65.

48. Harvey C, Axelrod A. Impact of medical care and compensation on employment of persons with spinal cord injury. *J Am Paraplegia Soc.* 1993;16:59. Abstract.

49. Bureau of Labor Statistics. *Employment and Earnings.* Washington, DC: U.S. Government Printing Office; 1989;36:1.

50. DeVivo MJ. The cost of spinal cord injury: A growing national dilemma. In: Apple DF Jr, Hudson LM, eds. *Spinal Cord Injury: The Model.* Atlanta: Georgia Regional Spinal Cord Injury Care System; 1990:109–113.

51. Kraus JF, Franti CE, Riggins RS, Richards D, Borhani NO. Incidence of traumatic spinal cord lesions. *J Chronic Dis.* 1975;28:471–492.

52. Rice DP, MacKenzie EJ, and Associates. *Cost of Injury in the United States: A Report to Congress.* San Francisco: Institute for Health and Aging, University of California, and Baltimore: Injury Prevention Center, Johns Hopkins University; 1989.

53. Richards JS. *Resources: A National Directory of Spinal Cord Injury Prevention Programs.* Birmingham, Ala: University of Alabama at Birmingham; 1990.

54. Graitcer PL, Maynard FM, eds. *Proceedings of the First Colloquium on Preventing Secondary Disabilities among People with Spinal Cord Injuries.* Atlanta: Centers for Disease Control; 1990.

55. DeVivo MJ, Richards JS. Community reintegration and quality of life following spinal cord injury. *Paraplegia.* 1992;30:108–112.

13

Effects of Age at Injury and the Aging Process

Robert R. Menter and Lesley M. Hudson

INTRODUCTION

Age and aging begin with conception. Normal aging involves at least three major lifelong developmental processes, all overlapping, but all distinctly different: the physiologic changes of the body itself, the individual's changing social roles, and issues of self-realization.[1,2]

Physiologic aging is manifested by a gradual decline in all body systems. At birth each organ system functions with enormous reserve capacity, making it very resilient to any damage. However, as time passes, the body's various organ systems lose their reserve capacity. Whether reflected by a decrease in the cardiac reserve, by a decrease in the skin's resiliency, or by decreased visual acuity, as the decades pass it takes less and less injury to damage or alter the system and more time to recover when an insult does occur.

The sociologic stages of childhood, teenaged years, adulthood, middle age, and old age represent the environment in which both physiologic decline and self-realization occur. Indeed, throughout these stages, the social environment of peers, family, and friends plays a crucial role. The expectations they all have and the examples they set—whether they be smoking, overeating, advocacy of wellness, high stress, low stress, spiritual growth—all act to speed up or slow down both the physiologic decline and spiritual growth processes.

Finally, it is the changes brought about by self-realization that result in a gradual growth in understanding, ultimately bringing balance to the individual's relationship with the world. A topic rarely discussed, self-realization is perhaps the most important of the aging factors, for it holds the potential for making

We express our appreciation to Susan Charlifue, MA, David Weitzenkamp, BA, Kathy Quick, and Kenneth Gerhart, MS, for their assistance in the statistical analysis and chapter preparation.

physiologic and sociologic changes less devastating. It includes the issues of developing values, ethics, morality, and ultimately finding meaning in life. This is the growing up of the mind, also referred to as spiritual growth.[3,4]

This three-dimensional model of aging is particularly useful in understanding and conceptualizing long-term spinal cord injury (SCI). A topic that only recently has come under close scrutiny, early indications are that aging with SCI encompasses a variety of changes, ranging from declines in health and physiologic function, to sociologic changes such as increasing financial stresses and changing relationships with other family members, to spiritual growth manifested by an ability to perceive life with a disability as a satisfying and quality life.

This chapter reviews some of the data that are beginning to accumulate that will help us understand those changes.

PHYSIOLOGIC DECLINE FOLLOWING SPINAL CORD INJURY: THE ROLES OF AGE AT ONSET, AGING WITH A DISABILITY, AND TYPE OF NEUROLOGIC INJURY

SCI may be viewed as one form of instant aging. With paralysis comes loss of sensation, loss of movement, loss of bone density, loss of bowel and bladder function, and other physiologic changes. To the extent that these impairments of body systems diminish otherwise available reserves, in a conceptual sense, the individual with a new SCI may be thought of as having "aged."

With this in mind, three general concepts emerge that are fundamental to understanding the impact of age and aging in SCI. First, the older the individual is at the time of the SCI onset, the less resilient he or she may be in adapting to the injury. Second, the years following the SCI may be associated with an acceleration of the aging process because of the diminished reserves spoken of above and because of the increased demands made on still-functioning body systems. Third, the type of neurologic injury (paraplegia, tetraplegia) and the associated neurologic completeness of the injury create very different patterns of change within the aging process.

Age at Onset

Although most SCIs are seen in young males who suffer severe and violent trauma as a result of risk-taking behaviors, the picture is very different for older Americans who sustain SCIs. This rapidly growing segment of the population, because of aging-associated spinal osteoarthritis, which decreases the space available for the spinal cord in the cervical spinal canal, is at particular risk for cervical-level SCIs. Moreover, these injuries frequently result from relatively minimal amounts of trauma sustained during what are seemingly routine, non–risk-taking activities—a fall from a stool or a low chair or involvement in a minor "fender bender" motor vehicle crash.

Indeed, data from the National Spinal Cord Injury Statistical Center (NSCISC) during the past two decades seem to support this. There has been an increase in the frequency of SCI among people over age 60; individuals with SCIs over the age of 60 now comprise 8.5% of the Database's cases, compared with 4.5% two decades ago. This percentage, however, very likely underestimates the true incidence of SCI among older persons. Not a population-based sample that mandatorily enrolls all SCI survivors within a given geographic area, the NSCISC reports only cases admitted to participating centers. In one population-based SCI surveillance program, the percentages are higher. Specifically, in Colorado, where the mean age of residents is very similar to that of the nation as a whole, the statewide SCI tracking program has found that SCI persons over age 60 comprise 12% of the sample.[5] The difference between Colorado's findings and NSCISC data raises the possibility that the Model SCI Care Systems do not receive people with elderly-onset SCI in the same pattern as younger SCI individuals. The neurologic profile of older SCI survivors may play a prime role, as evidence suggests that, on the whole, they sustain many more incomplete neurologic SCIs than do younger persons.[5,6] As a result, hospitals receiving and treating them may not believe that comprehensive rehabilitation is necessary and thus may be less aggressive in referring them to Model SCI Programs. Additionally, the elderly SCI person's own goals, motivation, and readiness to leave the home community also may play a role.

Despite the smaller percentage of older individuals in the NSCISC dataset, the actual numbers are large enough to have permitted extensive and meaningful examination not only of the causes of their injuries and their neurologic impairments, but also of their pre-existing conditions, their complications during initial hospitalization, and such outcomes as length of hospitalization, place of discharge, independence in care, and costs. DeVivo and his associates[6] at the NSCISC compared these variables across different age groupings. With respect to pre-existing conditions, they found that older persons—those over 45 years of age at the time of SCI onset— had significantly higher prevalences of diabetes, obesity, heart disease, and arthritis in comparison to younger SCI survivors. Additionally, these same older persons had lower levels of independence at the time of their discharge from the hospital[6]—a finding that is supported by the work of Yarkony et al.[7] and others. In addition, they were discharged to nursing homes more frequently than their counterparts with younger ages at onset.

Older-at-onset SCI survivors also are susceptible to certain medical complications following their SCIs. Table 13–1, based on NSCISC initial hospital admission data, illustrates this. After excluding the less-than-15 and over-75 age groupings—both of which have relatively few numbers—trends toward in-

Table 13-1 Results of National Database Form I Analysis: Percentage of Patients in Each Age Group Who Developed Select Medical Complications during Initial Hospitalization*

Complication	Age Group†					
	0–15	16–30	31–45	46–60	61–75	76+
Pneumonia	9.8	15.7	21.5	17.4	27.8	34.0
Pulmonary Embolus	1.6	3.1	4.5	3.5	9.0	3.8
Renal Stone	0.0	0.8	0.7	1.4	1.6	0.0
Gastrointestinal Hemorrhage	3.2	3.0	2.9	3.4	6.0	3.7
Pressure Sore	30.2	33.3	30.5	30.2	36.3	31.5
Heterotopic Ossification	1.6	4.7	6.6	4.3	5.9	0.0
Thrombophlebitis	7.9	12.6	17.5	15.1	15.2	1.9
Use of Ventilator	28.6	21.6	25.9	26.9	38.6	42.6

*Note: includes only individuals with day-of-injury admission to Model SCI System.
†Shading denotes statistical significance.

creased prevalences of pneumonia, pulmonary emboli, renal stones, gastrointestinal hemorrhage, and use of the ventilator are noted.

The Postinjury Years: Aging with a Disability

In addition to complications experienced during the initial hospitalization, new analyses of NSCISC follow-up data examined medical complications occurring over time, as well as rehospitalizations and operative procedures performed. Table 13–2 highlights a few of these with respect to the individual's age at the time of follow-up, the years since the injury itself, and the level and severity of the neurologic deficit. Before proceeding, some information about Table 13–2 and the analysis it depicts is necessary. First, with respect to age at time of follow-up, the youngest age group—those under 15 years old—represents a small and a unique population, very unlike the otherwise mature adult population; as a result, it has not been included in this analysis. Second, for the years post-SCI groupings, it is important to keep in mind that since the NSCISC Database started in 1973 there are only limited numbers of individuals who have been followed for more than 15 years since injury. Third, for the SCI groups represented in Table 13–2, the categories utilized are based on the Frankel classification system.[8] Specifically, cervical injuries with significant functional impairment (Frankel grades A, B, and C) comprise the first group; individuals with paraplegia graded as Frankel grade A, B, or C comprise the second; while

Table 13-2 Results of National Database Form II Analysis: Percentage of People Who Developed Select Medical Complications in Follow-Up Years*

Condition/Event	Age Group					Years Post-SCI Group				SCI Group		
	16–30	31–45	46–60	61–75	76+	1–5	6–10	11–15	16+	Para ABC	Tetra ABC	All D&E
Contracture	4.7	6.4	6.3	8.7	16.0	6.0	5.3	5.4	9.1	7.3	2.3	4.2
Spasticity	40.7	40.1	37.7	36.4	26.3	41.1	39.4	33.3	35.9	49.5	25.8	26.6
Reported Chills/Fever	14.3	15.0	11.1	9.7	10.4	14.3	13.1	14.3	13.3	15.2	16.8	5.4
Urinary Tract Infection	65.5	68.6	64.1	63.3	41.2	61.5	71.3	80.2	82.9	72.6	57.6	43.3
Renal Calculi	1.9	2.2	1.3	2.1	1.3	1.6	2.0	3.1	5.4	2.7	1.6	0.6
Pneumonia	1.5	1.8	2.3	2.8	8.2	1.9	1.7	1.6	1.7	2.0	2.1	0.7
Acquired Scoliosis	2.2	2.0	1.4	0.9	0.6	1.7	2.0	3.3	3.0	2.6	1.2	0.6
Pressure Sores	17.7	21.1	15.9	14.0	19.2	16.3	21.6	24.9	26.9	22.6	20.0	5.0
Closure of Pressure Sores	3.7	5.1	3.5	2.1	0.0	3.5	4.6	5.7	6.0	5.6	3.5	0.7
Rehospitalized	33.5	32.2	33.7	34.2	30.8	35.3	29.0	27.2	23.4	40.4	30.0	19.3
Mean Days Rehospitalized	8.6	8.8	9.6	9.3	6.1	9.6	7.0	7.3	5.7	11.2	8.6	3.7
Mean Days in Nursing Home	3.8	5.9	14.1	31.8	68.5	7.5	7.0	3.9	5.3	7.1	8.8	4.7

*Shading denotes statistical significance.

all individuals with significant functional preservation (Frankel grade D or E)—regardless of level of injury—are included in the third group. This grouping scheme, which is used throughout the remainder of this chapter, was selected because persons within each group tend to have functional abilities that are similar to those of other group members, yet unique and distinct from those of the other two groups. Indeed, one basic functional difference between these groups relates to extremity function. While members of the tetraplegia group often have the most impaired upper extremity function, it is persons with paraplegia who place the greatest demands on their neurologically intact arms, predisposing them to a "premature wearing out," while individuals with Frankel grades D and E, on the other hand, tend to be ambulatory, thus decreasing the load on normal or impaired upper extremities, but adding stress to possibly weakened lower extremities. Finally, with respect to Table 13–2 and those that follow it, shaded areas represent those changes or values that were found to be statistically significant.

Age at Time of Follow-Up

Turning first to the effects of the SCI survivor's age at the time of follow-up contact, it was noted that pneumonia, which was more prevalent among older persons during their initial hospitalizations, also increases with age in subsequent postinjury years. In follow-up it had increased from a low of 1.5% in the 16- to 30-year-old age group to a high of 8.2% in the 76+-year-old age group. Joint contracture also increased. Among adults who had completed their growth processes, these joint limitations increased in frequency from an incidence of 4.7% in the 16- to 30-year-old age group to 16.0% in the 76+ year-old age group. However, spasticity requiring treatment, and which is frequently associated with contracture, surprisingly decreased—from 40.7% in the 16- to 30-year-old age group to a low of 26.3% in the 76+-year-age-old group. Although it is possible that this seeming contradiction is simply a result of a tendency to stop reporting a problem that the individual has accepted as a "fact of life" with chronic SCI, further study is indicated in order to understand what, if any, relationships exist between contracture and spasticity over time.

Like spasticity, the prevalence of reported chills and fever and urinary tract infections (bacteriuria) had similar patterns of decline over time. The former dropped from 14.3% in the youngest group to 10.4% in the 76+-year-old group, while the prevalence of bacteriuria declined by over 24 percentage points. The better urologic outcomes of older individuals may be associated with the more incomplete neurologic injuries associated with older age.

Finally, of particular significance in this analysis by age at the time of follow-up is the number of days spent in nursing homes. These increased from a low of 3.8 days per year in the 16- to 30-year-old age group to 68.5 days per year in the

76+-year-old age group. This dramatic and steady increase is relevant both in comparing the outcomes of younger and older SCI survivors and in comparing outcomes for aging persons with SCI with those of their nondisabled counterparts. Moreover, to the extent that nursing home stays are associated with declining physical independence, another published report by DeVivo and his colleagues adds useful insight.[9] Also utilizing NSCISC follow-up data, they examined levels of independence after the initial hospitalizations across six age groups for classification. Particularly significant was the finding that persons in each successive age group beyond the 16- to 30-year-old grouping were less likely to be independent in self-care activities and more likely to be residing in nursing homes when contacted for annual follow-up.

Years Postinjury

Separate from chronologic age are the effects of the duration of the SCI. For example, although urinary tract infections (UTI) with bacteriuria decrease with age, they nonetheless show a steady increase with each 5-year increment postinjury. This increase is not accompanied by an increase in reported chills and fever but is accompanied by a parallel increase in renal calculi. From lows (UTI, 61.5%; renal calculi, 1.6%) in years 1 to 5 postinjury, prevalences increase to highs (UTI, 82.9%; renal calculi, 5.4%) in 16+-year postinjury.

Acquired scoliosis, which may be associated with spasticity, shows a steady increase with each subsequent 5-year postinjury interval, rising from a prevalence of 1.7% in the 1- to 5-year postinjury group to 3% in the 16+-year postinjury group.

Pressure sores and surgery to close them also demonstrate a steady increase with duration of the SCI. Comparing the 1 to 5 years and 16+ years postinjury groups, the prevalence of pressure sores increased from 16.3% to 26.9%, while related skin repair surgeries rose from 3.5% to 6%. Further analysis of the data relating to this devastating and costly SCI complication will be crucial for the identification of additional risk factors. Design and appropriate targeting of interventions in this area can greatly decrease individual inconvenience and suffering, improve quality of life, and result in dramatic savings of scarce health care resources.

In spite of these findings, both hospitalization frequency and the mean number of days hospitalized actually decrease as the time from the initial injury increases. While 35.3% of those in the 1- to 5-year postinjury group had been hospitalized during the preceding follow-up year, the percentage of the longest-injured group (16+ years) was considerably less—23.4%. The average length of stay of the longest injured group, at 5.7 days, was a statistically significant 3.9 days shorter than the mean for those in the 1- to 5-year postinjury group.

Interestingly, the number of days in a nursing home has shown an initial decrease in years 1 to 5, 6 to 10, and 11 to 15, but is beginning to show an increase in the 16+-year postinjury follow-up. While it is too early to show statistical significance, this percentage might be expected to increase because increasing years postinjury inevitably will lead to older age, which is typically associated with greater utilization of nursing homes.

Neurologic Impairment

Utilizing the three neurologic groupings described earlier, it can be seen from Table 13–2 that the type of SCI indeed influences the complications experienced during follow-up years. Those with functionally complete paraplegia (para ABC) report almost twice the spasticity of either of the other groups. The reasons for this are not clear, especially since the paraplegia group assumedly includes a number of individuals with flaccid paralysis. Certainly, closer examination is indicated.

The paraplegia group also reported more UTIs and both more and longer rehospitalizations during the postinjury years. The latter may be accounted for, at least in part, by their higher prevalence of pressure ulcers and the need for surgical closure. Although they had only slightly more pressure ulcers reported than those with functionally complete cervical injuries (tetra ABC), both of these groups report four times the number of ulcers as their counterparts with more neurologic preservation (all D and E). However, despite the higher hospitalization rate and longer average length of stay within the paraplegia group, this group's mean nursing home admissions, at 7.1 days, was still 1.7 days shorter than that for the tetraplegia group.

Overall, it was the group composed of those with the most neurologic preservation that reported the fewest complications. The only seeming exceptions were contracture and spasticity, for which these Frankel grade D and E individuals fell between the paraplegia and tetraplegia groups. Finally, despite the fact that the tetra ABC group can be thought of as the most disabled, this group seldom reported more complications over time than the paraplegia group, and when they did—as for pneumonia and chills/fever—the differences were relatively slight.

Tying It Together: The Combined Effects of Age, Years Postinjury, and
  Neurologic Impairment

To truly understand aging in the long-term SCI survivor, the three components discussed—age, duration of injury, and extent of neurologic impairment—must be merged and examined in terms of their impact on one another and their inter-relationships. Because long-term follow-up variables are limited in the NSCISC Database, a large-scale, ongoing study not described previously provides some of this synthesis.

A special collaborative effort initiated by 6 of the 13 centers participating in the Model Systems programs and led by the Rocky Mountain Regional SCI

System, this investigation involves longitudinal outcome assessment in which a comprehensive evaluation of multiple physiologic, psychologic, and sociologic variables, which go beyond those in the NSCISC Database, will be performed on every fifth-year anniversary following SCI injury. Examples include lipid testing, the performance of electrocardiography, and an extensive health-status and quality-of-life interview. Begun in 1991, 429 cases have been reviewed, of which 39.4% are 5 years postinjury, 32.4% are 10 years, and 26.2% are 15 years. Obviously, the first cases will not be eligible for their second review until 1996; thus, the selected variables presented in Table 13–3 reflect a one-point-in-time view by neurologic injury, by age at follow-up and by years postinjury at follow-up within each of three injury groupings. Table 13–3 values represent the mean value reported for continuous variables or the percentage reporting the presence of dichotomous variables. Within each injury grouping, multiple regression analyses were performed by age and years postinjury (linear regression for continuous variables and logistic regression for dichotomous variables) in order to isolate the separate effects of these two aging components. The means and percentages reported in Table 13–3 are shaded when statistically significant regression coefficients were identified.

Relevant findings, which seem to confirm clinical experience, already have been found in the areas of upper- and lower-extremity joint pain. Among persons with functionally complete paraplegia (para ABC), the percentage reporting upper-extremity joint pain increased significantly with years postinjury from 29.3% at 5 years postinjury to 54.2% at 15 years postinjury. More detailed logistic regression analysis indicated that shoulder pain was increasing at a rate of 20% per decade postinjury; elbow pain was increasing at a rate of 16% per decade postinjury; and wrist pain was increasing at the rate of 17% per decade postinjury. Persons with functionally incomplete SCIs at any level (all Frankel grade D) showed a pattern of increasing pain in both the upper and lower extremities with chronologic age. In the upper extremities, reports of pain increased from 11.1% among those under age 30, to 61.1% in those over age 45. Similarly, complaints of lower-extremity pain escalated from 33.3% to 77.8%. The more detailed logistic regression analysis indicated that the prevalence of hip pain was increasing at a rate of 7% per decade; the prevalence of knee pain was increasing at a rate of 11% per decade; and the prevalence of ankle pain was increasing at the rate of 7% per decade; while the combined prevalence of upper extremity pain was increasing at the rate of 11% per decade of chronologic age. The variable "feeling fatigued" was noticeably increased by age and most significant in the para ABC group, rising from 15.7% in the under-30-year age group to 40.5% in the over-45-year age group. The need for more help also increased. From lows in the under-30-year age group (para ABC 2.1%, all D 0.0%) to highs in the over-45-year age group (para ABC 19.1%, all D 27.8%),

Table 13–3 Collaborative Model SCI System Study of Aging Values of Selected Variables

Variable	Injury Class	Age*			Year Postinjury*		
		<30	*31–45*	*>45*	*5*	*10*	*15*
Upper Extremity Pain	Para ABC	27.5	47.1	47.6	29.3	50.0	54.2
(% Reporting)	Tetra ABC	42.6	40.7	32.3	45.0	38.3	34.7
	All D	11.1	38.5	61.1	28.6	56.3	43.8
Lower Extremity Pain†	Para ABC	19.6	17.7	9.5	20.7	16.7	8.3
(% Reporting)	Tetra ABC	12.8	15.4	22.6	16.7	16.7	14.3
	All D	33.3	34.6	77.8	47.6	50.0	50.0
Feeling Fatigued	Para ABC	15.7	24.7	40.5	20.7	35.4	25.0
(% Reporting)	Tetra ABC	29.8	38.5	38.7	43.3	33.3	30.6
	All D	22.2	11.5	33.3	23.8	6.3	31.3
More Help Needed	Para ABC	2.1	3.6	19.1	6.5	4.2	10.4
(% Reporting)	Tetra ABC	2.1	8.9	0.0	3.5	5.0	8.2
	All D	0.0	0.0	27.8	0.0	12.5	18.8
Total FIM Score	Para ABC	112.3	112.7	107.2	108.7	112.7	114.4
(Points [Max. 126])	Tetra ABC	81.7	73.6	83.6	76.0	77.2	81.9
	All D	109.8	111.7	107.7	112.8	97.6	118.7
Current Weight (lb)	Para ABC	161.6	166.3	175.9	168.2	162.1	172.3
	Tetra ABC	136.8	162.3	178.6	164.6	152.5	157.0
	All D	131.0	174.1	174.1	162.1	164.1	168.3
Systolic Blood Pressure†	Para ABC	115.4	121.0	130.1	119.6	122.5	124.4
(mm/Hg)	Tetra ABC	104.6	102.5	115.6	107.3	104.7	104.7
	All D	106.0	121.6	122.3	122.4	109.0	123.4
Diastolic Blood Pressure†	Para ABC	74.4	79.6	83.0	78.7	79.0	78.5
(mm/Hg)	Tetra ABC	67.5	67.9	75.9	69.7	70.6	67.1
	All D	69.7	76.0	77.8	78.9	70.7	73.7
High-Density Lipoproteins	Para ABC	47.8	38.7	25.2	42.6	37.5	39.6
(mg/dL)	Tetra ABC	41.7	37.0	37.8	36.0	42.4	37.0
	All D	46.5	57.6	46.0	54.4	44.2	40.6
Low-Density Lipoproteins†	Para ABC	113.8	126.3	131.6	130.2	123.1	105.2
(mg/dL)	Tetra ABC	96.2	96.8	123.4	109.9	90.7	103.0
	All D	86.1	105.8	110.3	107.7	99.2	90.4
Total Cholesterol (mg/dL)	Para ABC	178.5	180.7	192.0	193.2	180.3	162.6
	Tetra ABC	161.9	170.6	188.5	183.2	164.5	164.2
	All D	157.0	177.0	190.3	181.2	178.8	168.7
Glucose (mg/dL)	Para ABC	81.6	98.8	108.9	91.7	103.0	104.6
	Tetra ABC	79.6	94.6	94.2	90.3	86.0	98.7
	All D	83.0	94.2	109.2	95.1	103.0	97.0

*Shading denotes statistically significant regression coefficients.
†Indicates statistically significant differences by injury class.

increasing age seems to be accompanied by a perceived need for more help. Perhaps surprising is the finding that those with what are traditionally the most disabling of all spinal cord injuries (tetra ABC) showed no clear pattern of an increased need for help. This is very likely due to the reality that most individuals with functionally complete cervical injuries (tetra ABC) already had assistance from others, and gradual increases in the assistance they receive may not have been particularly noticeable or significant to them.

The Functional Independence Measure (FIM)[10] is an outcome assessment tool designed to measure more objectively the extent of disability and the need for assistance. Because it measures objective tasks and focuses on the burden of care, it is capable of detecting changes in function over time. As might be expected, among the para ABC group in the multicenter collaborative study, FIM scores significantly declined with respect to age. Those over age 45 had average scores that were four points less than those under age 30. At the same time, however, this same group's FIM scores increased with years postinjury. Those in the 5-year post-SCI group had an average FIM score of 108.7; those injured 15 years averaged 114.4. For the other two neurologic impairment groups—tetra ABC and all Frankel D—FIM scores did not differ significantly.

Blood pressure values—both systolic and diastolic—increased significantly in both para ABC and tetra ABC, as demonstrated on Table 13–3. Interestingly, it is the functionally incomplete group (all Frankel D) whose physiologic functioning is most like that of nondisabled people, where blood pressure changes were not significant.

Regarding lipids and glucose, two competing trends were noted. As expected, older persons had higher levels of total cholesterol, but persons 15 years postinjury had lower levels of total cholesterol than those injured only 5 years ago. Both of these competing trends were statistically significant for persons with tetraplegia, and the years postinjury effect was statistically significant among persons with paraplegia. Similar competing significant trends were also seen in low-density lipoprotein (LDL) among persons with paraplegia, where LDL levels increased with age but decreased with years post-injury. High-density lipoprotein (HDL) levels decreased significantly across the three age groups of persons with paraplegia from 47.8 for those under 30 to 25.2 for those over 45. This has some similarity to the findings of Bauman et al.,[11] who reported decreased total cholesterol and HDL in veterans with tetraplegia and paraplegia when compared with a control group of nondisabled veterans. Persons with Frankel grade D demonstrated a significant trend toward increasing glucose levels with chronologic age. The regression analysis indicated an average 11.0% increase in glucose levels per decade.

Another study, one that preceded the foregoing Model Systems collaborative study and was conducted by Whiteneck et al. in another population, also attempted to integrate the effects of aging, duration of injury, and severity of the neurologic impairment.[12] Also longitudinal in nature, it supports many of the Model Systems study's preliminary findings.

Initially published in 1992, this study reported on the mortality, morbidity, health, functional, and psychosocial outcomes of 834 individuals over 20 years postinjury.[12] It was conducted at two British SCI centers—The National Spinal Injuries Centre at Stoke Mandeville Hospital and the Regional Spinal Injuries Centre in Southport. Two tables from the study that review the incidence of follow-up diagnoses and procedures by age (Table 13–4) and by years postinjury (Table 13–5) are reproduced here.

This study found some conditions more strongly associated with age than with years postinjury. These included operations of the cardiac, internal, and nervous systems; pneumonia, atelectasis, respiratory infections, dyspepsia, and urinary tract infections; renal stones and failure; and fainting and headaches. There was also a variety of conditions more strongly associated with increasing years postinjury than with increasing age. This list comprised musculoskeletal problems such as tendon and joint procedures, muscle and joint pain and stiffness, and rectal abscesses and bleeding, as well as urinary problems among men. Last, there was a substantial number of conditions that appeared most frequently in both the oldest age group and in the group with the longest postinjury follow-up. These included a wide range of gastrointestinal problems and operations, hemorrhoids, nausea, and vomiting.

These analyses of the Model Systems Collaborative Aging Study and the British Aging Study indicate that aging with SCI is a complex phenomenon in which the relative impact of chronologic age and years postinjury differs depending on the outcome examined and the neurologic injury. Continuation of these investigations over time will add longitudinal data to help refine these early findings and help identify preventable consequences of aging with SCI that can be eliminated, lessened, or forestalled with effective interventions.

SOCIOLOGIC ROLE CHANGE AND SPIRITUAL GROWTH: THE MISSING PIECES

In introducing this chapter, a three-dimensional model of aging was described. Much of what has been discussed thus far has related to the first dimension: physiologic decline. Although this area as it relates to long-term SCI is itself in its investigational infancy, there has been even less empirical study of how changing sociologic roles, self-realization, and spiritual maturation contribute to the SCI survivors' successful—or unsuccessful—aging.

Table 13–4 British SCI Aging Study: Incidence of Follow-Up Diagnoses and Procedures by Age (Episodes per 100 Cases per Year)

	By Age at Episode				
	<30	30–39	40–49	50–59	60+
Diagnoses					
Infectious Disease/Neoplasm	1.7	2.9	4.7	6.1	11.1
CNS/Seizure	5.9	1.8	1.5	1.3	2.6
Fainting/Headache	1.9	2.7	2.1	1.9	4.9
Motor/Sensory Change	2.0	1.5	1.9	2.1	2.3
Disorder of Eye/Ear	0.4	1.5	1.7	3.5	7.7
Heart/Circulatory	2.0	2.9	5.2	8.1	19.3
Pneumonia/Atelectasis	1.6	1.7	1.9	3.4	5.4
Respiratory Infection	3.2	3.4	2.2	3.1	2.6
Gastrointestinal	5.3	7.7	9.0	8.9	15.3
Hemorrhoids	1.0	2.4	3.4	2.7	2.1
Rectal Abscess/Bleeding	1.3	2.5	3.5	2.9	2.1
UTI	19.7	20.1	19.0	17.1	27.8
GU Retention/Hydronephrosis	12.6	10.9	10.2	10.4	10.3
Renal Stone/Failure	3.4	4.8	3.8	6.0	8.3
Male GU Problem	2.1	2.6	4.8	3.8	4.7
Pressure Sore	25.5	20.4	22.0	24.5	27.4
Muscle/Joint Pain	5.2	6.9	11.8	9.0	10.2
Spasticity/Contracture	5.5	5.3	5.5	4.4	4.7
Fracture/Sprain/Amputation	1.7	2.7	2.4	2.5	3.0
Superficial Wound	2.8	1.9	1.7	1.5	2.1
Injury/Suicide	1.5	0.8	0.8	1.3	0.6
Operations					
Cardiac/Internal/CNS	4.9	6.6	5.1	6.4	5.7
Gastrointestinal	1.9	4.9	4.5	3.9	5.3
Genitourinary	10.0	8.7	9.7	12.1	12.1
Musculoskeletal	3.0	2.9	4.7	3.3	4.7

Source: Reprinted from Whiteneck, G., et al., Mortality, Morbidity, and Psychosocial Outcomes of Persons Spinal Cord Injured More Than 20 Years Ago, *Paraplegia*, Vol. 30, pp. 617–630, with permission of Churchill Livingstone, © 1992.

Changing Sociologic Roles

One key sociologic role—how disability affects relationships within the family—is beginning to gain the attention of researchers. Much of the attendant care that is provided to SCI survivors is provided by spouses and other family members. Issues relating to the physical aging, fatigue, and burnout of these caregivers are being brought to the forefront.[13] Issues relating the SCI survivor's contribution to the family unit—as a lover, parent, and wage earner—and as a

Table 13–5 British SCI Aging Study: Incidence of Follow-Up Procedures and Diagnoses (Episodes per 100 Cases per Year)

	By Years Postinjury			
	<10	*10–19*	*20–29*	*30+*
Diagnoses				
Infectious Disease/Neoplasm	2.4	4.4	7.3	10.7
CNS/Seizure	3.3	1.8	2.3	1.5
Fainting/Headache	2.0	3.0	2.6	1.8
Motor/Sensory Change	1.7	1.5	2.6	2.8
Disorder of Eye/Ear	0.8	1.1	5.4	10.3
Heart/Circulatory	2.9	5.4	10.0	14.2
Pneumonia/Atelectasis	2.4	2.3	2.4	2.0
Respiratory Infection	3.2	2.8	2.8	1.8
Gastrointestinal	7.1	8.7	9.9	14.4
Hemorrhoids	1.7	2.8	3.4	1.3
Rectal Abscess/Bleeding	1.5	2.9	4.4	3.3
UTI	17.3	22.8	22.0	13.8
GU Retention/Hydronephrosis	12.7	9.3	10.3	8.1
Renal Stone/Failure	3.7	5.5	5.4	6.3
Male GU Problem	2.8	3.1	4.6	7.2
Pressure Sore	27.7	20.1	19.4	16.6
Muscle/Joint Pain	5.8	7.0	11.3	16.0
Spasticity/Contracture	5.8	4.6	5.2	3.7
Fracture/Sprain/Amputation	1.9	2.6	3.2	3.3
Superficial Wound	2.5	1.8	1.4	0.9
Injury/Suicide	1.2	1.1	0.8	0.4
Operations				
Cardiac/Internal/CNS	6.8	4.5	6.6	4.6
Gastrointestinal	2.1	5.7	5.7	5.3
Genitourinary	8.9	9.5	12.2	17.3
Musculoskeletal	2.6	3.9	5.1	5.8

Source: Reprinted from Whiteneck, G., et al., Mortality, Morbidity, and Psychosocial Outcomes of Persons Spinal Cord Injured More Than 20 Years Ago, *Paraplegia,* Vol. 30, pp. 617–630, with permission of Churchill Livingstone, © 1992.

spender and user of family emotional, physical, and financial resources also are receiving increased scrutiny. At the same time, resource utilization and costs are becoming important on a larger sociologic level, particularly in light of changes within the health care system that affect availability, access, and costs of care. An early work in this area was completed by Menter et al, examining 205 long-term SCI survivors at the Rocky Mountain Regional Spinal Injury System.[14] Results indicated that the process of aging with SCI is accompanied by increasing disability, increased handicap, and increased costs of care—thus, increased impact on the survivor, on his or her family, and on society. In particular, in an attempt to combine the effects of increasing age with aging (years postinjury), the costs incurred by those individuals whose age plus years postinjury were under 50 were compared with the costs of those whose age plus years postinjury were over 50. It was found that costs for those in the latter group were nearly two times greater.[14]

In other studies, certain clear trends are appearing in the limited information available regarding costs for individuals with SCI over 20 years postinjury.[14-16] These trends show that at some point most individuals will require additional assistance to maintain their activity level. Various examples of additional assistance are lighter-weight wheelchairs, power wheelchairs in place of manual wheelchairs, transfer assistive devices, vans instead of cars for transportation, and increased amounts of attendant care. All of these are associated with considerable increase in costs. Unfortunately, no information can presently predict when the increases will occur and how dramatic they will be.

Self-Realization and Spiritual Growth

The final dimension of the aging model—spiritual change—also has been studied in only a limited manner. Although they address the issue somewhat indirectly, evidences that SCI survivors experience spiritual growth are accumulating. One of these evidences relates to perceived quality of life.

Often, our society casts aging as a negative process and getting older as undesirable. Almost always, our society views disability as an even more negative and undesirable phenomenon. Although both processes do result in some decline of physical function, decreasing independence, and greater need for assistance, society frequently loses sight of the bigger picture, which is life satisfaction. That many SCI survivors are able to find increasing satisfaction amid all of the "negatives" may be taken as evidence that life satisfaction is a growing, evolving process for them.

In the British study of individuals with SCI over 20 years postinjury by Whiteneck and associates,[12] two particular areas stood out in analysis. First, approximately three quarters of the subjects rated their current quality of life as either good or excellent on a five-point scale. A similar favorable response was reported retrospectively for a period 10 years ago; only 56%, however, reported that they would have given a favorable response 20 years ago. This seems to indicate an increase in life satisfaction over time. Second, those individuals with the greatest aging impact—over 50 years old and injured 30 or more years—reported the largest decline in quality of life. This suggests a pattern of increasing quality of life up to age 50 and 30 years postinjury, followed by a slight decline afterward. Similar findings were illustrated in an article by Krause and Crewe on the effects of chronologic age and time postinjury after SCI.[17] They noted, with one important exception (medical stability), the more time since injury, the more positive the adjustment. Their findings strongly suggest that SCI has its most devastating impact on the oldest persons and the persons with the least time since injury. Another study by Krause[18] reviewed adjustment following SCI over a 15-year period with an average follow-up of 24.3 years postinjury. Positive changes identified included increased sitting tolerance, more years of education, greater satisfaction with finances and employment, a higher percentage of persons working, and decreases in numbers of hospitalizations and days hospitalized.

CONCLUSION

Indeed, our intuition tells us, and the research reported throughout this chapter confirms, that aging with SCI is a complex phenomenon whereby chronologic age, years postinjury, and the type and severity of the neurologic injury itself interact with each other, both positively and negatively affecting the process of physiologic decline. Thus, the process of aging with an SCI may be accompanied by increasing physiologic decline, increasing disability, increasing handicap, and increasing costs of care. Yet, at the same time, these impact on and are impacted by the SCI survivor's own personal growth, perceptions of himself or herself, and his or her roles and relationships with not only the immediate family but the larger society as well. Initial research, although clearly just the tip of the iceberg, indicates that, like those of nondisabled persons, the lives of many SCI survivors can continue to be satisfying, meaningful, and rewarding into and beyond what we typically think of as "old age."

REFERENCES

1. Menter RR. Aging and spinal cord injury: Implications for existing model systems and future federal, state, and local health policy. In: Apple DF, Hudson LM, eds. *Spinal Cord Injury: The Model.* Atlanta: Georgia Regional Spinal Cord Injury Care System; 1990.

2. Menter RR. Spinal cord injury and aging: Exploring the unknown. *J Am Paraplegia Soc.* 1993; 16:179–189.

3. Jung C; Hall RFC, trans. *The Stages of Life. The Collected Works of Carl Jung.* Princeton, NJ: Princeton University Press; 1971.

4. Dossey L. *Meaning and Medicine.* New York: Bantam Books, Inc; 1991.

5. Colorado Department of Health. *1991 Annual Report of the Spinal Cord Injury Early Notification System.* Denver: Colorado Department of Health, Division of Prevention Programs; 1992.

6. DeVivo MJ, Kartus PL, Rutt RD, Stover SL, Fine PR. The influence of age at time of spinal cord injury on rehabilitation outcome. *Arch Neurol.* 1990; 687–691.

7. Yarkony GM, Roth EL, Heinemann AW, Lovell LL. Spinal cord injury rehabilitation outcome: The impact of age. *J Clin Epidemiol.* 1988;41:173–177.

8. Frankel HL, Hancock DO, Hyslop G, et al. The value of postural reduction in the initial management of closed injuries of the spine with paraplegia and tetraplegia. *Paraplegia.* 1969;7: 179–192.

9. DeVivo MJ, Shewchuk RM, Stover SL, Black KJ, Go BK. A cross-sectional study of the relationship between age and current health status for persons with spinal cord injuries. *Paraplegia.* 1992;30:820–827.

10. Data Management Service. *Guide for Use of the Uniform Data Set for Medical Rehabilitation: Uniform Data System for Medical Rehabilitation.* Buffalo, NY: State University of New York; 1987.

11. Bauman WA, Spungen AM, Zhong Y, Rothstein JL, Petry C, Gordon SK. Depressed serum high density lipoprotein cholesterol levels in veterans with spinal cord injury. *Paraplegia.* 1992;30:697–703.

12. Whiteneck G, Charlifue SW, Frankel H, et al. Mortality, morbidity, and psychosocial outcomes of persons spinal cord injured more than 20 years ago. *Paraplegia.* 1992;30:617–630.

13. Callahan D. Families as caregivers: The limits of morality. *Arch Phys Med Rehabil.* 1988;69:323–328.

14. Menter RR, Whiteneck GG, Charlifue SW, Gerhart K, Solnick SJ, Brooks CA. Impairment, disability, handicap, and medical expenses of persons aging with spinal cord injury. *Paraplegia.* 1991;29:613–619.

15. Menter RR. Aging with a spinal cord injury. *Phys Med Rehabil Med Clin North Am.* 1992;3:879–891.

16. Whiteneck G, Charlifue SW, Gerhart K, et al. *Aging with Spinal Cord Injury.* New York: Demos Publications; 1993.

17. Kraus JS, Crewe NM. Chronologic age, time since injury, and time of measurement: Effect on adjustment after spinal cord injury. *Arch Phys Med Rehabil.* 1991;72:91–100.

18. Kraus JS. Longitudinal changes in adjustment after spinal cord injury: A 15-year study. *Arch Phys Med Rehabil.* 1992;73:564–568.

14

Long-Term Survival and Causes of Death

Michael J. DeVivo and Samuel L. Stover

INTRODUCTION

During the past 50 years, both acute and long-term survival rates for persons with SCI have improved dramatically.[1–16] In fact, although the prognosis for some persons (particularly those injured later in life who sustain neurologically complete tetraplegia) remains relatively poor, the life expectancy of others (e.g., persons with neurologically incomplete motor functional injuries and normal bladder function who survive the initial effects of the injury) now approaches normal. For most individuals with SCI, however, life expectancy remains somewhat below normal.[15]

Mortality rates are significantly higher during the first year after injury than during subsequent years, particularly for more severely injured individuals.[6,12,15,17–20] Not surprisingly, the most significant prognostic factors related to survival are age and measures of injury severity such as neurologic level, degree of injury completeness, and ventilator dependency.[5,12–16,20–24] Given comparable age and injury severity, females and whites have slightly higher survival rates than males and nonwhites, but the difference is not as great as it would be in the absence of SCI.[15] Undoubtedly, the long-term quality of care received by persons with SCI as well as many psychosocial factors are also important determinants of survival, but these have received relatively little attention.[25,26]

Until recently, renal failure and other urinary tract complications were reported to be the leading causes of death among persons with SCI.[13,27–31] This led many clinicians and investigators to focus their attention and research efforts on management of the neurogenic bladder and prevention of renal failure. As a result, enormous progress has been made toward reducing urinary tract–related morbidity and mortality. Studies conducted more recently suggest that respiratory system complications, particularly pneumonia, have surpassed urinary tract complications as the leading underlying cause of both short- and long-term deaths among persons with tetraplegia.[8,9,22,32,33] Septicemia, suicide (particularly during the first several years), heart disease, and cancer are now the leading causes of death among persons with paraplegia.[8,16,24,32–36] Pulmonary emboli are also a leading cause of death early after SCI regardless of injury level.[32,33] Nonetheless, multiple inter-related causes play a role in many deaths, and although urinary tract complications are no longer among the leading underlying causes of death, they may still be a secondary or contributing cause, such as septicemia and, therefore, cannot be ignored.[32,33]

Historically, the Model Systems have placed a high priority on acquiring complete and accurate mortality information that has been an integral part of the National Database since its inception in 1973. This information includes the date of death, the primary (or underlying) cause of death, and up to four contributing causes of death. Causes are reported using ICD9CM codes after thorough review of all pertinent available records including hospital discharge summaries, death certificates, and autopsy reports. As a measure of the quality of cause of death information, a separate variable documents whether the reported cause was confirmed by autopsy.

Since collection of follow-up data is often difficult, the mortality information contained in the National Database is somewhat incomplete. As discussed in previous chapters, many individuals are ultimately lost to follow-up for a variety of reasons. Therefore, because of the high priority the Model Systems have placed on acquiring complete and accurate mortality data, considerable resources were expended to conduct periodic multisystem collaborative studies to supplement information contained in the National Database.[14,15,32,33] For these studies, each Model System made a special effort to identify the location of all former patients. Additional persons with traumatic SCI who did not meet the rigorous eligibility criteria for National Database inclusion but who were nonetheless injured since 1973, treated within 1 year of injury, and who survived at least 24 hours were also enrolled. The support of the Social Security Administration was enlisted to assist in identifying the survival status of persons who were otherwise lost to follow-up by searching its Master Beneficiary Record and Summary Earnings Record files for information on persons for whom benefit claims were submitted or for whom benefits were terminated because of death. By testing the accuracy of the Social Security Administration data with persons from the National Database whose survival status was already known, sensitivity (the ability to correctly identify people who were deceased) was found to be 92.4% and specificity (the ability to correctly identify people who were still alive) was found to be 99.5%.[15]

The information on long-term survival and causes of death reported in this chapter represents the merging of all data from the National Database, the collaborative studies, and the Social Security Administration. Although a few misclassifications of vital status will occur from using the Social Security Administration data, their impact on the results is negligible and far outweighed by the benefits of using these data to increase follow-up and identify deceased persons of whom the Model Systems were unaware. The overall data-merging process enhanced the quality of the data by increasing the study population size from 14,791 to 17,349 persons and increasing the length of follow-up for many of these individuals. However, the last collaborative study included follow-up only to the end of 1985, and the last Social Security Administration file search was conducted in 1989. Therefore, follow-up remains incomplete for many persons. For purposes of this report, all data collection ceased as of June 30, 1992.

LONG-TERM SURVIVAL

Cumulative survival was analyzed using standard Cutler-Ederer life table techniques.[37] In addition, the number of person-years of follow-up was calculated, with each person contributing 1 person-year for each year followed from injury until death, loss, or study termination.[38] Expected numbers of deaths and cumulative survival rates in the absence of SCI were calculated by applying U.S. population annual mortality rates to the actual follow-up period for each individual. These rates were published by the federal government for the year 1982 (the midyear of the study period) and were specific for age, sex, and race.[39]

The overall 18-year cumulative survival for persons injured since 1973 who survived at least 24 hours postinjury and were treated at a Model System within 1 year of injury was 74.6% (Figure 14–1). This compared with an expected cumulative survival in the absence of SCI of 92.4%.

Actual and expected mortality during each year after injury appears in Figure 14–2. The mortality rate for persons with SCI was 3.75% during the first postinjury year and 1.61% during the second postinjury year. Over the next 10 years, the mortality rate was approximately 1.2% per year (range 0.9% to 1.5%). After the 12th postinjury year, estimates of the annual mortality rate became increasingly unstable as sample sizes diminished. It does appear, however, that the annual mortality rate was beginning to increase as the population of persons with SCI aged. Annual expected mortality ranged from 0.4% to 0.5% per year.

Since the mean time from injury to admission to the Model System was 31 days, a small bias was introduced into the first-year mortality rate shown in Figure 14–2. This is because the number of persons who died between 24 hours after injury and time of System admission could not be determined. In a previous Model System study of postinjury survival from 1973 to 1985, first-year mortality increased to 6.3% when only persons admitted within 24 hours of injury were considered.[15] This bias would also have a small effect on the 18-year cumulative survival shown in Figure 14–1.

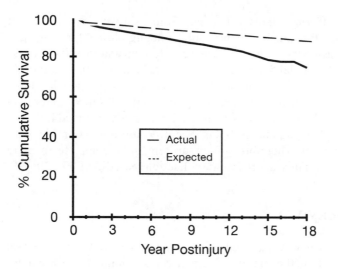

Figure 14–1 Cumulative Actual and Expected Survival for Persons with Spinal Cord Injuries Who Survive at Least 24 Hours Postinjury

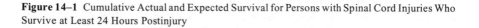

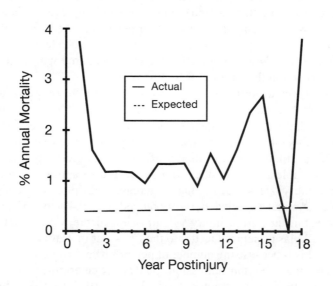

Figure 14–2 Actual and Expected Mortality during Each Year after Spinal Cord Injury for Persons Who Survive at Least 24 Hours Postinjury

As in previous studies, survival rates were strongly associated with neurologic level of injury, Frankel grade,[40] and age at injury.[5,12–16,20–24] In previous studies in which stratified (grouped) analyses were performed, the injury severity strata most often used were incomplete paraplegia, complete paraplegia, incomplete tetraplegia, and complete tetraplegia. The severity of neurologically incomplete lesions varies widely, however, with survival rates for persons who have only sensory sparing (Frankel grade B) or nonfunctional motor capability (Frankel grade C) below the injury level being closer to those of persons with neurologically complete lesions (Frankel grade A) than to persons with functional motor capability below the injury level (Frankel grade D). Moreover, among persons with tetraplegia, substantial differences in survival rates occur at each neurologic level.[15] Therefore, a more effective way to group persons with SCI that maximizes differences in survival rates is to create the following four groups: (1) injury level between C1 and C4 with Frankel grade A, B, or C; (2) injury level between C5 and C8 with Frankel grade A, B, or C; (3) thoracic, lumbar, or sacral injury with Frankel grade A, B, or C; and (4) Frankel grade D regardless of injury level.

Ten-year cumulative survival for each of these groups by age at injury appears in Figure 14–3. As can be seen, survival rates vary dramatically across strata. Persons in the oldest age group have relatively poor prognoses regardless of neurologic category. In fact, more than half of all persons in group 1 over 60 years of age at injury die within the first postinjury year. Older persons in group 1 who survive this initial high-risk period, however, have substantially improved survival rates thereafter. Conversely, cumulative 10-year survival rates are almost normal for persons in group 4 who are less than 46 years of age and persons in group 3 who are less than 31 years of age.

A simpler approach to quantifying long-term survival prospects for persons with SCI is to calculate a measure of average length of future survival. One such measure, commonly referred to as median survival, is the point in time at which 50% of the population has died. Because the Model System program did not begin until 1973, median survival has not yet been reached for several strata. Median survival time was 14.4 years for persons in group 1 (high tetraplegia, C1 to C4) between 31 and 45 years of age at injury, and 18.0 years for persons of comparable age in group 2 (low tetraplegia, C5 to C8). Median survival times for persons in these two neurologic groups who were between 46 and 60 years of age at injury were 6.7 and 13.3 years, respectively. Among persons over 60 years of age at injury, median survival times for the four neurologic groups were 0.9 years for group 1, 3.0 years for group 2, 7.7 years for group 3 (paraplegia), and 10.3 years for group 4 (Frankel grade D).

A second and perhaps more popular measure is life expectancy, which is defined as the arithmetic average (mean) remaining years of life for an individ-

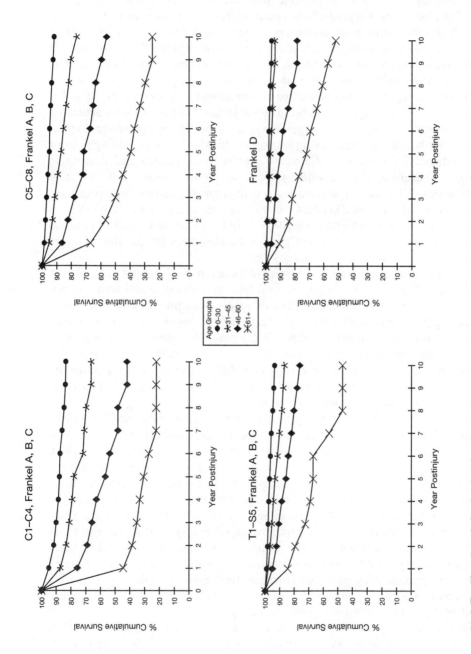

Figure 14–3 Ten-Year Cumulative Survival for Neurologic Groups by Age at Injury

ual. The process by which life expectancies for persons with SCI can be calculated has been discussed in detail elsewhere.[41] After determining the actual and expected number of deaths as discussed previously, the ratio of actual to expected deaths is calculated for each stratum. This is known as either the standardized mortality ratio (SMR) or the relative mortality ratio (RMR). An SMR of 1.0 implies that there is no increase in the mortality rate, whereas an SMR of 2.0 implies that the mortality rate for persons with SCIs in that stratum is twice the rate for the general population of comparable age, sex, and race. These ratios are sometimes multiplied by 100 and expressed as percentages so that an SMR of 1.5 would be expressed as 150% of normal. The annual probabilities of dying in the general population that appear in the standard life table published by the federal government are then multiplied by the appropriate SMR. These revised mortality probabilities are subtracted from 1.0 to get the corresponding survival probabilities that are then multiplied in a cumulative manner to arrive at the cumulative survival probability for each year after injury. Life expectancy (in years) is calculated as the sum of these cumulative survival probabilities.

Standardized mortality ratios for the Model System study population stratified by age at injury and neurologic group appear in Table 14–1. Because of the relatively high mortality experienced during the first postinjury year, a second set of SMRs was calculated with actual and expected deaths during the first postinjury year excluded. Although the exact pattern is somewhat inconsistent, in general, the SMR declines with advancing age and reduced injury severity. The SMR is consistently lower when the first postinjury year is excluded. It has also been demonstrated that the SMR decreases with advancing time after injury.[13]

Estimated life expectancies by age at injury and neurologic group for persons who survive at least 24 hours after injury appear in Table 14–2. These life expectancies are based on the SMR values with the first postinjury year included that appear in Table 14–1. Normal life expectancies for the general population taken from the standard life tables published by the federal government for the year 1988 (the most recent available) are included for comparison purposes.[42] These estimates of life expectancies are substantially higher than those that were published during the mid-1980s.[5,43,44] An individual in neurologic group 1 injured at 25 years of age now has a life expectancy that is 43.4% of normal, while the same individual in neurologic group 4 now has a life expectancy that is 83.9% of normal.

Estimates of life expectancy by current age and neurologic group for persons who survive the first postinjury year appear in Table 14–3. These estimates are based on the SMR values with the first postinjury year excluded that appear in Table 14–1. Figures for normal life expectancy are the same as those that appear in Table 14–2. Not surprisingly, given the difference in SMR values, the estimates appearing in Table 14–3 are uniformly higher than those shown in

Table 14–1   Standardized Mortality Ratios for Persons with Spinal Cord Injuries with First Postinjury Year Included and Excluded by Age at Injury and Neurologic Category

First Postinjury Year	Age at Injury	Standardized Mortality Ratio			
		C1–C4 (Frankel Grade A, B, C)	C5–C8 (Frankel Grade A, B, C)	T1–S5 (Frankel Grade A, B, C)	Frankel Grade D
Included	0–30	14.47	5.83	4.22	2.93
	31–45	16.98	7.85	4.27	2.04
	46–60	9.53	5.52	2.44	1.99
	61+	9.22	5.37	3.01	1.95
Excluded	0–30	10.94	5.07	3.86	2.58
	31–45	9.78	6.30	3.74	2.03
	46–60	5.24	3.83	1.96	1.66
	61+	3.07	3.07	2.21	1.68

Table 14–2. Nonetheless, these life expectancy estimates are still well below normal, particularly for more severely injured persons.

There is a common misconception, often expressed by many rehabilitation professionals, that as a result of recent medical advances, life expectancy for persons who survive the first postinjury year is either normal or reduced by at most 10%. While much progress has been made, there is clearly no justification for such statements. An individual in neurologic group 1 who has survived at least 1 year after injury and is now 25 years of age has a life expectancy that is 57.9% of normal, while the same individual in neurologic groups 2, 3, and 4 now has a life expectancy that is 67.2%, 79.1%, and 86.6% of normal, respectively.

While projections of life expectancy contained in Tables 14–2 and 14–3 are of great use in tracking progress in the overall medical management of persons with SCI, great caution should be exercised when applying these figures to individual cases for several reasons. First, considerable variability in injury severity exists within each neurologic group. This is particularly true for neurologic groups 1 and 4. For example, the tabulated life expectancies for persons in neurologic group 1 would be overestimates for individuals who were ventilator dependent and underestimates for persons who were not ventilator dependent. Second, the effects of gender, race, and other known determinants of general population survival are not considered. Moreover, the effects of numerous psychosocial factors and the anticipated lifetime quality of care are also not considered, although they are difficult to quantify. Therefore, more precise projections should be made for specific persons only by matching such characteristics of the individual as the exact neurologic level of injury and Frankel

Table 14–2 Life Expectancy for Persons with Spinal Cord Injuries Who Survive at Least 24 Hours Postinjury by Age at Injury and Neurologic Category

Age at Injury	Normal*	*Life Expectancy (Years)* C1–C4 (Frankel Grade A, B, C)	C5–C8 (Frankel Grade A, B, C)	T1–S5 (Frankel Grade A, B, C)	Frankel Grade D
5	70.8	37.3	47.7	55.7	61.4
10	65.9	32.9	43.1	51.0	56.6
15	61.0	28.5	38.4	46.3	51.8
20	56.3	25.3	34.3	42.1	47.5
25	51.6	22.4	30.5	38.1	43.3
30	46.9	19.3	26.5	34.0	39.0
35	42.2	16.5	22.9	30.0	34.6
40	37.6	14.2	19.5	26.2	30.3
45	33.0	12.2	16.4	22.6	26.0
50	28.6	9.7	13.1	18.7	21.9
55	24.4	7.3	10.2	15.0	18.1
60	20.5	5.0	7.8	11.6	14.8
65	16.9	3.5	5.8	8.9	11.8
70	13.6	2.2	4.0	6.7	9.0
75	10.7	1.3	2.7	4.8	6.7
80	8.1	0.3	1.6	3.2	4.6

*Normal values are from 1988 U.S. Life Tables for the general population.

grade, age, gender, race, ventilator status, length of postinjury survival to date, presence of pre-existing or unrelated concurrent medical conditions, motivation in self-care, and availability of good medical care to the largest possible sample population.

Finally, because of their uncertain nature, these projections cannot take into consideration possible future advances in medical treatment and prevention practices, not only for potentially fatal secondary medical complications related to SCI, but also for unrelated medical conditions such as cancer, heart disease, and stroke that nonetheless affect life expectancy for persons with SCIs. In fact, by using Cox proportional hazards regression analysis to control for confounding due to trends over time in age, gender, race, and neurologic category, a striking trend toward improving survival rates is clearly evident.[45] As seen in Table 14–4, the mortality rate for persons injured between 1976 and 1979 was 0.92 times the mortality rate for persons injured in the referent time period (1973-1975). Stated simply, this means that given comparable age, gender, race, and neurologic category, the mortality rate for 1976–1979 was 8% lower than the mortality rate for 1973–1975. Similarly, the mortality rate was reduced by 25%

Table 14–3   Life Expectancy for Persons with Spinal Cord Injuries Who Survive at Least 1 Year Postinjury by Current Age and Neurologic Category

	Life Expectancy (Years)				
Current Age	Normal*	C1–C4 (Frankel Grade A, B, C)	C5–C8 (Frankel Grade A, B, C)	T1–S5 (Frankel Grade A, B, C)	Frankel Grade D
5	70.8	45.0	52.0	59.5	63.0
10	65.9	40.5	47.3	53.7	58.2
15	61.0	36.1	42.6	49.0	53.4
20	56.3	32.8	38.6	44.8	49.0
25	51.6	29.9	34.7	40.8	44.7
30	46.9	26.8	30.7	36.7	40.5
35	42.2	23.7	27.0	32.7	36.1
40	37.6	20.9	23.6	28.8	31.7
45	33.0	18.4	20.4	25.1	27.5
50	28.6	15.5	17.0	21.2	23.4
55	24.4	12.8	13.8	17.3	19.5
60	20.5	11.0	11.2	13.8	15.9
65	16.9	8.8	8.8	10.9	13.2
70	13.6	6.6	6.6	8.3	10.4
75	10.7	4.7	4.7	6.1	8.0
80	8.1	3.1	3.1	4.2	6.1

*Normal values are from 1988 U.S. Life Tables for the general population.

for persons injured between 1980 and 1982, by 28% for persons injured between 1983 and 1985, by 37% for persons injured between 1986 and 1988, and by 42% for persons injured between 1989 and 1992 relative to persons injured between 1973 and 1975. This improvement represents one of the major accomplishments of the Model System program.

Table 14–4 also confirms the necessity for taking race and gender into account when projecting life expectancy for individuals with SCIs. While these factors are somewhat less important than neurologic category, the mortality rate for males is 27% higher than that for females, and the mortality rate for nonwhites is 19% higher than that for whites given comparable neurologic category, age, and injury year.

CAUSES OF DEATH

Why is life expectancy below normal, even for persons who survive the initial high-risk period immediately after injury? To answer this question, one must

Table 14–4 Results of Proportional Hazards Regression Analysis of Survival Following Spinal Cord Injury

Predictor	Relative Risk
Male	1.27
Female	1.00
Nonwhite	1.19
White	1.00
Each Year of Age	1.06
Neurologic Category	
C1–C4, Frankel Grade A, B, C	5.42
C5–C8, Frankel Grade A, B, C	2.72
T1–S5, Frankel Grade A, B, C	1.53
Frankel Grade D	1.00
Year of Injury	
1973–75	1.00
1976–79	0.92
1980–82	0.75
1983–85	0.72
1986–88	0.63
1989–92	0.58

consider cause-specific mortality rates for persons with SCI compared with those of the general population. The methodology for doing this is the same as was used to calculate the SMR values shown in Table 14–1 except that cause-specific mortality rates for the general population are used rather than overall mortality rates to determine the expected number of deaths from each cause. The general population mortality rates for each cause are also age-, sex-, and race-specific so that differences in these characteristics between the general and the SCI population can be controlled.[39] The expected number of deaths from each cause is then compared with the actual number of deaths from that cause to arrive at a separate SMR for each cause. A more detailed understanding of why life expectancy remains below normal can then be obtained by stratifying the cause-of-death analyses by age, neurologic group, and time postinjury. [32,33]

Before proceeding further, it is important to understand that when someone with SCI dies, multiple causes (sometimes even unrelated causes) may play a role in that death. The same is true for persons in the general population. The cause-specific mortality rates for the general population published by the National Center for Health Statistics, however, are based solely on the underlying cause of death. Contributing causes and incidental findings are not considered. For these purposes, the underlying cause of death is defined as the cause that initiated the sequence of events that directly led to the person's death. It is often different from the immediate cause of death. For example, if the death certificate lists cardiorespiratory arrest due to or as a consequence of pneumonia, then cardiorespiratory arrest would be the immediate cause of death and pneumonia would be the underlying cause of death. Although comparison of causes of death between the SCI and general population by calculating the SMR is therefore restricted to the underlying cause, frequencies and descriptive information about secondary or contributing causes among the SCI population are included to provide a more complete picture of the impact of particular causes on life expectancy.

The results of these analyses appear in Tables 14–5 through 14–9. Because most specific causes of death are relatively rare, particularly among younger-aged persons who comprise the largest segment of the SCI population, sample sizes preclude use of multivariate analyses, even though our study population includes over 17,000 persons. Therefore, age, neurologic group, and time postinjury were analyzed separately rather than jointly (Tables 14–7 through 14–9).

Pneumonia and Other Respiratory Diseases

The leading cause of death for persons with SCIs is pneumonia. Overall, 16.3% of all deaths of known cause were due to pneumonia (Table 14–5). Pneumonia was also listed as a contributing cause of an additional 21 deaths (1.5%). Pneumonia is the leading underlying cause of death in all age groups, ranging from 20.3% in the oldest age group to 12.8% in the youngest age group. It is the leading underlying cause of death in persons with high-level (C1 to C4) tetraplegia (24.7%) and persons with low-level (C5 to C8) tetraplegia (19.6%). Pneumonia is also the leading underlying cause of death during all postinjury time periods, ranging from 18.9% during the first postinjury year to 12.7% after the fifth postinjury year.

The actual number of deaths due to pneumonia was 35.6 times the expected number of deaths given the age, gender, race, and length of follow-up of these persons. The pneumonia SMR was particularly high for younger persons (SMR = 65.7) and persons with high-level tetraplegia (SMR = 151.7), and was highest during the first postinjury year (SMR = 83.8). Nonetheless, there were substantially more deaths due to pneumonia than expected for all groups and time periods.

In addition to pneumonia, there were 109 deaths due to other diseases of the respiratory system (58 underlying and 51 secondary). Combining these with the deaths due to pneumonia, respiratory system complications are the underlying cause of death in 20.4% of cases and, accounting for duplication, a secondary cause of death in an additional 3.5% of cases.

Table 14–5 Underlying and Secondary Causes of Death for Persons with Spinal Cord Injuries Who Survive at Least 24 Hours after Injury

Cause of Death*	Underlying Cause of Death[†]		Secondary Cause of Death[†]		Total	
	No.	%	No.	%	No.	%
Septicemia (038)	122	8.7	47	3.3	169	12.0
Cancer (140–239)	71	5.1	8	0.6	79	5.6
Diseases of the Nervous System (320–359)	30	2.1	28	2.0	58	4.1
Ischemic Heart Disease (410–414)	91	6.5	13	0.9	104	7.4
Diseases of Pulmonary Circulation (415–417)	113	8.1	3	0.2	116	8.3
Nonischemic Heart Disease (420–429)	171	12.2	60	4.3	231	16.5
Cerebrovascular Disease (430–438)	41	2.9	12	0.9	53	3.8
Diseases of Arteries (440–448)	17	1.2	16	1.1	33	2.4
Pneumonia and Influenza (480–487)	228	16.3	21	1.5	249	17.7
Other Respiratory Diseases (460–478, 490–519)	58	4.1	51	3.6	109	7.8
Diseases of the Digestive System (520–579)	67	4.8	28	2.0	95	6.8
Diseases of the Urinary System (580–599)	49	3.5	73	5.2	122	8.7
Symptoms and Ill-Defined Conditions (780–799)	102	7.3	112	8.0	214	15.3
Unintentional Injuries (E800–E949)	72	5.1	—	—	72	5.1
Suicide (E950–E959)	80	5.7	—	—	80	5.7
Homicide and Legal Intervention (E960–E978)	15	1.1	—	—	15	1.1
All Other External Causes (E980–E999)	32	2.3	—	—	32	2.3
Residual (All Others)	44	3.1	70	5.0	114	8.1
Total Deaths of Known Cause	1403	100.0				
Unknown	198	—				
Total Deaths	1601					

*ICD-9-CM codes are in parentheses.
[†]All percentages are based on 1403 deaths of known cause.

Of the 109 deaths due to other diseases of the respiratory system, there were 12 cases of pulmonary congestion (11.0%); 10 cases of pulmonary collapse (9.2%); 9 cases of acute pulmonary edema (8.3%); 8 cases each of lung abscess and pneumothorax (7.3%); 6 cases each of pleurisy and emphysema (5.5%); 5 cases of bronchitis (4.6%); 4 cases each of asthma and pulmonary insufficiency (3.7%); 2 cases each of pulmonary fibrosis, empyema, and mediastinitis

Table 14–6   Standardized Mortality Ratios for Underlying Cause of Death among Persons with Spinal Cord Injuries Who Survive at Least 24 Hours Postinjury

Cause of Death	Actual Deaths	Expected Deaths	SMR
Septicemia	122	1.9	64.2
Cancer	71	82.0	0.9
Diseases of the Nervous System	30	5.1	5.9
Ischemic Heart Disease	91	78.4	1.2
Diseases of Pulmonary Circulation	113	2.4	47.1
Nonischemic Heart Disease	171	26.7	6.4
Cerebrovascular Disease	41	18.6	2.2
Diseases of Arteries	17	5.0	3.4
Pneumonia and Influenza	228	6.4	35.6
Other Respiratory Diseases	58	12.8	4.5
Diseases of the Digestive System	67	17.8	3.8
Diseases of the Urinary System	49	4.5	10.9
Symptoms and Ill-Defined Conditions	102	7.4	13.8
Unintentional Injuries	72	51.8	1.4
Suicide	80	16.6	4.8
Homicide and Legal Intervention	15	21.8	0.7
All Other External Causes	32	2.3	13.9
Residual	44	23.2	1.9
Unknown	198		

(1.8%); 1 case each of asphyxiation, tracheostomy complications, chronic airway obstruction, upper respiratory infection, and sinusitis (0.9%); and 26 unspecified cases of lung or respiratory system diseases (23.9%).

Pulmonary Embolus

There were 113 deaths for which the underlying cause was coded as a disease of pulmonary circulation (8.1% of all deaths of known cause). All of these deaths were the result of a pulmonary embolus that usually occurs secondary to deep venous thrombosis. Pulmonary embolus was also listed as a secondary cause of death in 3 cases (0.2%). Therefore, respiratory diseases plus pulmonary emboli account for 28.4% of all underlying causes of death in this population, and when secondary causes of death are included, respiratory disease plus pulmonary emboli can be said to contribute to 31.9% of all deaths. Pulmonary emboli were among the leading underlying causes of death for persons in the younger and middle age groups (9.4% and 10.1% of all deaths of known cause, respectively). Pulmonary emboli were the third leading underlying cause of

Table 14-7 Underlying Cause of Death for Persons with Spinal Cord Injuries Who Survive at Least 24 Hours after Injury, by Age

Cause of Death	Age ≤30 Years			Age 31–60 Years			Age ≥61 Years		
	Actual Deaths	Expected Deaths	SMR	Actual Deaths	Expected Deaths	SMR	Actual Deaths	Expected Deaths	SMR
Septicemia	28	0.2	140.0	63	0.8	78.8	31	0.9	34.4
Cancer	6	4.8	1.3	32	38.6	0.8	33	38.6	0.9
Diseases of the Nervous System	12	1.5	8.0	10	2.2	4.5	8	1.5	5.3
Ischemic Heart Disease	7	1.2	5.8	42	32.5	1.3	42	44.7	0.9
Diseases of Pulmonary Circulation	34	0.3	113.3	63	1.1	57.3	16	1.0	16.0
Nonischemic Heart Disease	33	1.7	19.4	60	11.6	5.2	78	13.4	5.8
Cerebrovascular Disease	11	0.8	13.8	16	6.5	2.5	14	11.3	1.2
Diseases of Arteries	2	0.1	20.0	4	1.3	3.1	11	3.5	3.1
Pneumonia and Influenza	46	0.7	65.7	97	2.4	40.4	85	3.4	25.0
Other Respiratory Diseases	11	0.8	13.8	28	4.3	6.5	19	7.7	2.5
Diseases of the Digestive System	18	1.8	10.0	36	10.8	3.3	13	5.2	2.5
Diseases of the Urinary System	12	0.3	40.0	23	1.7	13.5	14	2.5	5.6
Symptoms and Ill-Defined Conditions	24	2.0	12.0	44	3.5	12.6	34	1.9	17.9
Unintentional Injuries	35	31.5	1.1	32	17.2	1.9	5	3.1	1.6
Suicide	40	9.2	4.3	36	6.4	5.6	4	0.9	4.4
Homicide and Legal Intervention	11	12.5	0.9	4	8.9	0.4	0	0.5	0.0
All Other External Causes	16	1.2	13.3	13	1.0	13.0	3	0.1	30.0
Residual	14	3.9	3.6	21	10.3	2.0	9	8.9	1.0
Unknown	49			87			62		

Table 14–8 Underlying Cause of Death for Persons with Spinal Cord Injuries Who Survive at Least 24 Hours after Injury, by Neurologic Category

Cause of Death	C1–C4, Frankel Grade ABC			C5–C8, Frankel Grade ABC		
	Actual Deaths	Expected Deaths	SMR	Actual Deaths	Expected Deaths	SMR
Septicemia	27	0.2	135.0	39	0.4	97.5
Cancer	4	7.0	0.6	14	17.1	0.8
Diseases of the Nervous System	15	0.5	30.0	9	1.2	7.5
Ischemic Heart Disease	17	6.7	2.5	22	16.1	1.4
Diseases of Pulmonary Circulation	21	0.2	105.0	32	0.5	64.0
Nonischemic Heart Disease	56	2.5	22.4	54	5.7	9.5
Cerebrovascular Disease	14	1.8	7.8	11	3.9	2.8
Diseases of Arteries	2	0.5	4.0	4	1.1	3.6
Pneumonia and Influenza	91	0.6	151.7	88	1.5	58.7
Other Respiratory Disease	18	1.1	16.4	26	2.7	9.6
Diseases of Digestive System	21	1.5	14.0	17	4.0	4.3
Diseases of Urinary System	10	0.4	25.0	19	1.0	19.0
Symptoms and Ill-Defined Conditions	44	0.7	62.9	37	1.8	20.6
Unintentional Injuries	11	5.5	2.0	26	14.6	1.8
Suicide	3	1.7	1.8	22	4.6	4.8
Homicide and Legal Intervention	0	2.3	0.0	4	5.8	0.7
All Other External Causes	3	0.2	15.0	9	0.6	15.0
Residual	11	2.2	5.0	17	5.1	3.3
Unknown	46			53		

	T1–S5, Frankel Grade ABC			Frankel Grade D		
Septicemia	46	0.5	92.0	10	0.7	14.3
Cancer	31	25.6	1.2	22	32.2	0.7
Diseases of the Nervous System	3	1.7	1.8	3	1.7	1.8
Ischemic Heart Disease	29	23.4	1.2	23	32.2	0.7
Dieases of Pulmonary Circulation	34	0.7	48.6	26	0.9	28.9
Nonischemic Heart Disease	27	7.9	3.4	34	10.6	3.2
Cerebrovascular Disease	7	5.2	1.3	9	7.7	1.2
Diseases of Arteries	8	1.3	6.2	3	2.1	1.4
Pneumonia and Influenza	23	1.8	12.8	26	2.5	10.4
Other Respiratory Disease	9	3.8	2.4	5	5.2	1.0

continues

Table 14–8 continued

	T1–S5, Frankel Grade ABC			Frankel Grade D		
Diseases of Digestive System	16	6.1	2.6	13	6.3	2.1
Diseases of Urinary System	15	1.3	11.5	5	1.8	2.8
Symptoms and Ill-Defined Conditions	9	2.5	3.6	12	2.4	5.0
Unintentional Injuries	18	18.1	1.0	17	13.6	1.3
Suicide	40	5.9	6.8	15	4.4	3.4
Homicide and Legal Intervention	6	8.5	0.7	5	5.3	0.9
All Other External Causes	15	0.8	18.8	5	0.6	8.3
Residual	12	7.7	1.6	4	8.4	0.5
Unknown	57			42		

death for persons with paraplegia (9.8%), tied for the second leading underlying cause of death for persons with Frankel grade D lesions (11.0%), and the third leading underlying cause of death during the first postinjury year (14.6%). However, the frequency of deaths due to pulmonary emboli decreased substantially with advancing time after injury, accounting for only 2.5% of deaths after the fifth postinjury year.

Overall, pulmonary embolus had the second highest SMR among all causes of death. The actual number of deaths due to pulmonary emboli was 47.1 times the expected number of deaths given age, gender, race, and length of follow-up of these persons. The pulmonary embolus SMR was particularly high for both younger persons (SMR = 113.3) and persons in the middle age group (SMR = 57.3). The pulmonary embolus SMR decreased substantially with decreasing injury severity, ranging from 105.0 for persons with high-level tetraplegia to 28.9 for persons in the Frankel grade D group. Nonetheless, pulmonary embolus had the highest SMR among persons in the Frankel grade D group, the second highest SMR among persons with paraplegia or low-level tetraplegia, and the third highest SMR among persons with high-level tetraplegia. Pulmonary embolus had the highest SMR during the first postinjury year (SMR = 210.0) and the third highest SMR during postinjury years 2 through 5 (SMR = 19.1).

Diseases of the Urinary System

Diseases of the urinary system now account for only a small percentage of underlying causes of death in this population. Overall, there were 49 deaths for which the underlying cause was a disease of the urinary tract (3.5% of all deaths

Table 14–9 Underlying Cause of Death for Persons with Spinal Cord Injuries Who Survive at Least 24 Hours Postinjury, by Length of Postinjury Survival

Cause of Death	Survival <1 Year			Survival 1–5 Years			Survival >5 Years		
	Actual Deaths	Expected Deaths	SMR	Actual Deaths	Expected Deaths	SMR	Actual Deaths	Expected Deaths	SMR
Septicemia	38	0.4	95.0	56	0.9	62.2	28	0.6	46.7
Cancer	12	14.7	0.8	33	37.7	0.9	26	29.6	0.9
Diseases of the Nervous System	22	1.0	22.0	4	2.4	1.7	4	1.7	2.4
Ischemic Heart Disease	30	14.5	2.1	42	35.8	1.2	19	28.1	0.7
Diseases of Pulmonary Circulation	84	0.4	210.0	21	1.1	19.1	8	0.9	8.9
Nonischemic Heart Disease	89	5.8	15.3	48	10.1	4.8	34	10.8	3.1
Cerebrovascular Disease	17	3.6	4.7	16	8.5	1.9	8	6.5	1.2
Diseases of Arteries	6	1.0	6.0	7	2.3	3.0	4	1.7	2.3
Pneumonia and Influenza	109	1.3	83.8	79	3.0	26.3	40	2.1	19.0
Other Respiratory Diseases	34	2.4	14.2	16	5.9	2.7	8	4.5	1.8
Diseases of the Digestive System	24	3.1	7.7	25	8.2	3.0	18	6.5	2.8
Diseases of the Urinary System	14	0.9	15.6	20	2.1	9.5	15	1.5	10.0
Symptoms and Ill-Defined Conditions	56	1.3	43.1	32	3.5	9.1	14	2.6	5.4
Unintentional Injuries	11	9.5	1.2	32	25.8	1.2	29	16.5	1.8
Suicide	13	2.6	5.0	49	8.0	6.1	18	6.0	3.0
Homicide and Legal Intervention	1	4.1	0.2	7	14.9	0.5	7	2.8	2.5
All Other External Causes	3	0.4	7.5	12	1.1	10.9	17	0.8	21.3
Residual	13	3.8	3.4	14	8.7	1.6	17	10.7	1.6
Unknown	36			89			73		

of known cause). However, diseases of the urinary system were listed as a secondary contributing cause of death for an additional 73 persons (5.2%), making this the most frequent secondary cause of death among persons with SCIs.

Of 122 deaths for which diseases of the urinary system were either the underlying or secondary cause, only 13 were due to renal failure (10.7%). There were 40 urinary tract infections (32.8%), most of which were listed as secondary causes of death. There were 19 cases of glomerulonephritis (15.6%); two cases of kidney stones (1.6%); one case each of kidney cyst, cystitis, and unspecified bladder disease (0.8%); and 45 cases of unspecified kidney disease (36.9%).

The actual number of deaths due to diseases of the urinary system was 10.9 times the expected number of deaths given age, gender, race, and length of follow-up of these persons. The SMR for diseases of the urinary system decreased with advancing age and with decreasing injury severity. However, no trend in the SMR for diseases of the urinary system was observed by time postinjury.

Septicemia

Septicemia is the third leading underlying cause of death for persons with SCIs. Overall, there were 122 deaths for which the underlying cause was septicemia (8.7% of all deaths of known cause). Septicemia is usually secondary to an infection occurring in any of several organ systems of the body. Unfortunately, the source of septicemia is often not documented on death certificates. Among the 122 deaths where septicemia was listed as the underlying cause, 27 cases were actually secondary to pressure sores (22.1%). These deaths were included in the septicemia category rather than in a newly created category for diseases of the skin. The source of 55 cases of septicemia was not documented (45.1%), while the remaining 40 cases were included in this category because they had multiple possible sources listed as contributing causes of death (32.8%).

In addition, septicemia was listed as a secondary cause of death for 47 cases (3.3%). Of these, 23 were secondary to urinary tract infections (48.9%), 18 were secondary to respiratory infections (38.3%), and 6 were secondary to peritoneal infections (12.8%). This generally agrees with others who reported that urinary tract infections were the source of bacteremia in 47% of cases.[46]

Septicemia is tied for the second leading underlying cause of death in the middle-aged-group (10.1%), the leading underlying cause of death among persons with paraplegia (13.2%), the third leading underlying cause of death among persons with low-level tetraplegia (8.7%), and the second leading underlying cause of death between 1 and 5 years postinjury (10.9%). Overall, septicemia has the highest SMR of any cause of death in this population (SMR = 64.2). It has the highest SMR across all age groups, the second highest SMR among persons with either high-level tetraplegia or Frankel grade D lesions, the highest SMR among persons with either low-level tetraplegia or paraplegia, the highest SMR after the first postinjury year, and the second highest SMR during the first postinjury year.

Many of these deaths might be preventable with appropriate skin care, proper supplies and equipment, routine long-term follow-up, and improved compliance with therapeutic regimens. Therefore, increased emphasis should be placed on patient education, particularly in the areas of proper skin care and bladder management. Regular home visits by skilled personnel trained to identify and manage problems before they become life-threatening may also prove beneficial for some persons with SCIs. Nonetheless, many infections are probably not preventable in this population. Therefore, prompt and appropriate treatment of infections when they occur in these organ systems is also important in preventing septicemia.

Diseases of the Digestive System

There were 67 deaths for which diseases of the digestive system were listed as the underlying cause (4.8% of all deaths of known cause). In addition, diseases of the digestive system were listed as a secondary contributing cause of death in 28 cases (2.0%). Of the 95 total cases in which diseases of the digestive system were cited as either the underlying or a contributing cause of death, 39 (41.1%) were cases of peritonitis or gastrointestinal hemorrhage usually secondary to perforated and/or hemorrhaging ulcers; 25 (26.3%) were diseases of the liver (usually alcoholic cirrhosis); 16 (16.8%) were intestinal disorders, including obstructions, adhesions, fistulas, and enteritis; 5 (5.3%) were pancreatic diseases; 5 (5.3%) were unspecified vascular insufficiencies; and there was 1 case each of obstructed inguinal hernia, unspecified disorder of gastric motility, unspecified disorder of the esophagus, unspecified disorder of the stomach, and acute appendicitis (1.1%).

Diseases of the digestive system were not among the leading underlying causes of death for any age, neurologic, or time postinjury group. Nonetheless, there were 3.8 times more deaths due to diseases of the digestive system than expected in this population. While this is not an exceptionally high SMR compared with other causes, it does suggest that digestive system complications cannot be ignored as a contributor to reduced life expectancies in this population, particularly among young persons for whom the SMR was 10.0 and among persons with high-level tetraplegia for whom the SMR reached 14.0.

Unintentional Injuries, Suicide, and Homicide

By definition, all deaths in these categories begin with a traumatic event. Therefore, these events will always constitute the underlying cause rather than a secondary cause of death.

There were 72 deaths due to unintentional injuries that occurred subsequent to the event that caused the SCI (5.1% of all deaths of known cause). This was only slightly more than the expected number of deaths from this cause (SMR = 1.4). Unintentional injuries were not among the leading underlying causes of death for any neurologic group or time postinjury. However, they were the third leading underlying cause of death for persons in the youngest age group (9.7%). This is not surprising, since unintentional injuries are the leading cause of death in the younger-aged general population.[42]

Recently, attention has been focused on the relatively high rate of suicide in this population.[34-36] The data presented in Tables 14–5 through 14–9 confirm this disturbing trend. There were 80 confirmed suicides in this population (5.7% of all deaths of known cause). Suicide was the second leading underlying cause of death among persons in the youngest age group (11.1%), the second leading underlying cause of death for persons with paraplegia (11.5%), and the third leading underlying cause of death between the first and fifth postinjury years (9.6%). Conversely, suicide was rare among persons with high-level tetraplegia.

The overall SMR for suicide was 4.8. The highest suicide SMR was for persons with paraplegia (SMR = 6.8). The suicide SMR was higher during the first 5 years than later postinjury. These trends are similar to those reported previously.[36] Additional analyses and discussion of the issue of suicide in this population appears in Chapter 10, and other reports have also been published.[34-36]

Very few persons in this population were homicide victims (1.1% of all deaths of known cause). Moreover, the number of homicides was slightly below that which was expected given the age, gender, race, and length of postinjury follow-up for this population (SMR = 0.7).

There were 32 deaths due to "all other external causes." These are invariably cases of fatal injuries that were sustained from events of uncertain circumstances. Since there were 72 confirmed unintentional injuries, 80 confirmed suicides, and 15 confirmed homicides, it might be assumed that approximately these same proportions should apply to the 32 cases of uncertain circumstances. If that were true, then these 32 cases would include 14 deaths due to unintentional injuries, 15 suicides, and 3 homicides. This would increase the overall SMR to 1.7 for unintentional injuries, 5.7 for suicide, and 0.8 for homicide.

Cardiovascular, Cerebrovascular, and Arterial Diseases

Nonischemic heart disease is the second leading underlying cause of death in this population, while ischemic heart disease ranks sixth. Combining these two categories, heart disease accounts for 18.7% of all deaths of known cause, ranking second only to pneumonia and other diseases of the respiratory system as the underlying cause of death. In addition, there were 71 deaths (5.1%) for which heart disease was listed as a secondary contributing cause (58 nonischemic, 11 ischemic, and 2 with both). After eliminating duplication among the underlying and secondary causes, heart disease contributes to 22.4% of all deaths.

If both ischemic disease and nonischemic disease are combined, then heart disease is the second leading underlying cause of death among persons with tetraplegia and the leading underlying cause of death among persons with paraplegia and persons with Frankel grade D injuries. Heart disease would also be the second leading underlying cause of death during the first 5 postinjury years, and the leading underlying cause of death thereafter.

Interestingly, there is no significant increased risk of mortality due to ischemic heart disease in this population (SMR = 1.2). However, it is possible that follow-up is not yet long enough for significant increases in mortality due to ischemic heart disease to appear. There is a significant increase in mortality due to nonischemic heart disease (SMR = 6.4) that requires further scrutiny.

Among the 231 deaths for which nonischemic heart disease was either the underlying or secondary cause, 98 (42.4%) were classified as cardiac arrests not otherwise specified (ICD9CM code 427.5). The remaining 133 causes of death in this category included 71 cases of congestive and other heart failure, 40 cases of cardiac dysrhythmia, 19 cases of ill-defined heart disease, two cases of endocardial disorders, and one case of cardiomyopathy.

Closer inspection of the 98 deaths coded as cardiac arrests not otherwise specified revealed that this category was often used in cases where the cause of death appeared uncertain. These are virtually always listed as immediate causes of death with no secondary cause listed. These deaths often occur during the first postinjury year. Many of these individuals are young and have no previous history of heart disease, and only 30% of these cases were autopsied. It is likely that several of these cases represent sudden death secondary to vagal arrest rather than intrinsic heart disease, particularly among persons with high-level tetraplegia.[47] Therefore, the true number of deaths due to nonischemic heart disease is probably considerably overestimated. Nonetheless, even if all suspect deaths were excluded from the nonischemic heart disease category, there would still be almost three times as many deaths remaining as expected.

Unlike ischemic heart disease, there is a small increase in mortality due to cerebrovascular disease (SMR = 2.2). Overall, cerebrovascular disease was the underlying cause of 2.9% of all deaths of known cause. Cerebrovascular disease also contributed as a secondary cause to 12 additional deaths (0.9%). Cerebrovascular disease was not among the leading underlying causes of death for any study group, and SMR values were consistently small by comparison with other causes.

Diseases of the arteries were also a relatively rare underlying cause of death (1.2% of all deaths of known cause). However, the overall SMR was somewhat elevated (SMR = 3.4). Among older persons, the usual cause of death in this category was arteriosclerosis, while among younger persons aneurysms were the usual cause. Diseases of the arteries were also listed as a secondary contributing cause of death for 16 cases (1.1%). In almost all of these secondary cases, heart disease or cerebrovascular disease was listed as the underlying cause of death.

Although the SMRs for heart disease, cerebrovascular disease, and diseases of the arteries are not particularly high relative to those of other causes, there are nonetheless a substantial number of excess deaths due to these combined causes. Therefore, these data suggest that smoking cessation, changing diet, and increasing exercise to the extent possible would have an even greater impact on life expectancy of persons with SCIs than they would in the general population.

Cancer

Cancer mortality rates do not appear to be increased among persons with SCI. Overall, 5.1% of all deaths of known cause were due to cancer. Cancer was also listed as a contributing cause of an additional eight deaths (0.6%). Of 79 deaths where cancer was either the underlying or a contributing cause, 27 were metastatic lung disease (34.2%). There were six prostate cancers (7.6%); five colorectal cancers (6.3%); four pancreatic malignancies (5.1%); three each of the brain, esophagus, bladder, and connective and soft tissue of the head, face, and neck (3.8%); two each of liver, kidneys, endocrine glands, leukemia, and multiple myeloma (2.5%); and one each of urinary system (unspecified), endometrium, ovary, breast, bone, peritoneum, melanoma, and other malignant neoplasm of the skin (1.3%). The remaining seven cases were disseminated or unspecified malignancies (8.9%). This pattern of cancers seems consistent with what one would expect in the general population of comparable age, sex, and race. Cancer would be expected to increase as a cause of death as the population is followed longer and ages.

Other Causes of Death

There were 30 deaths for which the underlying cause was listed as a disease of the nervous system (2.1%). In addition, diseases of the nervous system were listed as a secondary contributing cause of death in 28 other cases (2.0%). These figures do not include any persons with ICD9CM code 344 (other paralytic syndromes) because these codes typically are used to represent the SCI itself. Four cases of meningitis, three cases of abscesses, and two cases of epilepsy were documented. The exact nature of the remaining 49 cases was unspecified.

Interestingly, most of these deaths occur among persons with high-level tetraplegia during the first postinjury year. In fact, although the overall SMR is 5.9, the SMR for persons with high-level tetraplegia is 30.0, and the SMR for the first postinjury year is 22.0. Given the unspecified nature of most of these reported deaths, there may be some overestimation of deaths in this category due to potentially inappropriate use of these nonspecific central nervous system codes in cases when either the exact cause of death is unknown or the death occurs very shortly after injury and is attributed to the injury itself. Autopsies were performed on only 30% of cases for which diseases of the nervous system were the underlying cause.

Another indicator of the relatively poor quality of information contained on many death certificates is the exceptionally high rate of reported deaths due to symptoms and ill-defined conditions. Overall, symptoms and ill-defined conditions were listed as the underlying cause of death in 7.3% of cases and as a secondary contributing cause in an additional 8.0% of cases. The SMR for symptoms and ill-defined conditions was 13.8; however, once again, most of these deaths occur during the first postinjury year (SMR = 43.1) and among persons with high-level tetraplegia (SMR = 62.9). Most of these cases are coded in the respiratory arrest (ICD9CM code = 799.1) subcategory of "other ill-defined and unknown causes of morbidity and mortality." Therefore, many of these cases might be more appropriately classified in the "other respiratory disease" category described previously. If so, this would substantially increase the percentage of total deaths due to diseases of the respiratory system.

Finally, there were 44 deaths for which the underlying cause was "none of the above" (3.1% of all deaths of known cause). In addition, 70 other cases had residual secondary causes of death (5.0%). The most frequent residual cause of death was infectious diseases (n = 20), followed by diabetes mellitus (n = 15), nutritional deficiencies (n = 12), unspecified diseases of the circulatory system (n = 12), acquired immune deficiency syndrome (n = 8), hyperosmolality (n = 7), hypertension (n = 6), osteomyelitis (n = 5), coagulation defects (n = 5), and assorted others (n = 24). Because these causes were listed slightly more frequently than expected as the underlying cause of death (SMR = 1.9), it appears that many of these deaths were probably related to SCI.

Cause of Death Data Limitations and Biases

Cause of death information was unavailable for 198 persons (12.4% of deaths). These are often persons who are not actively followed by the Model System but who instead either return to the care of their local community physician or receive little or no care. Frequently, these deaths are identified only through Social Security Administration records that provide dates and locations of death but not causes.

Acquisition of death certificates is often unrevealing. Unfortunately, attributing cause of death on death certificates simply to SCI or the original event that caused the injury without identifying the secondary complications that actually caused death is relatively common, even when the individual has survived several years after the injury. As a result, the percentage of deaths due to unknown causes is relatively high. Moreover, as in the general population, autopsies are not always performed on persons with SCI, even when cause of death is uncertain. In fact, only 38% of the causes of death appearing in Tables 14–5 through 14–9 were confirmed by autopsy.

Because the person-years that these individuals with unknown causes of death survived until the time of their deaths were included in the calculation of expected deaths, the cause-specific SMRs are slightly underestimated. In general, the higher the SMR, the greater the underestimation due to unknown causes is likely to be. Therefore, the greatest impact would probably be on the SMR for septicemia. For example, if the 198 deaths of unknown cause were allocated in accordance with the distribution of known causes of death, then 17 additional deaths would be expected to have resulted from septicemia, thereby bringing the total number of actual deaths to 139 and raising its overall SMR from 64.2 to 73.2. However, adding an anticipated 10 cancer deaths from the 198 deaths of unknown cause would only change the cancer SMR from 0.9 to 1.0.

The SMR will also be underestimated to a somewhat greater degree in the strata that have higher percentages of unknown causes of death. For example, only 5.9% of deaths during the first postinjury year resulted from unknown causes, whereas 18.9% of deaths occurring more than 5 years after injury had unknown causes.

CONCLUSION

In comparing these results with our previous studies of 7- and 12-year survival, it is clear that mortality rates have continued to decline and that corresponding life expectancies have increased.[14,15,43,44] In fact, the sequential results of these studies confirm the improvement in survival rates reflected in Table 14–4. Interestingly, this appears to have occurred largely due to a decline in the overall SMR for septicemia from 140.7 in our first study to 82.2 in our second study and 64.2 currently.[32,33] For persons in the youngest age group (defined originally as less than or equal to age 25), the SMR for septicemia has declined from 500 in our first study to 388.9 in our second study and 140 currently.[32,33] Nonetheless, the SMR for septicemia remains higher than that of any other cause of death in this population. Overall SMR values for other causes are relatively consistent with the results of our 12-year study, except for a slight increase in unspecified external causes of death.[33]

Because life expectancy is affected more by deaths occurring early after SCI rather than later, the causes of death that appear to have the greatest impact on reduced life expectancy for this population are pneumonia, pulmonary emboli, and septicemia (Table 14–9). With the development of improved methods of prevention and management of these three secondary complications, life expectancies should continue to improve.

The dramatic reduction in mortality due to diseases of the urinary tract clearly demonstrates the value of clinical emphasis and research in the prevention of secondary complications and deaths. The respiratory system has not received the attention that the urinary tract has received over the past years. Therefore, although other types of potentially fatal secondary medical complications that continue to occur among persons with SCI cannot be ignored, these data strongly suggest that increased clinical attention, research, and dissemination activities should be focused on the respiratory system in much the same way they have been focused on the urinary tract.

REFERENCES

1. Poer DH. Newer concepts in the treatment of paralyzed patients due to war-time injuries of the spinal cord. *Ann Surg.* 1946;123:510–516.

2. Burke MH, Hicks AF, Robbins M, Kessler H. Survival of patients with injuries to the spinal cord. *JAMA.* 1960;172:121–124.

3. Freed MM, Bakst HJ, Barrie DL. Life expectancy, survival rates, and causes of death in civilian patients with spinal cord trauma. *Arch Phys Med Rehabil.* 1966;47:457–463.

4. Geisler WO, Jousse AT, Wynne-Jones M. Survival in traumatic transverse myelitis. *Paraplegia.* 1977;14:262–275.

5. Geisler WO, Jousse AT, Wynne-Jones M, Breithaupt D. Survival in traumatic spinal cord injury. *Paraplegia.* 1983;21:364–373.

6. Mesard L, Carmody A, Mannarino E, Ruge D. Survival after spinal cord trauma. *Arch Neurol.* 1978;35:78–83.

7. Hackler RH. A 25 year prospective mortality study in the spinal cord injured patient: Comparison with the long-term living paraplegic. *J Urol.* 1977;117:486–488.

8. Frisbie JH, Kache A. Increasing survival and changing causes of death in myelopathy patients. *J Am Paraplegia Soc.* 1983;6:51–56.

9. Carter RE. Experiences with high tetraplegics. *Paraplegia.* 1979;17:140–146.

10. Hardy AG. Survival periods in traumatic tetraplegia. *Paraplegia.* 1976;14:41–46.

11. Ravichandran G, Silver JR. Survival following traumatic tetraplegia. *Paraplegia.* 1982;20:264–269.

12. Kraus JF, Franti CE, Borhani NO, Riggins RS. Survival with an acute spinal cord injury. *J Chronic Dis.* 1979;32:269-283.

13. Whiteneck GG, Charlifue SW, Frankel HL, et al. Mortality, morbidity, and psychosocial outcomes of persons spinal cord injured more than 20 years ago. *Paraplegia.* 1992;30:617–630.

14. DeVivo MJ, Kartus PL, Stover SL, Rutt RD, Fine PR. Seven-year survival following spinal cord injury. *Arch Neurol.* 1987;44:872–875.

15. DeVivo MJ, Stover SL, Black KJ. Prognostic factors for 12-year survival after spinal cord injury. *Arch Phys Med Rehabil.* 1992;73:156–162.

16. Samsa GP, Patrick CH, Feussner JR. Long-term survival of veterans with traumatic spinal cord injury. *Arch Neurol.* 1993;50:909–914.

17. Minaire P, Demolin P, Bourret J, et al. Life expectancy following spinal cord injury: A ten-year survey in the Rhone-Alpes region, France, 1969–1980. *Paraplegia.* 1983;21:11–15.

18. Griffin MR, O'Fallon WM, Opitz JL, Kurland LT. Mortality, survival and prevalence: Traumatic spinal cord injury in Olmsted County, Minnesota, 1935–1981. *J Chronic Dis.* 1985;38: 643–653.

19. Burney RE, Maio RF, Maynard F, Karunas R. Incidence, characteristics and outcome of spinal cord injury at trauma centers in North America. *Arch Surg.* 1993;128:596–599.

20. Daverat P, Gagnon M, Dartigues JF, Mazaux JM, Barat M. Initial factors predicting survival in patients with a spinal cord injury. *J Neurol Neurosurg Psychiatry.* 1989;52:403–406.

21. Webb DR, Fitzpatrick JM, O'Flynn JD. A 15-year follow-up of 406 consecutive spinal cord injuries. *Br J Urol.* 1984;56:614–617.

22. Kiwerski J, Weiss M, Chrostowska T. Analysis of mortality of patients after cervical spine trauma. *Paraplegia.* 1981;19:347–351.

23. Sneddon DG, Bedbrook G. Survival following traumatic tetraplegia. *Paraplegia.* 1982;20:201–207.

24. Le CT, Price M. Survival from spinal cord injury. *J Chronic Dis.* 1982;35:487–492.

25. Kraus JS, Crewe NM. Prediction of long-term survival of persons with spinal cord injury: An 11-year prospective study. *Rehabil Psychol.* 1987;32:205–213.

26. Kraus JS, Kjorsvig JM. Mortality after spinal cord injury: A four-year prospective study. *Arch Phys Med Rehabil.* 1992;73:558–563.

27. Barber KE, Cross RR Jr. The urinary tract as a cause of death in paraplegia. *J Urol.* 1952;67:494–502.

28. Bunts RC. Preservation of renal function in the paraplegic. *J Urol.* 1959;81:720–727.

29. Dietrick RB, Russi S. Tabulation and review of autopsy findings in fifty five paraplegics. *JAMA.* 1958;166:41–44.

30. Nyquist RH, Bors E. Mortality and survival in traumatic myelopathy during nineteen years, from 1946 to 1965. *Paraplegia.* 1967;5:22–48.

31. Tribe CR. Causes of death in the early and late stages of paraplegia. *Paraplegia.* 1963;1: 19–47.

32. DeVivo MJ, Kartus PL, Stover SL, Rutt RD, Fine PR. Cause of death for patients with spinal cord injuries. *Arch Intern Med.* 1989;149:1761–1766.

33. DeVivo MJ, Black KJ, Stover SL. Causes of death during the first 12 years after spinal cord injury. *Arch Phys Med Rehabil.* 1993;74:248–254.

34. Ducharme SH, Freed MM, Oates C, Ramos MU. The role of self-destruction in spinal cord injury mortality. *Model Systems' SCI Digest.* 1981;2(4):29–38.

35. Charlifue SW, Gerhart KA. Behavioral and demographic predictors of suicide after traumatic spinal cord injury. *Arch Phys Med Rehabil.* 1991;72:488–492.

36. DeVivo MJ, Black KJ, Richards JS, Stover SL. Suicide following spinal cord injury. *Paraplegia.* 1991;29:620–627.

37. Cutler SJ, Ederer F. Maximum utilization of the life table method in analyzing survival. *J Chronic Dis.* 1958;8:699–712.

38. Lilienfeld AM, Lilienfeld DE. *Foundations of Epidemiology.* New York: Oxford University Press; 1980.

39. *Vital Statistics of the United States, 1982.* Vol. 2: *Mortality.* Hyattsville, Md: National Center for Health Statistics; 1986.

40. Frankel HL, Hancock DO, Hyslop G, et al. The value of postural reduction in the initial management of closed injuries to the spine with paraplegia and tetraplegia. *Paraplegia.* 1969;7: 179–192.

41. Smart CN, Sanders CR. The costs of motor vehicle related SCI. Washington, DC: Insurance Institute for Highway Safety; 1976.

42. *Vital Statistics of the United States, 1988.* Vol. 2: *Mortality.* Hyattsville, Md: National Center for Health Statistics; 1992.

43. Stover SL, Fine PR, eds. *Spinal Cord Injury: The Facts and Figures.* Birmingham, Ala: University of Alabama at Birmingham; 1986.

44. Stover SL, Fine PR. The epidemiology and economics of spinal cord injury. *Paraplegia.* 1987;25:225–228.

45. Cox DR. Regression models and life tables. *J R Stat Soc.* 1972;34(B):187–220.

46. Montgomerie JZ, Chan E, Gilmore DS, Canawati HN, Sapico FL. Low mortality among patients with spinal cord injury and bacteremia. *Rev Infect Dis.* 1991;13:867–871.

47. Carter RE. Experience with ventilator dependent patients. *Paraplegia.* 1993;31:150–153.

15

System Benefits

Samuel L. Stover, Karyl M. Hall, Joel A. DeLisa,
and William H. Donovan

NATIONAL INTEREST AND DEVELOPMENT OF THE MODEL SYSTEMS PROGRAM

An important benefit of the Model SCI Systems has been the stimulation of national interest in the care and well-being of persons with SCI. Through the efforts of Dr. John S. Young, Dr. J. Paul Thomas, Dr. James F. Garrett, and others, the federal government funded the first Model System in 1970. This unique and exciting concept was expanded to include seven additional Model Systems in 1972 and 1973.[1] In an effort to improve communication, education, and research, the directors of the initial Model Systems and other interested persons met on several occasions and eventually formally organized the American Spinal Injury Association (ASIA) in 1975. Presentations by professionals from these Model Systems at the ASIA annual scientific meetings and other national conferences provided visibility and further stimulated interest in the subject of SCI. The Model Systems established both short- and long-term training programs for professionals, as well as other educational materials (see Appendix B). The establishment of the National Spinal Cord Injury Data Research Center (NSCIDRC) in Phoenix, Arizona, in 1975 was a milestone in an effort to collect uniform data.[2] The Model Systems' initial success led to federal funding of as many as 17 Model Systems during 1984 and 1985. The Model Systems program became the catalyst for the development of other well-organized SCI centers throughout the United States, which in turn also provided improved care by teams of professionals knowledgeable in SCI. Those who have experienced the last two or three decades of SCI care recognize the dramatic advances in the care of persons with SCI as a result of the federal initiatives and the Model Systems concept.

RESEARCH ACTIVITIES

Funding of the Model Systems and data collection activities also sparked an interest in research initially targeted toward reducing complications and improving care. This movement then stimulated interest in learning more about the basic science of spinal cord physiology and injury. Efforts to understand spinal cord neuroregeneration and learn more about prevention of spinal cord neural damage immediately after injury were included. Consumer groups began to advocate for additional dollars for research through private organizations and the National Institutes of Health, which then also became sponsors of research in both acute management of SCI and nerve regeneration. The Centers for Disease Control selected SCI as the first surveillance effort in its Injury Control Program. Meanwhile, the Model Systems were active in a wide range of research. The Model Systems have now published about 1000 articles in peer-reviewed journals with topics ranging from basic science to costs and outcome.[3]

CLINICAL BENEFITS

A gradual decline in the percentage of complete injuries with a corresponding increase in incomplete injuries suggests that improvements in emergency medical services and acute care are resulting in more sparing of neurologic function. Incomplete injuries increased from 44.3% between 1973 and 1977 to as high as 56.7% between 1987 and 1989 (see Figure 3–11). This proportional increase in the number of persons with incomplete injuries is one of the benefits of increased awareness of a possible SCI at the injury site by emergency medical personnel. Greater recognition of a possible SCI by such personnel allows for improved emergency medical services at the scene of the accident and for proper immobilization and handling of these patients until they are stabilized in the acute care facility. Any preservation of neurologic function below the level of SCI can improve the prognosis for additional neurologic recovery.

One of the benefits of an organized system of care should be the reduction of secondary medical complications. For all secondary complications, the benefits of early admission are often underestimated. The occurrence of medical complications in the delayed-admission group are not as well documented as are those for persons who are admitted to the Model Systems within 24 hours. For this reason, comparisons of most of the secondary complications of early versus delayed admissions were not considered reliable unless the complication was still evident at the time of delayed admission to the Model System.

As presented in Chapter 6, persons admitted to a Model System within 24 hours had significantly fewer pressure ulcers during the initial hospitalization, compared with persons who had delayed admissions. The severity of the ulcers was also less. In a previous study it was shown that early admission to one of the Model Systems helped to prevent the development of grade II or greater pressure ulcers, which developed during acute care.[4] This difference was statistically significant for persons with complete and incomplete tetraplegia, as well as complete paraplegia. Over the years there has also been a downward trend in the proportion of early-admission patients who develop pressure ulcers, indicating improved care and greater success in prevention. In Chapter 8, there is also evidence that joint contractures that restrict function occur significantly less frequently in persons admitted within 24 hours (3.7%) than in persons who are admitted between 2 and 60 days after injury (5.4%).

Reduced Length of Hospitalization and Hospital Charges

The initial mean length of hospital stay has decreased considerably since the Model System Program was started. For all patients, the length of hospital stay decreased from 144.8 days during the period 1973–1977 to 77.5 days during the period 1989–1992. To look at this trend more carefully, a uniform sample of patients who were admitted to the Model Systems within 24 hours of injury was studied so that almost all costs were accrued within Model System facilities. The total length of initial hospital stay decreased from 147 to 82 days over the same time period, a 55.8% decrease. The length of stay in the acute care hospital decreased from 25.1 days to 19 days and the length of stay in the rehabilitation hospital decreased from 122 days to 63 days. This most likely reflects improved efficiency of both acute care and rehabilitation service delivery.

Comparison of data from the Uniform Data System of Medical Rehabilitation with one of the Model Systems (University of Alabama at Birmingham) for traumatic SCI revealed that the length of initial rehabilitation hospital stay for the Model System was only 52.7% of that for the nation in 1991 and 60.0% in 1992.[5]

Prevention of complications is also important in decreasing the length of hospital stay. A decrease in medical complications and hospital length of stay would suggest that the patient was in better medical condition at discharge and better prepared to return to the community and society. Recent additional factors that may influence length of stay include third-party coverage allowed per hospital stay and various other limits imposed by managed care. The decline in hospital length of stay, however, started long before some of these factors were an issue.

If length of hospital stay had remained as long in 1991 as it was in 1974, the average charges would have increased by 118% above the overall health care inflation rate. In constant 1992 dollars, average Model System hospital charges actually rose approximately 22% from 1974 to 1991 (Figure 15–1). A relative

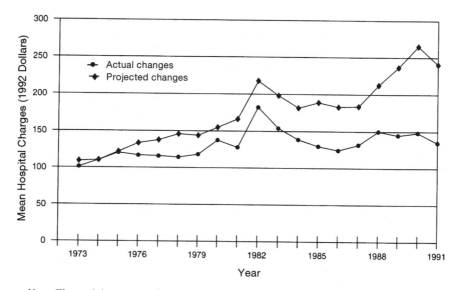

Note: The peak in average charges that occurred during 1982 and 1983 is a statistical artifact resulting in large part from a hiatus in data collection during the transition from the National SCI Data Research Center to the National SCI Statistical Center in which one Model System enrolled into the Database only persons with high-level tetraplegia who were participating in a special collaborative study.

Figure 15–1 Mean Projected and Actual Hospital Charges by Year of Injury, Based on Annual Charge per Day Estimates and 1974 Length of Hospital Stay.

decrease in the initial hospital-billed charges for SCI illustrates cost-effectiveness benefits of the Model Systems approach. Despite the marked increase in hospital care costs over the past two decades, the decreased length of hospital stay in the acute hospital and rehabilitation facility have partially compensated for the rise in daily charges. If one looks only at patients admitted within 24 hours, the average hospital charges for acute care and rehabilitation increased from $110,240 in 1974 to $134,653 in 1991 (adjusted for inflation to 1992 dollars, using the medical care component of the Consumer Price Index). This increase occurred in spite of the decrease in the mean hospital length of stay from 147 days to only 82 days over that same period.

The costs of hospitalization are responsible for approximately 80% of the total cost during the early phase after SCI.[2] Service intensity required for persons with SCI at the Model Systems has increased. The percentage of persons requiring ventilator assistance increased from 13.7% to 25.2% from 1974 to 1991. The fact that average charges increased by only 22% more than the overall health care inflation rate while ventilator usage nearly doubled can be attributed to the improved treatment efficiency of Model Systems that resulted in the substantial reduction in length of stay noted previously.

A comparison of charges was made between persons admitted to a federally designated Model System within 24 hours of injury with persons having delayed admissions to a Model System that included all charges from the referring acute care hospital. After controlling for neurologic category, year of injury, and specific Model System where care was received, there was an average savings associated with early Model System admission of $4998 (in 1992 dollars) per person. If that amount of money could be saved on a conservatively estimated 8000 new SCI persons annually, then savings would be approximately $40 million per year.

Increased Efficiency of Functional Independence Gain per Day

The Functional Index Measure (FIM) has become an accepted instrument to measure functional gains during rehabilitation. Persons admitted to one of the Model Systems (University of Alabama at Birmingham) had lower admission (FIM) scores in 1991, 54.3, compared with the nation, 63.0, reported by the Uniform Data System for Medical Rehabilitation.[5] The range of possible FIM scores is 18 (lowest function) to 126 (completely independent function). At the time of hospital discharge, the FIM scores were still somewhat lower for the Model System, 79.4, compared with the nation, 91.2. Similar figures were reported during 1992.[5] Even though the FIM change during rehabilitation was slightly less and still lower at the time of initial hospital discharge, the reduced length of stay allowed a much greater efficiency of FIM gain per day of hospitalization compared with the nation.[5] In an independent study, Heinemann et al.,[6] using the modified Barthel Index, showed that the daily rate of functional gains was significantly greater for persons with SCI admitted early to their Model System.

Increased Discharge to Home and Community

Data provided in Chapter 10 show that only 4.0% of persons were discharged from Model Systems to nursing homes or custodial care facilities. This has remained relatively constant over the past years. Certainly, one of the benefits of an organized system of care should include the ability of persons with SCI to return to their homes and communities. In the Model Systems, 92.3% are actually initially discharged to private residences in the community. These data compare favorably with data reported by the Uniform Data System in which the percentage of persons with traumatic SCI having community discharges averaged 82% during 1990–1992.[5] Community discharge in the Uniform Data System is defined as including living arrangements in the home, board and care, and transitional living. The Model Systems 92.3% includes discharges only to private residences. Additionally, since the Uniform Data System's figures include several of the Model Systems, the greater percentage of discharges to the community by the Model Systems would also tend to improve the data from the Uniform Data System. The difference would be even greater if the Model Systems were excluded.

Gibson compared the ratio of community to long-term care facilities from three different studies.[7] The community/long-term care ratio for the Model Systems in a subset analysis during 1988–1989 was 34.0:1. In a study of rehabilitation centers by the Rand Corporation[8] in 1984 the ratio was 4.7:1, and in data from the Uniform Data Systems during 1988–1989 the ratio was 22.3:1. Although the population studied may not be completely comparable, the studies tend to document the benefit of a well-organized system of care in discharge planning and outcome.

Decreased Rehospitalization

Chapter 12 provides data to show that the frequency of rehospitalizations has declined significantly since the beginning of the Model Systems program. This would also suggest that the number of severe secondary complications has decreased over the years. From 1973 to 1975, the average days for all patients rehospitalized was 11.7, which has decreased to 4.4 days between 1986 and 1989. The number of average rehospitalizations each year per person was 0.61 from 1973 to 1975, compared with 0.31 from 1986 to 1989. There has also been a 4.5-day decrease in the length of hospitalization over the same time periods, most recently being 14.2 average days per rehospitalization. The decreased number and length of rehospitalizations may to some extent be consistent with changing reimbursement practices; however, it is also likely the result of improved follow-up programs and improved care that reduce the incidence of postdischarge medical complications.

Improving Survival Rates

Chapter 14 provides evidence of improving survival rates. The mortality rate was reduced by 42% for persons injured between 1989 and 1992 relative to persons injured between 1973 and 1975. One of the primary reasons for this decline in mortality rates appears to be the decrease in the risk of septicemia.[9,10]

This also suggests that improved long-term follow-up helps to prevent secondary complications and to treat them more appropriately if they occur. There is also evidence that persons who are admitted early to a Model System have improved survival rates compared with persons treated at non-System hospitals.[4]

Referral Patterns

With conservative estimates, Gibson reported that the Model Systems "capture" approximately 15% of all new cases of SCI in the United States.[7] The estimated capture rate of the referral networks ranged from 67% to 74% within the individual Model System catchment areas, suggesting that the Model Systems are recognized for their high quality of care.

Increased Health Professional Interest

Increased interest by a whole team of health professionals in improving the care of persons with SCI, along with adequate support and follow-up systems developed by the Model Systems, is also an extremely important benefit. As reported in Chapter 10, the neurologic impairment is not nearly as important as the "quality of rehabilitation, the social support system, and possibly the personality and mind-set of persons with spinal cord injury themselves that determine coping and ultimately satisfaction with life after injury" [11–13] Persons with inadequate acute care, rehabilitation, community integration, and follow-up and who have recurring complications cannot be expected to achieve readily a personally acceptable level of function in society.

Since a vast majority of SCI persons discharged from the Model Systems live at home rather than in institutions, access to community health care resources is very important. Continuing long-term follow-up of patients admitted to the Model Systems includes not only regular re-evaluation in the clinic, but also other follow-up services that are of value to persons with SCI.

Health Promotion and Education

An important service is health promotion. It remains trite but true to say that participation in exercise, education, or vocational training programs or even an occupation requires good health. Fitness programs that have become popular with the able-bodied population should also be available for the disabled. Similarly, education plays an important role in health promotion for the person with SCI. Information on health promotion is routinely provided during the initial rehabilitation at an SCI center but might not have been fully remembered. The opportunity to hear this material again, as well as new information since the patient was discharged, is available on a recurring basis through Model Systems direction or sponsorship. This information is disseminated in the form of conferences for consumers, as well as books, educational films, and pamphlets (see Appendix B).

Peer counselor programs are also available in many of the Model Systems to encourage persons in coping with SCI. It has often been said that individuals with SCI learn as much from each other as they do from professionals.

Regular Follow-Up, Early Illness Intervention, and Prevention of Complications

The primary SCI physician who cares for the patient during the initial hospitalization provides and directs ongoing care, periodic examinations, laboratory tests, and other evaluations as needed. Periodic examinations are important to determine the health status of a population that is vulnerable to certain medical complications, some of which can begin occultly, and to assess compliance with prescribed treatment. Compliance has been shown to be problematic for many persons with SCI for various reasons. Not surprisingly, in one survey, 30% of SCI persons were found to be noncompliant with regard to taking prescribed medications.[14] Patients over the age of 60 are particularly vulnerable to medical complications requiring rehospitalization and nursing home placement.[15]

Certain specialist consultations may also be needed at this time, and appropriate referrals are important in providing efficient care. In addition, an annual evaluation of equipment, particularly wheelchair(s), adaptive equipment, and pressure relief devices, is necessary. Assessment of psychosocial problems and vocational goals is also required to determine whether changes caused by age, living conditions, or family relationships require professional help.

The complications referred to in earlier chapters must be treated if they develop despite one's best efforts to prevent them. Even though there has been a significant reduction in urinary tract complications in general, and as a cause of death in recent years, one survey revealed that 44% of patients on intermittent catheterization were hospitalized at least once in a 5-year period for urologic complications.[16] This study helped to illustrate the importance of having knowledgeable medical professionals who are accessible to the SCI population and are familiar with their unique problems. Complications related to the aging process, whether one is disabled or not, such as degenerative arthritis of the cervical spine or joints of the upper extremities, are common in the SCI population and only add to their existing disability.[17]

People often do not achieve all of their functional expectations during their first hospitalization, either because of the constraining effects of external immobilizing devices or other limitations. The Model System enables them to improve through further training and education on either an inpatient or outpatient basis. Assessment of psychosocial problems and vocational goals is also required to determine whether changes caused by age, living conditions, or family relationships would benefit from professional assistance. As the person's equipment wears out, the Model System provides ongoing prescriptions for replacement of wheelchairs, cushions, bathroom equipment, and devices intended to improve performance in activities of daily living. The Model System provides training to compensate for declining functions and endurance as a result of the aging process, intervening illnesses, or complications.

Persons with disabilities certainly are more likely to encounter more obstacles and stresses than the average able-bodied person. The Model System provides not only the training and equipment to overcome the physical barriers and challenges but also the psychologic strategies to confront stresses appropriately.

REFERENCES

1. Thomas JP. Definition of the model system of spinal cord injury care. In: Apple DF, Hudson LM, eds. *Spinal Cord Injury: The Model*. Atlanta: Georgia Regional Spinal Cord Injury Care System, Shepherd Center for Treatment of Spinal Injuries, Inc; 1990;7–9.

2. Young JS, Burns PE, Bowen AM, McCutchen R. *Spinal Cord Injury Statistics: Experience of Regional Model Spinal Cord Injury Systems*. Phoenix, Ariz: Good Samaritan Medical Center; 1982.

3. Ditunno JF, Stover SL, Donovan WH, Waters RL, Sniezek JE. Research and training benefits of the model system. In: Apple DF, Hudson LM, eds. *Spinal Cord Injury: The Model*. Atlanta: Georgia Regional Spinal Cord Injury Care System, Shepherd Center for Treatment of Spinal Injuries, Inc; 1990;85–105.

4. DeVivo MJ, Kartus PL, Stover SL, Fine PR. Benefits of early admission to an organized spinal cord injury care system. *Paraplegia*. 1990;28:545–555.

5. Granger CV, Hamilton BB. The uniform data system for medical rehabilitation report of first admissions for 1992. *Am J Phys Med Rehabil*. 1994;73:51–55.

6. Heinemann AW, Yarkony GM, Roth EJ, et al. Functional outcome following spinal cord injury: A comparison of specialized spinal cord injury center vs. general hospital short-term care. *Arch Neurol*. 1989;46:1098–1102.

7. Gibson CJ. Criteria for evaluating performance of the system. In: Apple DF, Hudson LM, eds. *Spinal Cord Injury: The Model*. Atlanta: Georgia Regional Spinal Cord Injury Care System, Shepherd Center for Treatment of Spinal Injuries, Inc; 1990;45–48.

8. Hosek S, Kane R, Carney M. *Charges and Outcomes for Rehabilitative Care*. Santa Monica, Calif: Rand Corporation; 1986.

9. DeVivo MJ, Kartus PL, Stover SL, Rutt RD, Fine PR. Cause of death for patients with spinal cord injuries. *Arch Intern Med*. 1989;149:1761–1766.

10. DeVivo MJ, Black KJ, Stover SL. Causes of death during the first 12 years after spinal cord injury. *Arch Phys Med Rehabil*. 1993;74:248–254.

11. Cushman LA, Hassett J. Spinal cord injury: 10 and 15 years after. *Paraplegia.* 1992;30: 690–696.

12. Lundquist C, Siosteen A, Blomstrand C, Lind B, Sullivan M. Spinal cord injuries: Clinical functional and emotional status. *Spine.* 1991;16:78–83.

13. MacDonald MR, Nielson WR, Cameron MGP. Depression and activity patterns of spinal cord injured persons living in the community. *Arch Phys Med Rehabil.* 1987;68:339–343.

14. Harrison C, Kurick J. Community reintegration of SCI persons: Problems and perceptions. *SCI Nursing.* 1989;6(3):44–47.

15. DeVivo MJ, Kartus PL, Rutt RD, Stover SL, Fine PR. The influence of age at time of spinal cord injury on rehabilitation outcome. *Arch Neurol.* 1990;47:687–691.

16. Maynard FM, Glass J. Management of the neuropathic bladder by clean intermittent catheterization: 5 year outcomes. *Paraplegia.* 1987;25(2):106–110.

17. Sie I, Waters RL, Adkins R. Upper extremity disability due to lower extremity paralysis in paraplegia. *Curr Orthop.* 1991;5(2).

Implications for the Future

Theodore M. Cole

Systematic generation of patient-based research data separates the investigator from the clinician. Analysis of the data identifies the scientist within. Research dissemination is the hallmark of the educator. Well-argued data are the tools that help the clinician to improve treatment strategies for persons with spinal cord injury. Together they close the circle at the point where it began—the patient.

This volume points the way to future development of the system of care that was begun 24 years ago in Phoenix, Arizona, and is now presented here for careful scrutiny. The reports herein demonstrate the accomplishments of over 20 years of multicenter data collection. They set the expectation that much more can be learned from the researchers, the data, and especially the persons with spinal cord injury (SCI) who participated in and responded to the Model System of care.

All of these accomplishments are prologue to the contributions that the Model SCI Systems can offer in the future. The major priorities that research can address will focus on consumers or constituents who represent the multicultural diversity of America's citizens. They will gain from the widest possible dissemination of research results that the several projects and this publication can reach. They will gain the most when primary prevention strategies finally reduce the frequency of this often-devastating disability.

IMPLICATION 1: CONTINUE TO USE AND REFINE THE SCI DATABASE

The model projects will continue to evaluate the system of care during a time of change in health care. The information they generate is the result of careful work by hundreds of clinicians and scientists. The original dataset has undergone continual refinement, refocusing, and abridging in order to concentrate on the most important and reliable data that the researchers could collect. The epidemiologic and clinical nature of the information will help to discover and promote optimum care. The trail from the past and through the present leads into the future precisely at the time when it is essential that we see clearly. The world of SCI care is now fully engaged with the disciplines of acute medicine and surgery.

Although the health care team is not the product of the SCI Model Systems, it nonetheless was greatly benefited by them. At more than 20 SCI centers in many regions of the United States, SCI specialists and researchers collaborated effectively, within and between institutions and professions. This was no small accomplishment during a time when medicine and health care were more characterized by fragmentation than by coordinated efforts.

What we learn together will help us understand strategies of care provision and payment in order to allocate expensive resources prudently and effectively. Future data can be compared with past data so that we can understand causal relationships of health care changes. Therefore, an immediate implication for the future is the preservation of the lineage of SCI research data and their continued refinement for clinicians and policymakers alike.

IMPLICATION 2: DISSEMINATE RESEARCH INFORMATION

More than 1000 publications in medical and related professional journals have stemmed from the SCI research that this project spawned over the last 20 years. In 1989 a consensus conference was held in Washington, DC, to showcase new information that the project had produced.[1] At that time 500 publications had appeared in peer-reviewed journals.

Equally important has been the corollary benefit of interaction between medical and scientific workers in the field. This interaction has led to personal exchanges that cannot be duplicated through journals and books. Arguably, the American Spinal Injury Association (ASIA) would not have come to such quick or bright success had it not been for the SCI Model System. Through members of ASIA who belonged to other organizations, the Model Systems in the United States have gained acclaim among policymakers, professionals, and persons with tetraplegia or paraplegia themselves. Through exchanges at scientific meetings, we have learned that clinical correlates such as heterotopic ossification and contracture, discharge location and treatment choices, and etiology and socioeconomic variables assist us to provide better care and prevent complications. They have helped shift the outcomes from early death due to renal failure to the expectation that a person can live to an age when cancer, heart disease, and degenerative diseases account for more of the documented outcomes. Now we can show that 92.3% of persons with SCI will reside in private residences after discharge. Research dissemination is a major accomplishment of the SCI Model System.[2] (See also Appendix B for a listing of publications and other educational materials.)

IMPLICATION 3: APPLY RESEARCH INFORMATION TO CLINICAL SETTINGS

Research results are now being applied in clinical settings across the land. However, the bulk of persons with SCI still receive part or all of their care outside of a truly coordinated system or one that utilizes the breadth and depth of knowledge gained from the Model Systems SCI Project. Therefore, it is imperative that further application of research results be applied to the clinical settings. An example is the use of prophylactic techniques to prevent worsening of an acute neurologic injury immediately after onset. The large number of subjects created by the collaborative projects elevates heretofore anecdotal observations to the level of statistical significance. An example is the incidence of post-traumatic myelopathy.

New predictive models allow us to anticipate the person who is less likely to return to work and, therefore, to offer timely interventions. Other models predict the person likely to develop pressure ulcers. They allow us to take preventive steps. We can now reduce hospital length of stay through better teamwork at the bedside. In fact, models of organization and structure have been transferred from the SCI projects to colleagues in the fields of traumatic brain injury, burns, and trauma.[3,4] These colleagues have replicated the SCI model of care and shown its transferability. Now others are considering the same approach in the treatment of cancer and pulmonary and chronic diseases.[5]

IMPLICATION 4: FORMULATE NEW RESEARCH HYPOTHESES

We have answered the original research question by demonstrating that a system of care from emergency detection and evacuation to lifelong follow-up has advantages not only to persons with SCI but also to those who pay the bill, those who formulate policy, and those who provide care. All have gained enormously. New hypotheses are being formed that can be studied with the rich database of information we are collecting from individuals and groups. For example, we are determining the ways in which the normal aging process in persons with SCI can be modified in order to prolong survival and enhance quality of life. We must identify those gender-specific characteristics of women that fundamentally alter their need for or response to treatment. We must understand how to identify and/or modify employment situations so that women as well as men in different socioeconomic segments of society can equally enjoy postinjury employment. As we plan capitated, managed, competitive health care systems, we must specify the differences in risk factors, course of injury, and treatment choices that are unique to the regional segmentation of the United States. We must study the neurophysiology of the axial nervous system so that we can find new information that helps us in the long-term treatment of spasticity patterns, different levels and severity of spinal cord lesions, and variable responses to treatment or age. We must continue to experiment with the model system of care so as to reduce further the costs of treating this classic, although relatively infrequent, disability. We must improve patient outcomes with more innovative systems of SCI care. We must change where necessary the nature of SCI care so as to reduce the mounting frequency of suicide as an outcome. We must address minority-group issues to learn more effective ways to reduce incidence and secondary complications and improve postdischarge outcomes. Throughout many of these future plans, we must learn how best to include consumers in the decision-making process.

IMPLICATION 5: SEEK FURTHER DEVELOPMENTS IN SYSTEM OF CARE

The system of care that the collaborative centers have pioneered for persons with spinal cord injury must be further developed. Changing social and medical circumstances will adversely affect some SCI outcomes, such as discharge locations and ability to participate in long-term follow-up. Earlier rehabilitation discharges will require better education programs for patients and families. Intensive outpatient care will necessitate large increases in outpatient treatment centers and a method to transport patients from home to treatment locations. Therefore, the system must respond to societal needs that are different from those that existed 24 years ago when the first collaborating centers created a new paradigm in health care. With impending health care reform, we must not assume that the costs of hospitalization are 80% of total costs during the early phase after SCI. We must gain more information about personal assistance services in order to guide future health policy that will allocate cost between acute rehabilitation and annual expenditures for attendant care.

We must further refine our understanding of community integration and personal services in order to allocate more effectively the health care dollar to benefit the SCI person. The growing network of SCI health care facilities must enhance understanding of their role in promotion and fitness, both physical and emotional, on behalf of persons with SCI. Centers must develop cost-effective educational programs for individuals and their families. We must grapple with the very difficult constructs of social evolution and spiritual maturation in order to include them in tomorrow's expectations for an improved system of care. The Model Systems must conduct the studies to help determine whether a center should be a one-stop location for all needs or should play a role in conjunction with other community providers. The centers must develop and then disseminate the expertise that will allow better primary care services to children and adults with spinal cord injuries.

IMPLICATION 6: DEVELOP AN ENVIRONMENT IN WHICH HEALTH POLICY RESEARCH QUESTIONS CAN BE STUDIED

The etiology and epidemiology of spinal cord injury continues to change over time. The Model Centers must continue to monitor these changes in order to rationalize the anticipated changes in health reform. Access to medical rehabilitation continues to stand as one of the most needed yet unmet aspects of health care. The Model Centers must study various subpopulations (e.g., older persons and persons with mental illness) to evaluate their ability to access medical rehabilitation. Outcomes and effectiveness of treatment are on everyone's mind today. The Model Centers must continue to evaluate the relationship between resource consumption and outcome. They must also evaluate the intensity of service and its impact on outcome.

We must appreciate the qualities that the patient brings to the health care setting by evaluating the patient's contribution, as well as the contribution of the rehabilitation process to the eventual outcome. We must better understand the comparative outcomes of rehabilitation delivered in various rehabilitation settings. We must evaluate the rate of medical complications associated with not only full rehabilitation but minimal or no rehabilitation at all. Within the centers, it is likely that information can be generated that will help develop practice guidelines for all professions involved in SCI service delivery.

An adequate definition of quality of life continues to elude us. However, it is most likely that from the construct of model systems will emerge an operational definition responsive to the perspective and experiences of persons with spinal cord injury. Only then will we be able to measure and evaluate it and track people from the onset of their spinal injury in all settings. America is experiencing a growing tension between those who advocate for disability rights and others who advocate for health care rationing. The Model Systems offer the best possible environment in which to test continually the validity of both sides of that issue.

Finally, as we enter into an era in which every disabled American is promised the hope embodied in the Americans with Disabilities Act, the Model Systems can contribute substantially to the medical, economic, social, recreational, educational, and employment promises of the American society of the twenty-first century.

REFERENCES

1. Apple DF, Hudson LM, eds. *Spinal Cord Injury: The Model.* Atlanta: Georgia Regional Spinal Cord Injury Care System, Shepherd Center for Treatment of Spinal Injuries, Inc; 1990.

2. Stover SL, Fine PR. *Spinal Cord Injury: The Facts and Figures.* Birmingham, Ala: University of Alabama; 1986.

3. *Federal Register,* 57:75, April 17, 1992, 14291.

4. *Federal Register*, 57:233, December 3, 1992, 57283.

5. Report of a Workshop on Pulmonary Rehabilitation Research, April 26-28. Bethesda, Md: National Institutes of Health. In press.

Appendix A

Glossary

This glossary includes only selected terms that are not readily found in other sources, or definitions of data collection variables that may differ, for data collection purposes, from those in standard medical dictionaries.

Aspiration: Aspiration of oral or gastric contents leading to pulmonary complications requiring treatment.

Associated injuries: Selected major injuries occurring at the same time as the spinal cord injury.

Amputation—Amputation that is secondary to trauma occurring at the same time as the spinal cord injury, or surgical amputation during the immediate postinjury period as a result of the initial injury, including arms, legs, fingers, toes, and hip disarticulations.

Brachial plexus injury—Injury to the brachial plexus, including upper plexus (Erb-Duchenne), defined as damage to 5th and 6th cervical roots or upper trunk; lower plexus (Klumpke), defined as damage to 8th cervical and 1st thoracic roots of lower trunk; and middle plexus, defined as damage to middle trunk.

Fracture(s) —Break of a bone including both open and closed fractures at any location.

Head injury—Documented head injury sufficient to affect cognitive and/or emotional functioning, including contusion; concussion; subarachnoid, subdural, and extradural hemorrhage; intracranial injury of other unspecified nature; and anoxic brain injury. Suspected brain injuries are documented with a separate code and are included in the analyses.

Loss of consciousness—Documented loss of consciousness of any duration.

Major burn—Third-degree burn on more than 10% of the body area.

Peripheral nerve injury—Injury to a nerve outside the spinal canal, including but not limited to radial, median, ulnar, musculocutaneous, axillary, femoral, obturator, sciatic, common peroneal, and tibial nerves.

Traumatic pneumothorax and/or hemothorax—Occurrence of air and/or fluid within the pleural space, which can be demonstrated radiographically, that requires chest tube intervention.

Atelectasis: State of airlessness within the lung, diagnosed radiographically. Radiographic diagnosis of lobar or diffuse atelectasis is taken from the recorded radiograph interpretation.

Autonomic dysreflexia: Sympathetic response to stimulation below the level of injury that requires any intervention. Response is marked by symptoms such as hypertension, sweating above the lesion level, "goose bumps," nasal stuffiness, and/or headache.

Bacteriuria: Bacteria isolated from the urine irrespective of collection method or presence of symptoms.

Cardiopulmonary arrest: Cessation of respiration and/or heartbeat requiring resuscitation but not resulting in death.

Contributing cause of death: Secondary complication that is present at the time of death and is at least partly responsible for that death.

Cumulative survival rate: Proportion of persons surviving longer than a given time period.

Deep venous thrombosis: Occlusion of the venous system of the lower extremity. Deep venous thrombosis, when diagnosed, was either confirmed by specific diagnostic procedures, such as ^{125}I labeled fibrogen uptake, impedance plethysmography (IPG), Doppler sonography or venography, etc., or was chemically identified but not confirmed by such procedures.

Department of vocational rehabilitation client status: Specifies whether the person at the specific time point considered was active on the state department of vocational rehabilitation caseload—in any of the evaluation or service categories.

Direct costs: Charges that are the direct result of the injury, incurred either by the person with spinal cord injury or his or her responsible third party regardless of the amount that is actually paid.

Discount rate: Assumed rate of return on investments over and above the rate of inflation that is used to convert future charges or losses into current dollars.

Education: Highest level of formal education that a person has completed at a specific time point, per self-report. Trade or technical schools are disregarded.

Etiology: Causes of spinal cord injury which include several categories:

Air sports—includes parachuting, parasailing

All other penetrating wounds—includes stabbing, impalement

All-terrain vehicle (ATV) and all-terrain cycle (ATC)—includes both three-wheeled and four-wheeled vehicles

Auto accident—includes jeep, truck, dune buggy, bus

Bicycle—includes tricycles and unicycles

Explosion—includes bomb, grenade, dynamite, gasoline

Fall: includes jumping, being pushed

Field sports—includes field hockey, lacrosse, soccer, rugby

Gymnastics—includes all gymnastic activities other than trampoline, break-dancing

Hit by falling/flying object—includes ditch cave-in, avalanche, rock slide

Medical/surgical complication—Impairment of spinal cord function resulting from adverse effects of medical, surgical, or diagnostic procedures and treatment for non–spinal cord conditions

Motorcycle accident—includes 2-wheeled, motorized vehicles such as mopeds, motorized dirt bikes

Other sport, unclassified—includes auto racing, glider kite, slide, swimming

Other vehicular, unclassified—includes tractor, bulldozer, go-cart, steam roller, train, road grader, forklift

Other winter sports—includes sled, snow tube, toboggan

Other unclassified—includes lightning, kick from an animal, machinery accidents (excludes falls, hits from falling/flying objects)

Personal contact—includes hits from a blunt object

Rodeo—includes bronco/bull riding

Track and field—includes pole vault, high jump, vault

Expected deaths: Number of deaths in a given population, anticipated over a given time period, based on the age, sex, and race of the population members coupled with general population mortality rates.

Frankel grade: Tool for measuring the completeness of SCI. The grade of A was applied to a complete injury; B to an injury with sparing of sensation only, without sparing of voluntary motor activity; C to an injury in which there was some preserved but nonfunctional voluntary motor activity; D to an injury with preserved functional motor activity; and E to an injury with normal motor and sensory function.

Functional index measure (FIM): An 18-item, 7-level scale of independent performance in self-care, sphincter control, transfers, locomotion, communication, and social cognition as developed by the Uniform Data System Data Management Service, State University of New York at Buffalo, Buffalo, New York.

Heterotopic ossification: Bone formation in abnormal soft tissue locations documented by radiograph or bone scan about the hip and/or knee restricting flexion to less than 90°.

Indirect costs: Forgone wages and associated fringe benefits that directly result from the spinal cord injury.

Joint contracture: Reduction in joint range of motion severe enough to have warranted or recommended specific stretching exercises.

Life expectancy: Arithmetic average (mean) remaining years of life for a group of comparable individuals.

Marital status: Self-reported marital status. "Separated" includes legal separations and living apart from one's marital partner. Common-law status is disregarded.

Median survival time: Point at which 50% of the population has died.

Motor index score: Calculated by summing the motor scores for each of the 10 pairs of key muscles. Since there are 10 such pairs, with a maximum individual score of 5, the maximum possible motor index score is 100.

Myocardial infarction: Coronary artery insufficiency producing necrosis of the myocardium, confirmed by electrocardiogram and/or enzyme changes.

Neurologic impairment category: Gross descriptor of the level and completeness of SCI, with four categories combining a description of level (tetraplegia or paraplegia) and completeness (complete or incomplete).

Neurologic level: Most caudal level with intact motor and sensory function bilaterally. All levels above the neurologic level also have intact motor and sensory function. A level can also be specified for each side, and a level can be specified separately for motor and sensory function.

Paraplegia: Impairment or loss of motor and/or sensory function in the thoracic, lumbar, or sacral (but not cervical) segments of the spinal cord, secondary to damage of neural elements within the spinal canal.

Paraplegia/tetraplegia complete/incomplete: Persons classified as "paraplegia-minimal deficit" are combined with the "paraplegia-incomplete" group. The same is true for the "tetraplegia-minimal" deficit group. Persons with "minimal deficit-level unspecified" are included in the analysis of the overall group, but are not shown separately in tabulations.

Place of residence: Place where the person is actually residing and may not be the legal residence. "Nursing home" includes various types of facilities providing custodial chronic disease care. "Hospital" includes mental hospital. "Private residence" includes house, apartment, mobile home, etc. "Other," which includes group living facilities (e.g., dormitory), correctional institution, hotel or motel, and other nonmedical residences that are not private, is combined with "private" into the category "community resident."

Pneumonia: State of lung tissue inflammation of infectious etiology with radiographic demonstration of parenchymal disease.

Pre-existing conditions: Selected major (pre-SCI) medical problems identified upon initial admission to the SCI Care System, which have the capacity to inhibit or impair the rehabilitation potential of a person with SCI.

History of ankylosing spondylitis, rheumatoid arthritis—Includes history of any of the following conditions (related to the spinal column): Strümpell-Marie spondylitis, Strümpell-Marie disease, Bekhterev's disease, pelvospondylitis ossificans, and rheumatoid spondylitis. Findings must be documented by a physician.

History of calculus of kidney or ureter—Abnormal concretion in the kidney or ureter. Calculi first identified in the bladder are not presumed to have originated elsewhere and are therefore excluded.

History of cervical spondylosis—Includes cervical spondylosis, cervical osteoarthritis, and degenerative arthritis of the cervical spinal. Documented by a physician.

History of chronic obstructive pulmonary disease (COPD)—Positive history of pulmonary emphysema, bronchial asthma, and/or chronic bronchitis.

History of diabetes mellitus—Metabolic disorder of carbohydrate metabolism requiring therapy by daily insulin and/or hypoglycemic agents. Diabetes controlled only by diet is not included.

History of degenerative joint disease—Includes any degenerative joint disease of rheumatoid arthritis in areas *exclusive* of the spine.

History of heart disease—History of any of the following conditions: acute pericarditis, acute and subacute endocarditis, acute myocarditis, other diseases of the pericardium, valvular heart disease (excluding endocarditis classified as bacterial, rheumatic, or syphilitic), cardiomyelopathy, conduction disorders, cardiac dysrhythmias, heart failure, ill-defined descriptions and complications of heart disease, angina pectoris, and other acute and sub-acute forms of ischemia.

History of hypertension—Sustained elevation of blood pressure for which treatment with antihypertensive medication was recommended, regardless of whether treatment was actually received.

History of spinal canal stenosis—Reduction of the cross-sectional area of the spinal canal caused by spondylopathy secondary to disc disease that is either congenital or acquired. It includes persons with neurologic loss secondary to acute trauma who do not have a fracture or dislocation of the spinal column but who have gross radiographic evidence of cervical or thoracic spondylopathy corresponding to the zone of injury. Must be documented by a physician.

Present value of lifetime direct costs: Dollar amount needed to be set aside today to meet the average expenses of the person with spinal cord injury that are directly related to his or her injury over his or her remaining lifetime.

Present value of lifetime indirect costs: Average value in current dollars of all future wages and fringe benefits that will be lost as a direct result of the spinal cord injury.

Pressure ulcers: Breakdown of the skin due to pressure and shear. Also called decubitus ulcers, ischemic ulcers, bed sores.

Primary occupational, educational, or training status: Activity that a person considers to be his or her *primary* activity. "Working" includes active in the competitive labor market, including the military. "Other" includes on-the-job training, sheltered workshop, medical leave, etc. Only those who state they are working are considered employed. "Unemployed" is used frequently by persons who are not looking for work. "Retired" presumably includes only those retired for age.

Pulmonary embolus: Condition resulting when a pulmonary artery becomes acutely obstructed by a clot formed upstream from the pulmonary arterial vascular tree. Pulmonary embolus, when diagnosed, is either confirmed by specific diagnostic procedures, such as ventilation-perfusion lung scan, pulmonary angiogram, or by other techniques, or clinically identified but not confirmed by such procedures.

Relative mortality ratio (RMR): Another name for the standardized mortality ratio.

Secondary cause of death: Another name for a contributing cause of death.

Spasticity: Involuntary movement or resistance to passive movement that is severe enough to have warranted a trial of medication, continuation of medication, or surgical treatment.

Sponsor of care: Third party, such as a private insurance company, Medicare, etc., that is responsible for paying all or part of the health care charges incurred by the person with a spinal cord injury.

Standardized mortality ratio: Ratio of the actual number of deaths occurring in a group of individuals in a given time period to the expected number of deaths in that same group over that same time period. The ratio is based on the age, sex, and race of the group members coupled with general population mortality rates.

Suicide: Death reported to have been caused, on purpose, by a person himself or herself.

Tetraplegia: Impairment or loss of motor and/or sensory function in the cervical segments of the spinal cord due to damage of the neural elements within the spinal cord.

Underlying cause of death: Cause that initiated the sequence of events that directly led to a person's death.

Urinary tract infection: Microbial invasion of any of the tissues of the urinary tract, as documented by a colony count of (a) 1-100,000 colonies; or (b) over 100,000 colonies.

Ventilatory failure: Necessity for partial or total ventilatory support for a period of at least seven consecutive days.

Appendix B

Publications and Educational Programs Prepared by the Model Systems

Karen A. Hart

PRESENTATIONS MADE BY PERSONNEL
FROM 13 MODEL SYSTEMS 1990–1994

Model System	1990	1991	1992	1993	Thru 6/94	Total
Georgia Regional SCI Systems	13	69	90	36	56	264
Midwest Regional SCI System	24	48	51	25	NR*	148
Mount Sinai Model SCI System	6	23	31	27	21	108
Northern California SCI System	17	14	18	24	4	77
Northern New Jersey SCI System	30	77	88	122	57	374
Northwest Regional SCI System	8	45	32	40	8	133
Regional SCI Care System of Southern California	9	17	27	18	4	75
Regional SCI Center of Delaware Valley	17	72	71	74	62	296
Rocky Mountain SCI Center	9	33	16	78	5	141
Southeastern Michigan SCI System	11	39	9	14	1	74
Texas Regional SCI System	28	97	78	80	35	318
UAB Model Regional SCI Care System	8	21	26	78	15	148
University of Michigan Model SCI Care System	3	14	24	26	6	73
Total	183	569	561	642	274	2,229

*No report.

WRITTEN AND MEDIA RESOURCES PRODUCED BY
13 MODEL SYSTEMS 1990–1994

CATEGORY I: SCI Overview

Title*	Model System	Format	Date
Compendia of SCI Educational Resources: Audio/Visual and Unpublished Written Materials	Texas Regional Model SCI System The Institute for Rehabilitation and Research, Houston	Soft-bound Book	01/01/91
From Medical Rehab thru Employment: An Update on SCI—Rehab Resource Guide	UAB Model Regional SCI System Spain Rehabilitation Center	Soft-bound Book	01/20/92
Handbook for Patients and Families	Georgia Regional SCI System Shepherd Spinal Center	Booklet	12/01/91
Information Kit for Prospective Patients	Georgia Regional SCI System Shepherd Spinal Center	Information Packet	08/01/91
Learning about Spinal Cord Injury	UAB Model Regional SCI System Spain Rehabilitation Center	Booklet	01/01/92
Let's Get Started	Regional SCI Care System of Southern California, Rancho Los Amigos Medical Center	Videotape ½"	01/01/91
Spinal Column Magazine	Georgia Regional SCI System Shepherd Spinal Center	Magazine	Quarterly
The Challenged Life: Spinal Cord Injury	Midwest Regional SCI System Rehab. Institute of Chicago	Videotape ½"	01/23/92
Information tapes on SCI topics via telephone access	Texas Regional Model SCI System The Institute for Rehabilitation and Research, Houston	Audiotapes (7)	12/31/93

---

*Some titles will repeat, since subject matter covers more than one category. These resources can be accessed by calling 713-797-5945.

CATEGORY II: Emergency Care Immediately Post-SCI

None

CATEGORY III: Acute Care of SCI

A Community Campaign for Preventing SCI & TBI— Grades 5–6	UAB Model Regional SCI System Spain Rehabilitation Center	Booklet	08/01/91
A Community Campaign for Preventing SCI & TBI— PSAs	UAB Model Regional SCI System Spain Rehabilitation Center	Public Service Announce- ment	01/01/91
A Community Campaign for Preventing SCI & TBI— Poster	UAB Model Regional SCI System Spain Rehabilitation Center	Poster	08/01/91
A Community Campaign for Preventing SCI & TBI— Preschool–Kindergarten	UAB Model Regional SCI System Spain Rehabilitation Center	Information Packet	01/01/91
A Community Campaign for Preventing SCI & TBI— Grades 1–2	UAB Model Regional SCI System Spain Rehabilitation Center	Information Packet	08/01/91
A Community Campaign for Preventing SCI & TBI— Grades 3–4	UAB Model Regional SCI System Spain Rehabilitation Center	Information Packet	08/01/91
Anatomy and Physiology of the Spinal Cord	Northern California Regional SCI System, Rehab. Nursing	Videotape ½"	11/01/91
Research Update— Concomitant Traumatic Brain Injury and Spinal Cord Injury	UAB Model Regional SCI System Spain Rehabilitation Center	Newsletter	04/01/91
The Care of the High Quadriplegic Patient	Georgia Regional SCI System Shepherd Spinal Center	Manual Workbook Slide/Sound	01/01/94

CATEGORY IV: Medical and Nursing Management and Medical Complications

Autonomic Dysreflexia	UAB Model Regional SCI System Spain Rehabilitation Center	Poster	11/01/91

Busting Loose to Independence through Personal Attendant Services	Texas Regional Model SCI System The Institute for Rehabilitation and Research, Houston	Audiotapes	12/01/90
Continence Clinic Fact Sheet	Georgia Regional SCI System Shepherd Spinal Center	Fact Sheet	11/01/91
Continence Educational/ Informational Sheet	Georgia Regional SCI System Shepherd Spinal Center	Fact Sheet	11/01/91
Critical Pathways, Part I	Northern California SCI System Santa Clara Valley Medical Center	Booklet	11/01/92
Drugs Most Frequently Used at Shepherd Spinal Center	Georgia Regional SCI System Shepherd Spinal Center	Pamphlet	01/01/91
Maintaining Healthy Skin, Part I	Northern Regional SCI System University of Washington	Pamphlet	01/01/91
Maintaining Healthy Skin, Part II	Northwest Regional SCI System University of Washington	Pamphlet	01/01/92
Medical Alert for Autonomic Dysreflexia	Northwest Regional SCI System University of Washington	Other	07/01/92
Partners in Independence: The Personal Care Attendant's Role in Pressure Sore Prevention	Texas Regional Model SCI System The Institute for Rehabilitation and Research, Houston	Videotape ½"	01/01/90
Pressure Ulcer Treatment Practice Guidelines— Pilot Site Reviewer	Regional SCI Center of Delaware Valley, Thomas Jefferson University, Philadelphia	Pamphlet	01/01/94
Research Update— Occurrence & Management of UTIs Following Spinal Cord Injury	UAB Model Regional SCI System Spain Rehabilitation Center	Newsletter	04/01/92
Respiratory Care of the Spinal Cord Injured Person	Georgia Regional SCI System Shepherd Spinal Center	Information Packet	01/20/92

Skin Care and Documentation	Northern California SCI System San Jose, California	Information Packet	10/01/92
Spinal Cord Injury: A Manual for Healthy Living	Texas Regional Model SCI System The Institute for Rehabilitation and Research, Houston	Manual/ Workbook	01/01/93
Starting Over: Part I—Skin Care	Regional SCI Care System of Southern California, Rancho Los Amigos Medical Center	Videotape ½"	01/01/91
Starting Over: Part II— Autonomic Dysreflexia	Regional SCI Care System of Southern California, Rancho Los Amigos Medical Center	Videotape ½"	01/01/91
Starting Over: Part III— Bowel Care	Regional SCI Care System of Southern California, Rancho Los Amigos Medical Center	Videotape ½"	01/01/91
Suprapubic Catheter: The Surgical Procedure	Rocky Mountain SCI System Craig Hospital, Denver	Videotape ½"	09/01/90
Taking Care of Pressure Sores	Northwest Regional SCI System University of Washington	Pamphlet	11/19/91
The Introduction to the Skin Protection Program on the SCI Unit at SCVMC	Northern California SCI System Santa Clara Valley Medical Center	Videotape ½"	10/01/92
Taking Care of Your Bowels: The Basics	Northwest Regional SCI System University of Washington	Pamphlet	07/01/94
Taking Care of Your Bowels: Ensuring Success	Northwest Regional SCI System University of Washington	Pamphlet	09/01/94

CATEGORY V: *Therapeutic Rehabilitation Management of SCI*

Assessment of Head and Neck Control and Functional Potential of the High Quad	Regional SCI Care System of Southern California, Rancho Los Amigos Medical Center	Videotape ½"	01/01/91
From Medical Rehab thru Employment: An Update on SCI—Rehab Resource Guide	UAB Model Regional SCI System Spain Rehabilitation Center	Soft-bound Book	01/01/91
Training Vignettes for FIM Plus FAM/Rationale for Training Vignettes	Northern California SCI System, Santa Clara Valley Medical Center	Manual/ Workbook	05/01/93

CATEGORY VI: *Psycho-Social—Vocational Management of SCI*

From Medical Rehab thru Employment: An Update on SCI—Rehab Resource Guide	UAB Model Regional SCI System Spain Rehabilitation Center	Soft-bound Book	01/01/91
Learning about Spinal Cord Injury	UAB Model Regional SCI System Spain Rehabilitation Center	Booklet	01/01/92
Peer Support Program	Georgia Regional SCI System Shepherd Spinal Center	Pamphlet	09/20/91
Rain, Rain Go Away	Rocky Mountain SCI System Craig Hospital, Denver	Videotape ½"	04/01/91
Return to Productivity	Georgia Regional SCI System Shepherd Spinal Center	Manual/ Workbook	06/01/91
Social Skills for the 90s— Coping with SCI in Social Situations	Georgia Regional SCI System Shepherd Spinal Center	Videotape ½"	01/01/90
Work in Progress	Georgia Regional SCI System Shepherd Spinal Center	Videotape ½"	06/01/92
Pastoral Services	Georgia Regional SCI System Shepherd Spinal Center	Pamphlet	01/01/94

CATEGORY VII: Sexuality and SCI

| Spinal Cord Injury Info-Sheet #3—Sexuality in Males with Spinal Cord Injury | UAB Model Regional SCI System Spain Rehabilitation Center | Fact Sheet | 01/01/94 |

CATEGORY VIII: Equipment and Aids for Persons with SCI

From Medical Rehab thru Employment: An Update on SCI—Rehab Resource Guide	UAB Model Regional SCI System Spain Rehabilitation Center	Soft-bound Book	01/01/91
Seating Fact Sheet	Georgia Regional SCI System Shepherd Spinal Center	Fact Sheet	12/01/91
Use, Care, and Maintenance of the Electrical Wheelchair	Northern California SCI System Santa Clara Valley Medical Center	Videotape ½"	07/01/91

CATEGORY IX: Environmental Modifications/Accessibility

| Accessible Community | Georgia Regional SCI System Shepherd Spinal Center | Pamphlet | 07/01/93 |
| Becoming God's Accessible Community | Georgia Regional SCI System through the Commission on Disability Concerns—CCMA, Atlanta | Pamphlet | 07/01/93 |

CATEGORY X: Lifelong Issues

A Guide for Personal Assistants to People with Spinal Cord Injury	UAB Model Regional SCI System Spain Rehabilitation Center	Booklet	01/01/92
ADA Brochure	Georgia Regional SCI System Shepherd Spinal Center	Fact Sheet	12/01/91
Adapted Golf	Georgia Regional SCI System Shepherd Spinal Center	Videotape ½"	06/01/93
Annual Health Evaluation and Monitoring Program	Northwest Regional SCI System University of Washington	Pamphlet	01/01/91

Cord Communicator	Southeastern Michigan SCI System Rehabilitation Institute of Detroit	Newsletter	Quarterly
From Medical Rehab thru Employment: An Update on SCI—Rehab Resource Guide	UAB Model Regional SCI System Spain Rehabilitation Center	Soft-bound Book	01/01/91
HealthWorks	Texas Regional Model SCI System The Institute for Rehabilitation and Research, Houston	Newsletter	Quarterly
Patient Education Handbook	Regional SCI Care System of Southern California, Rancho Los Amigos Medical Center	Manual/ Workbook	01/01/90
Progression	Midwest Regional SCI Care System, Rehabilitation Institute of Chicago	Newsletter	3 Years
Pushin' On	UAB Model Regional SCI System Spain Rehabilitation Center	Newsletter	Quarterly
Recreation Resource Guide for Individuals with Spinal Cord Injury	UAB Model Regional SCI System Spain Rehabilitation Center	Booklet	01/01/93
Spinal Cord Injury Info-Sheet—Locating Information about SCI—#1 and #2	UAB Model Regional SCI System Spain Rehabilitation Center	Fact Sheet	12/01/93
Spinal Cord Injury Update	Northwest Regional SCI System University of Washington	Newsletter	Quarterly

CATEGORY XI: Research in SCI

None

CATEGORY XII: Special SCI Issues

| A Community Campaign for Preventing SCI & TBI—Grades 5–6 | UAB Model Regional SCI System Spain Rehabilitation Center | Information Packet | 08/01/91 |

A Community Campaign for Preventing SCI & TBI— PSAs	UAB Model Regional SCI System Spain Rehabilitation Center	Public Service Announce- ment	01/01/91
A Community Campaign for Preventing SCI & TBI— Poster	UAB Model Regional SCI System Spain Rehabilitation Center	Poster	08/01/91
A Community Campaign for Preventing SCI & TBI— Preschool—Kindergarten	UAB Model Regional SCI System Spain Rehabilitation Center	Information Packet	01/01/91
A Community Campaign for Preventing SCI & TBI— Grades 1–2	UAB Model Regional SCI System Spain Rehabilitation Center	Information Packet	08/01/91
A Community Campaign for Preventing SCI & TBI— Grades 3–4	UAB Model Regional SCI System Spain Rehabilitation Center	Information Packet	08/01/91
Accessible Faith	Georgia Regional SCI System Shepherd Spinal Center	Pamphlet	04/01/91
Choices	Georgia Regional SCI System Shepherd Spinal Center	Videotape ½"	01/01/90
Diving Choices	Georgia Regional SCI System Shepherd Spinal Center	Videotape ½"	01/01/92
My House Shall Be for All People	Georgia Regional SCI System Shepherd Spinal Center	Videotape ½"	12/01/92
Speedway Sam—A Book about Spinal Cord Injury for Children	UAB Model Regional SCI System Spain Rehabilitation Center	Booklet	01/01/91
The Gift of Hospitality	Georgia Regional SCI System Shepherd Spinal Center	Pamphlet	11/01/93

Index